DATE DUE

Stress,
Immune Function,
and Health

Stress, Immune Function, and Health

The Connection

Bruce S. Rabin, M.D., Ph.D.

Professor of Pathology and Psychiatry
Director, Clinical Immunopathology Laboratory
Director, Brain, Behavior, and Immunity Center
University of Pittsburgh School of Medicine
and University of Pittsburgh Medical Center
Pittsburgh, PA

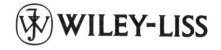

A John Wiley & Sons, Inc., Publication

New York • Chichester • Weinheim • Brisbane • Singapore • Toronto

Library of Congress Cataloging-in-Publication Data:

Rabin, Bruce S., 1941–
     Stress, immune function, and health : the connection / Bruce S.
     Rabin.
             p.   cm.
     Includes bibliographical reference and index.
     ISBN 0-471-24181-4 (cloth : alk. paper)
     1. Psychoneuroimmunology.   2. Stress (Psychology)—Immunological
aspects.   3. Stress (Physiology)—Immunological aspects.
4. Immunologic diseases—Psychosomatic aspects. I. Title.
[DNLM: 1. Immune System—physiology.   2. Immune System—
physiopathology.   3. Stress—complications.   4. Stress—immunology.
5. Psychoneuroimmunology.   QW 504R116s   1999]
QP356.47.R33   1999
616.07′9—dc21
DNLM/DLC
for Library of Congress   98-30128
                                                                    CIP
Printed in the United States of America.

10 9 8 7 6 5 4 3 2 1

To my children, Andy, Alison, and Rita, who I want to be healthy, productive, and happy. The joy they have provided me has contributed to my health and happiness.

To my grand-daughters, Micah Sara Rabin and Daniella Rachel Rabin. The world has become a better place because you are a part of it. I know that you will contribute to the betterment of all who know you.

The support and encouragement of my parents was essential to the completion of this book. They served as role models for how to become chronologically older while continuing to contribute to the welfare of others. Unfortunately for all who knew him, my 88 year old father passed away on October 9, 1998, after a brief illness. His last words were "I'm fine."

Contents

Foreword

The last 10 years have seen an explosion of research on the relationships between the brain and immune system. Much of this work has focused on the implications of psychological and social factors for our health. Psychological and physical stressors have been found to alter both humoral and cellular immune function. These changes have been attributed to direct central nervous system innervation of the immune system, to stress-elicited changes in circulating levels of hormones, and to stress-elicited coping behaviors such as smoking and poor diet that can also modify function of the immune system. Moreover, stress has also been associated with the deterioration of immune-related health outcomes, such as decreased host resistance to infection and the onset and exacerbation of autoimmune diseases. This book presents an unusually comprehensive and readable summary and integration of the various scientific disciplines that study brain–immune system–health interactions.

This very exciting area of basic and clinical research underscores the potential importance of stress reduction and stress coping as a component of preventive medicine. The subject has been reported on in numerous edited multicontributor publications. However, this volume differs in that it is a single-authored book written by a card-carrying physician/immunologist/scientist who actively contributes to both basic and clinical science. It will be of interest to researchers and health care workers whose areas of interest include the brain and the immune system, the brain and health, or the immune system and health.

The book begins with a thorough description of the components and function of the immune system, along with examples of how the function of the various immune components can be altered by stress. This review of the immune system will be of interest not only to individuals who are unfamiliar with immunology, but also to immunologists, as numerous examples from experimental animal and human studies are provided that document alterations of immune system function resulting from exposure to stress.

Following the overview of the immune system, the book discusses other basic science aspects of brain–immune interaction. Topics include the brain structures that regulate the function of the immune system, stressor-induced change in immune function, and hormones whose release is altered by stress, with subsequent implications for immune function. Throughout, examples from the research literature are provided, as well as cautions regarding the proper use of controls and the interpretation of experimental data.

The first five chapters of this book form a fairly complete, up-to-date discussion of the current understanding of brain–immune system interaction. Indeed, these chapters could form the basis of an undergraduate or graduate course in psychoneuroimmunology. The subsequent chapters turn to topics of more clinical and applied interest.

Chapter 6 discusses the clinical aspects of psychoneuroimmunology as related to autoimmune diseases, infectious diseases, and malignancies. The effects of stress on the onset and course of immune-mediated diseases are presented. In each case, the mechanisms responsible for these associations are discussed. This results in a cautious interpretation of the data in relation to what we know, and what we do not know, about the proven clinical significance of stress.

Chapter 7 discusses the role the brain can play in altering response to stressful events. The emphasis is on social and psychological factors that act to protect people from the detrimental effects of such events. The potential role of personality characteristics, such as optimism, of support provided by the social environment, and of persons' belief systems in promoting health is discussed. The author speculates as to how such factors might influence response to stressful events through brain regulation of hormonal response.

The final two chapters present interesting discussions of how stressful life events and stress hormones might influence the health and behaviors of the very young and the elderly. These chapters provide stimulating and thoughtful discussion of our social environment and its effect on health. Strong arguments for the importance of preventive medicine are made in regard to both enhancing the quality of health and controlling health care expenditures.

The science of psychoneuroimmunology has progressed to the point where its findings have important health implications. This book makes a significant contribution to the understanding and importance of mind–body medicine. It will be found useful as a text both for undergraduate and graduate psychoneuroimmunology courses and for all who are interested in the mind–body–health interaction.

Sheldon Cohen, Ph.D.
Carnegie Mellon University

Stephen Manuck, Ph.D.
University of Pittsburgh

Acknowledgments

I have received input, guidance, and education from the many who have helped develop my understanding of the interactions between the mind, the immune system, and health. Sheldon Cohen and Steve Manuck continue to help me develop an appreciation of the importance of psychoneuroimmunology on health. Other Pittsburgh colleagues who have provided needed intellectual activation include Alex Kusnecov, Michael Pezzone, Alan Sved, Matt Muldoon, Stefi Rassnick, and Niall Moyna. In Columbus, Ron Glaser and Jan Kiecolt-Glaser continue to provide important friendship and research contributions. George Solomon in Los Angeles and Bob Ader in Rochester have made significant contributions to the development and growth of psychoneuroimmunology.

The many students who have spent time with me have made significant contributions to my education and continue to motivate me to better understand the mind–body–health connection. I am also grateful to my principal teachers of immunology, Noel Rose and Felix Milgrom, for teaching me the basics and giving me the insights that have allowed me to understand the importance of the relationship between the immune system, the brain, and health.

Fred Altman and Leonard Mitnick, program directors at the National Institute of Mental Health, have helped the science of psychoneuroimmunology by working hard to secure grant funds for young and established investigators. Without them, the quality of the science would not be as advanced as it is today.

Thanks to all.

1

Introduction and Organization

When I had my thirtieth birthday, I began to have what I then considered to be meaningful thoughts about growing older. How long would I live? Would I be healthy or sick as I aged? Would I maintain my mental faculties? Would my existence have been meaningful by having improved the quality of other peoples' lives? I wanted to remain healthy and functional as I aged.

I soon realized that a way to contribute to my own successful aging process (which I define as being functional, self-sufficient, and making contributions that would maintain or improve the quality of life of others) was to find ways to keep other people healthy as they aged chronologically. As a medical research scientist, I wanted to use my professional career to dissociate chronological age from biological age. Indeed, the definition of age became of concern to me, as I never wanted to feel as old as my chronological age would indicate. Therefore, I have attempted to define age in a more meaningful manner.

One obvious way to define age is by stating the number of years that a person has lived: chronological age. However, the number provides no information regarding how physically or mentally fit someone is. A person can be 70 years old and physically and mentally fit, or age 70 and debilitated.

A better way to define age would be based on physiology. For example, if two people were to develop hypertension at the same time, their physiological age would be the same, regardless of their chronological age. Without intervention therapies, the subsequent duration and quality of life might be similar. They would be of similar physiologic ages.

Another way to look at age is on a psychological basis. Psychological age relates to how people feel about themselves and how they respond to how others feel about them. If we have a young psychological age and feel youthful, can we influence our physiological age? Is there a potential different effect on health when looking in a mirror and saying that you look great but feel awful, as opposed to looking in a mirror and saying that you don't look so good but feel wonderful? Probably.

The final way that I have considered looking at age is to define age on an immunological basis. If your immune system is working well and is protecting you from infectious diseases, the immune system can be considered youthful. If the immune system is not working well and you are predisposed to the development of infectious diseases, the immune system may be older. Indeed, the function of the immune system decreases in many individuals as they get older. If the immune system can be maintained at a youthful level, there may be less disease as we age.

Having decided that the maintenance of better quality health could be achieved by maintaining the immune system at a young age, I had to evaluate ways that this could be achieved. There are at least two areas of our lives that can have an impact on the function of the immune system: what we eat and how much stress we experience.

The concept that I use to explain this association of immune function with diet or stress is very simple but accurate. Imagine the body as a test tube that contains *tissue culture medium* (TCM). This medium is the fluid that supplies nutrients that are used to grow cells and tissues in glass or plastic bottles or small plastic chambers. TCM is a liquid that contains amino acids, sugars, vitamins, minerals, and hormones, and is supplemented with serum (the liquid part of clotted blood). There are hundreds of different tissue culture media, each having a different composition, available for purchase. Selecting the proper TCM for growth of a particular cell or tissue is an art and a science. Sometimes it is just trial and error.

Finding the right TCM to support the growth and function of a cell of interest to an investigator is very important. Different cells grow better or less well in different TCM. If our bodies are test tubes containing TCM, the chemical and hormonal composition of the TCM will have an influence on the growth and function of our cells and tissues. Not every composition of the TCM will support each tissue equally well.

In the body, TCM is the plasma (the liquid component of blood) that is present in blood vessels and in the extravascular spaces of the body, where it bathes all cells and tissues. The composition of plasma is not fixed, it varies. When seeing a physician for a routine checkup, a patient is often told to fast for approximately 12 hours before reporting to have a blood specimen obtained for evaluation. Obviously, the content of a meal will have an effect on the composition of blood. Certainly, numerous guidelines are being proposed regarding the amount of fat, fiber, vitamins, minerals, carbohydrates, and proteins that can optimize health. Therefore, diet can influence the composition of the TCM (plasma).

Diet can also have an influence on the function of the immune system. Indeed, there are dramatic examples in experimental animal systems where dietary modification has enhanced life span, reduced the likelihood of onset of immune-mediated diseases, and maintained the function of the immune system. Therefore, one approach to my concern about healthy aging could have been to study the quantity and quality of nutrition in regard to maintaining optimal immune function during chronological aging.

The second possible approach to healthy aging involves the study of stress and the capacity of the hormonal response to stress to alter the function of the immune system. Psychological or physical stress alters the composition of the TCM (plasma) and alters the way in which the immune system functions.

I was fortunate to be located at an academic center where faculty at the University of Pittsburgh and Carnegie Mellon University had interests in the effects of psychological stress on influencing the quality of an individuals health. This influenced my decision to pursue studies of the effect of stress on immune function and health. Working with Sheldon Cohen and Steven Manuck, we developed experimental approaches that contributed to the understanding of how psychological stress was able to modify the function of the immune system and alter susceptibility to immune mediated disease.

Most of the experimental work with which I have been involved has been published in the scientific literature. Thus, the work has been appropriately added to the wealth of information that is helping to better understand the mind–body–health connection. This is a meaningful reward for a scientist. However, I was not satisfied that the importance of the work that we and others were doing was being appropriately disseminated. Once I was convinced that the mind–body–health connection was real and did have an impact on the quality of an individual's health, I also realized that, at a time when the health delivery system is undergoing important changes, it becomes increasingly important for all people to become more responsible for the quality of their own health. Thus, this book provides the means of communicating the importance of the interaction between the mind, the body, and health, to other concerned scientists. My goal is to provide the information so that those who read this book will personally benefit, but additionally, so that those who are involved in the management of the health of others will become more aware of the capabilities of individuals to influence their own health. The message needs to be disseminated.

Indeed, in some ways we already are aware of the importance of preventive medicine. Many people are directing increased attention to the quality of their diet. Cholesterol is a household word. We are beginning to appreciate that cardiovascular disease can possibly be influenced by what we eat and whether we lead a physically active or sedentary lifestyle. By eating what we are being told is a healthy diet and exercising regularly, we are practicing preventive medicine.

If the amount of cholesterol in our blood is associated with an increased risk of developing heart disease, it would seem logical, and even easy and desirable, to reduce the amount of high cholesterol foods that we eat. If we were entirely logical and serious about it, there would be changes at the food store: bacon, sour cream, and super creamy ice cream would disappear. But, as we well know, this has not happened. We are complex creatures who do not always do what is in our best interest.

The most common causes of death in the United States are heart disease, cancer, strokes, accidents, lung disease, diabetes, suicide, liver disease, and acquired immunodeficiency syndrome (AIDS). It is possible to identify several factors, including behavioral activities, that contribute to the leading causes of death. Included are improper diet, smoking, physical inactivity, alcohol ingestion, infectious agents, trauma, unsafe sexual behavior, and the use of illicit drugs. If we could modify our exposure and susceptibility to factors that shorten the life span (whether self-induced or through the environment), it is likely that not only can we lengthen the number of years that we live but, more importantly, we could improve the quality of our lives *as we age*. Included in the improved quality of life would be (1) less dependence on the health care system, as there would be less need for it, and (2) gaining the potential of contributing to society (if we so wish), or (3) simply more enjoyment during the years of our lives after we stop working.

One way we may be capable of improving the quality of our health is learning to cope with the stressors that are increasingly part of our lives. This implies that stress is harmful, which is true. The definition of stress will vary with the individual. However, a unifying theme is that stress is a situation that occurs in one's local environment that produces behavioral and biologic alterations in the individual. When a situation produces stress that becomes apparent as behavioral and biologic alterations, it is usually as a result of the inability of the individual to effectively cope with the stressor. Coping is the ability to manage and to overcome the problems and difficulties associated with the stressor. If coping is successful, the stressor may not influence the body in a manner that may predispose to disease. However, if the ability to cope is unsuccessful, changes may occur that have an effect on health.

The scientific studies presented in this book comprise the scientific discipline of psychoneuroimmunology. Psychoneuroimmunology is the study of how (1) psychological factors that an individual experiences and that activate neurons in the brain (2) modify the production and release of neuropeptides and endocrine hormones that (3) alter the function of the immune system, which then (4) increases the susceptibility of an individual to diseases that are normally prevented by a healthy functioning immune system. Dr. George Solomon and Dr. Robert Ader deserve acknowledgment and thanks for their pioneering efforts to move the field from the realm of popular culture to a true scientific discipline with importance to all.

The chapters of the book have been selected to provide an understanding of many important components of psychoneuroimmunology.

Chapter 1 provides an introduction of the reason for this book and the difficulties inherent in asking people to engage in behaviors that may be beneficial to health at a later time in their life.

Chapter 2 presents an overview of the components of the immune system and how they function, as well as studies that show alteration of immune function by psychological stress. This chapter begins to develop the concept of the body as a test tube filled with TCM whose composition determines how well or how poorly the immune system does what it is supposed to do.

Writing Chapter 2 presented problems of scientific evolution that you need to be aware of. In the basic science of immunology, our understanding of how the immune system functions is constantly changing. Researchers continue to delve into the intricacies of newly identified populations of lymphocytes and the functional properties of lymphocytes, new cytokines are discovered, our understanding of the interactions between cells and cytokines are modified, and our understanding of the importance of the complement system is expanded. In the clinical applications of immunology, we are gaining new insights into why autoimmune diseases develop, how resistance to infectious diseases is achieved, and how the immune system resists the spontaneous development of malignancy. However, our detailed understanding of these clinical conditions depends on a more complete understanding of the development and function of the immune system. Thus, as the understanding of the immune system evolves, it is likely that our understanding of psychoneuroimmunology will also evolve. Psychoneuroimmunologists are dependent on the research efforts of basic and clinical immunologists and we look forward to continued interaction with them as we develop a better understanding of how the function of the immune system is modified by influences of the brain. Thus, Chapter 2 is a work in progress.

Chapter 3 presents information regarding how specific areas of the brain that perceive the presence of a stressor are able to communicate with the cells of the immune system. The communication is through the release of soluble molecules directly from the nervous system or from endocrine tissues responding to signals form the nervous system. Examples of modification of brain areas and its effect on immune function are provided. The identification of the pathways of communication between the brain and the immune system are important to the development of procedures (either behavioral modifications or possibly pharmacological interventions) that have the potential of providing the means of ameliorating the stressor effects on immune function and health.

Chapter 4 presents data from studies establishing the ability of stress to alter the function of the immune system. This chapter describes the quantitative and qualitative changes that occur in the various components of the immune system. Proper functioning of each component is essential for the proper response that will eliminate infectious microorganisms and prevent the activation of responses against an individual's own tissue. However, it is important to be aware of the multitude of effects of stress that can modify the function of the immune system. When experiencing stress, our sleep patterns and eating patterns may change. Increased amounts of alcohol may be consumed. We may not see physicians when we suspect that we might have a medical problem. Thus, stress-related changes in health practices may contribute to stressor-induced increased risk of the development of disease.

How changes in behavior interact with stress-induced changes in the function of the immune system to increase the risk of disease development or exacerbation of a disease needs to be carefully evaluated. As described in Chapter 4, experiencing an acute or chronic stress does not produce dramatic changes in the quantitative or qualitative aspects of any single component of the immune system. However, a minimal change in several components of the immune system may interact to predispose to the development of disease.

Chapter 5 describes the effect on the immune system of neuropeptides and hormones whose concentration is increased by stress. As emphasized in this chapter, many studies incubating cells of the immune system, injecting hormones into an experimental subject, or blocking the effect of a hormone in vivo, are done with single hormones. However, the reality of the effect of stress on hormones is that the concentration of multiple hormones is changed in plasma by stress. The functional activities that are changed are dependent on the simultaneous effect of all the hormones that bind to receptors on a cell.

Chapter 6 presents information regarding the effect of stress on disease categories whose onset or course, or both, are mediated by stress. Infectious and autoimmune diseases fall within this category. Malignant diseases also are likely to be influenced by the function of the immune system.

The first six chapters establish the basis for consideration that the brain can influence the function of the immune system, which then can alter susceptibility to disease. Chapter 7 discusses behaviors and beliefs that can ameliorate the effect of stress from altering the function of the immune system. It is likely that the behaviors discussed have their beneficial effect by interfering with activation of the stress-responsive areas of the brain. If the behaviors are able to reduce the extent of disease-enhancing immune system alteration induced by stress, they will provide a significant modality for preventive medicine. If people can be kept healthy, particularly as they age, not only will the quality of their lives be optimized, but a significant reduction in the utilization of health care resources may be achieved. It is much better to prevent illness than to treat it. This is the concept that motivated me to work in the area of psychoneuroimmunology. Indeed, I believe that significant improvements in the quality of life can be achieved by appropriate behavioral modifications.

Chapter 8 takes a slight diversion and discusses the effect of stress during pregnancy and the early period of development on behaviors and immune function of the offspring. This is an extremely important area of concern, as we seem to be entering a time when there are increasing levels of stress in many peoples' lives. If there is an impact of stress on the mental and physical health of children, isn't there a need to recognize this, firmly establish that it exists, and then develop interventions to prevent it?

The final chapter discusses the difficulty of studying the immune system in older individuals. The older population contains a mixture of individuals whose immune system works at different levels of competency. It is likely that those whose immune system works at a higher level of efficiency will have a longer duration of life due to better health. This emphasizes the importance of adopting behaviors that will contribute to the optimization of immune function throughout life.

It is important to emphasize, before you read the following chapters, that psychoneuroimmunology is a science in progress. Until there is a complete understanding of how the immune system functions and how the immune system maintains health, we will not have a definitive understanding of the mind–body–health connection. However, even without that definitive understanding, a wealth of well-conducted scientific studies establishes that psychological stress can alter the function of the immune system and that psychological stress can alter susceptibility to immune-mediated disease.

One important factor, restated throughout the book, is that the response of individuals to stress will differ depending on factors experienced in utero, during the early formative years, adolescence, and adult life. Not every individual will have the same hormonal responses and immune alterations when exposed to a stressor.

One area not addressed in this book (and probably one that I am not qualified to comment on, but why should that stop me) is who, besides the individual, bears the responsibility for implementing the resources that can be used to help people cope with the stress present in their lives. We need increased attention to facilities and activities that promote social interactions, exercise, light-heartedness, and belief systems that will help with coping with stress. If some simple behaviors can contribute to preventive medicine, we need to find ways to make these behaviors more accessible and acceptable to all who would use them.

It is important to attract health care workers who have the interest and capabilities of working in this science. This will require the funding of research to further advance the science of mind–body–medicine and the development of training programs for health care workers who want to participate in preventive medicine programs. Recognition of the importance of the application of preventive medicine to long term health should lead to the development of a health care system that will attract outstanding health care workers to the practice of preventive medicine.

Who needs to be more aware of the importance of stress and buffering the effects of stress on altering the function of the immune system and health? Medical students, physicians, nurses, clinical psychologists, social workers, hospital administrators, anyone who supervises someone else, elementary school teachers, high school teachers, nursery school teachers, dentists, bosses, mothers, fathers, brothers, sisters, and grandparents. We need to have more classes taught in high schools, colleges, and professional schools. We need to have more people trained in psychoneuroimmunology so that they can teach the courses. And we need to bring more researchers into psychoneuroimmunology programs.

Of course, being made aware of the benefits of a behavior does not mean that we will engage in that behavior. Why is it so difficult for many people to engage in activities that will have a beneficial effect on the quality of their health? If a high quality of health leads to a high quality of life as you get older, why wouldn't you *want* to engage in behaviors that promote good health during the aging process? One reason may be that you don't believe that anything you do when you are in your 20s, 30s, 40s, or even 60s, can have a beneficial effect 10, 20, or more years later. Certainly, that is a legitimate concern. How do you know that taking vitamin E every day will help reduce the risk of your developing heart disease or cancer? You don't know that you will benefit.

What you are being asked to do is to change your behavior on the basis of epidemiological studies. Epidemiology looks at the relationship between various factors in our environment and various behaviors that we engage in, and then relates these to the onset and severity of disease. However, epidemiology has its problems. Data from epidemiology studies report averages regarding whether a behavior that you engage in increases your risk of developing a disease.

Yet, not every individual who engages in a particular behavior, or who fails to engage in a particular behavior, will develop the disease or be protected from developing the disease being studied. You do not know that you will be one of those who benefits from changing your behavior or whose health is harmed by a specific behavior.

What is lacking is an immediate reinforcement. Something that occurs when you change your behavior that gives you information that indicates to you that you have done something that will definitely benefit your health, quality of life, or longevity.

You may ask the question, "Why should I give up something that I enjoy for a possible benefit 30 years from now?" You are an individual, not an average and, when dealing with the average, there are some below the average and some above the average. How do you know that a specific modification of behavior will place you above the average. You don't!

Changing behaviors to promote a better quality of life as we age is difficult, and it is because it is difficult that we tend to resist making changes in our behaviors. Certainly, the average quality of life for a large population of people may be improved if the information contained in this book contributes to a reduced risk of immune-mediated disease. But no one can guarantee that any one specific individual will benefit.

One can argue that one has a complicated life and that one prefers not to pay attention to activities that might possibly be beneficial, especially because there is no guarantee that changing an aspect of one's lifestyle will prove beneficial. To this I can only say that when someone has died and is being eulogized, no one will say that this person was special because he worked himself to death and didn't take care of his health needs. No one will say that he was a special person because he didn't take vacations or find time to read a book or just look at the trees. Rather, they will likely say that he was a jerk who didn't know how to relax and who lost an opportunity to enjoy many of the pleasures that we can experience as healthy, active individuals.

I'll take the long-term reward of using behaviors and social interactions to optimize my chances of living a healthy life, regardless of how long it is. Longevity only has meaning if it is associated with the highest quality of health that I can achieve.

My hope is that this book will contribute to the growing awareness of the health benefits that can be achieved by buffering the effects of stress on the immune system and health. This may lead to a decreased need for the use of health care services, which could result in more funding for medical research. It is hoped that we will pay as much attention to our physical health while aging as we do to our retirement income. As a physician, it is my responsibility to work to promote better health. This book is one of my contributions.

2
Overview of the Function of the Immune System

To assist those not familiar with the immune system, the following glossary is offered as a quick overview to help to begin to develop an understanding of the immune system. An essential part of the process of learning immunology is becoming familiar with the terminology. That is a lesson I am taught each year by first-year medical students at the University of Pittsburgh School of Medicine. I assure the students that even though it is confusing in the beginning, the immune system will be understood by the end of the course. I also assure you that you will be immunologically competent by the end of this book.

GLOSSARY OF FREQUENTLY USED TERMS

activated lymphocyte   when a T or B lymphocyte has interacted with antigen and antigen-presenting cells, the lymphocyte will be able to function by producing antibody (a property of B lymphocytes), killing a cell infected with a virus (a property of CD8 T lymphocytes), or mediating either a delayed hypersensitivity response or helping B lymphocytes produce antibody (a property of CD4 T lymphocytes). The activated T lymphocytes circulate through parenchymal tissue hunting for the antigen to which they are sensitized. Activated antibody-producing B lymphocytes may mature to plasma cells that are found in bone marrow or lymph nodes.

After looking at the first term in the glossary, the problems of understanding immunology for those not familiar with the subject should be clear. To explain *activated lymphocyte,* I used *T or B lymphocyte, antigen-presenting cells, CD8, delayed hyper-sensitivity, antibody, parenchymal tissue, antigen,* and *plasma cell.* Describing the terminology of immunology requires the use of terms that are not yet defined. Thus, the beginning of understanding is slow. However, as you go through the glossary and this chapter the terminology of immunology will be used repeatedly and clarified.

active immunity   the body is stimulated to: (1) produce an immune response to an infectious agent such as a bacteria, virus, or fungus, or (2) produce an immune response to something an individual is immunized or vaccinated against. An example is being immunized against tetanus, polio, or hepatitis.

allergy   a specific and rapid immune reactivity to an antigen that causes constriction of smooth muscle, dilation of blood vessels, and mucous secretion. Allergic reactions are mediated by the IgE class of immunoglobulin, and the clinical aspects are often mediated by chemical mediators (such as histamine) released from mast cells located in tissue.

anaphylaxis   when an animal receives two injections of an antigen, it is assumed that the first injection will lead to the production of antibody, bringing about protection against harmful effects of the second injection. However, in some cases, the second injection leads to fluid accumulations in tissue, constriction of airways, and possibly death. Because the first injection of antigen does not produce protection, *anaphylaxis* means "to be without protection." Anaphylactic reactions are caused by the IgE class of antibody or by immune complex formation.

antibody   also called gamma-globulins or immunoglobulins. An antibody is a protein that will combine with the antigen that caused the antibody to be produced. Antibodies have *specificity,* in that they combine most strongly with the particular antigen that stimulated their production. Antibodies are produced by a type of white blood cell called a *B lymphocyte.* Each B lymphocyte can only produce a single type of antibody, but the B lymphocyte will produce thousands of that particular antibody molecule each second. Antibodies bind to antigens located outside the tissue cells. When you are immunized against tetanus, several events take place: (1) you are injected with an antigen that is a soluble product released from the bacteria that causes the disease, tetanus. Tetanus is caused by a protein, often called "tetanus toxin," that is released by bacteria. The toxin attaches to and damages nerves involved in muscle movement. As a result muscles may experience spasm (contraction) with a frequent complication being "lockjaw." The toxin that is used for immunization is treated so that antibodies are produced against it but the toxin cannot damage nerves. The altered toxin is called a "toxoid." (2) when injected into tissue, the tetanus toxoid is carried to a lymph node where B lymphocytes begin to produce antibody to the toxoid. (3) the antibody circulates throughout the body in the blood and in the fluids that bath the tissues of the body. If some tetanus toxin gains entrance to the body, the antibody will neutralize it so that the toxin cannot attach to and damage nerves.

antigen   a substance that activates the immune system to produce a specific response that will react against the antigen that activated the immune response. An antigen is usually something that is foreign to the body such as an infectious agent. When immunized against tetanus, tetanus is the antigen. When the immune system reacts against an antigen it may neutralize its ability to damage the body or the immune system may actually cause the antigen (eg, a bacteria) to be killed.

antigenic determinant this is a localized region on the surface of an antigen, which can be recognized by an antibody. A single antigen molecule may have multiple antigenic determinants, each called an "epitope." Therefore, a single molecule of antigen may stimulate synthesis of several different antibodies, each of which will bind to a separate epitope (antigenic site) on the molecule of antigen.

antigen-presenting cell for an immune reaction to occur, several steps take place. One of the first steps is the presentation of the antigen to a type of lymphocyte called the CD4 T cell. This step is carried out by a cell called an "antigen-presenting cell." The antigen-presenting cell is a cell that (1) ingests proteins and digests them into small peptides (approximately 10–15 amino acids long), (2) synthesizes molecules called "MHC II," (3) binds the peptides derived from large proteins into a groove on the MHC II molecule and expresses the class II MHC molecule with the peptide in its groove on the surface of the antigen-presenting cell, (4) orients the MHC II molecule so that the peptide derived from the antigen is accessible to the T cell receptor of CD4 T lymphocytes, (5) expresses costimulatory molecules that will activate the CD4 T lymphocyte that have bound to a peptide in a MHC molecule. The important antigen-presenting cells involved with activation of the immune response are dendritic cells and B lymphocytes. After an immune response has been initiated and the immune system is ridding the body of foreign infectious agents, the important antigen-presenting cells (APCs) are any tissue cells that have been infected and tissue macrophages.

apoptosis a process by which a cell kills itself upon receiving an activation signal from another cell.

atopy the manifestation of an allergic reaction. A subject who has hay fever is said to be "atopic" or to have "atopy."

attenuated attenuation reduces the ability of an infectious agent to cause infection while still being able to stimulate the immune system. If a virus is altered so that it stimulates an immune response without producing an infection, the virus is designated as being attenuated.

autoimmunity an immune reaction that is directed against an individual's own tissue. The immune reaction may damage tissue and cause disease.

bone marrow the central portion of bones that is the source of all red and white blood cells. There are stem cells in the marrow which, under the influence of several hormones and cytokines, mature to the various populations of blood cells. Some of the cells that arise in the marrow mature in other organs, for example T lymphocytes mature in the thymus gland.

B lymphocyte a white blood cell that releases a protein molecule that is designated an antibody. B lymphocytes present a single specificity of antibody molecule on their surface. Every antibody molecule on a single B lymphocyte is identical (they have the same specificity for a single antigenic determinant). When the B lymphocyte encounters the antigen to which the antibody molecule binds, the B lymphocyte is selected for activation. Activation of the B lymphocyte depends on the lymphocyte presenting the antigen on its surface in special presentation molecules which allows the B lymphocyte to interact with an appropriately activated T lymphocyte that is reactive to the same antigen.

bursa derived   chickens have an organ called the bursa of Fabricius. In the chicken, the bursa is responsible for the development of the B lymphocyte population. There is no single equivalent organ in humans. The term "bursa derived" usually refers to B lymphocytes. Some use the definition of the B in "B lymphocyte" as indicating "bone marrow."

cell-mediated immunity   the activity of T lymphocytes that function to eliminate infectious agents located within a cell. Cellular immunity does not involve the production of antibody. The T lymphocytes are able to identify tissue cells that have an infectious agent within the cell because the tissue cell places a portion of the infectious agent on its surface in MHC molecules. When the T lymphocyte identifies an infected cell, the T lymphocytes initiate reactions that will kill the infected cell.

CD marker   molecules on the surface of cells that are used to identify types of tissue cells. Many of these molecules have had their function identified. Antibodies can be produced to the CD molecules, allowing them to be classified as antigens. CD membrane molecules are identified by antibodies that bind to the CD molecule. All antibodies that identify the same membrane molecule are grouped together and given a numerical CD definition. As an example, the CD3 marker is present on all T lymphocytes, the CD4 marker is present on all helper/inducer T lymphocytes, and the CD8 marker is present on all cytotoxic T lymphocytes.

clonal selection   each lymphocyte is capable of responding to a single antigen. Each lymphocyte has a different receptor specificity. The selective activation by an antigen of those lymphocytes which can respond to the antigen is referred to as "clonal selection." A clone of lymphocytes is the expansion (by cell division) of the single lymphocyte that responded to the antigen.

complement   the term applied to a group of sequentially interacting serum proteins that participate in mediating an inflammatory response in tissue. Activated complement attracts polymorphonuclear leukocytes and allows cells and fluids to escape from blood vessels and enter tissue. Complement promotes the ingestion of insoluble particles, including bacteria, by phagocytic cells. Fully functional complement can place holes in cell membranes.

costimulatory molecule   a lymphocyte that has never interacted with an antigen requires at least two different types of interaction with an antigen-presenting cell for the lymphocyte to become activated. One of the events is related to the specificity of the lymphocyte receptor molecule for antigen. When the lymphocyte's antigen receptor recognizes its specific antigen, a reaction occurs that allows that particular lymphocyte to become activated. Actual activation requires an interaction between a second molecule on the lymphocyte surface and a molecule on the surface of another cell. This second interaction, which has no specificity for antigen, is called "costimulation," and the molecule on the antigen-presenting cell is the "costimulatory molecule." An example of costimulation is provided by CD28 and B7. CD28 is a molecule on T-cell membranes that binds to the B7 molecule on the membrane of APCs. This interaction provides what is termed "costimulation" to a T cell whose antigen receptor has bound to a peptide being presented in the MHC molecule of the antigen-presenting cell. Costimulation allows the T cell to become activated and to develop effector functions. Other combinations of molecules interacting between two lymphocyte populations are also necessary for costimulation. For example, a CD40 molecule on a B lymphocyte must bind to a CD40L molecule on a helper T cell for the T cell to provide helper function to get the B cell to initiate antibody production by the B cell. Costimulation molecules do not have specificity, meaning that they are identical on each cell in an individual.

cytokine   one of numerous proteins made by a cell that can influence the activity of other cells. Cytokines bind to cytokine receptors on cells with different receptors binding different cytokines. Lymphocytes and antigen-presenting cells produce cytokines that, depending on the particular cytokine and the cell that it binds to, may either up-regulate or down-regulate the activity of other immune cells. Cytokines are also involved in the regulation of endocrine hormone production and contribute to the modulation of activity of the central nervous system. A variety of cells, other than cells of the immune system, produce cytokines. The nomenclature used to identify cytokines is "interleukin," followed by a number. For example, "interleukin-2" is a cytokine produced by CD4 lymphocytes with the biological property of promoting division of T lymphocytes.

cytotoxic T lymphocytes   a class of T lymphocytes that have the capability of recognizing when a tissue cells has been infected with a virus, a bacteria that is viable within the tissue cell, or a tissue cell which may have become malignant. Cytotoxic T lymphocytes have a molecule on their surface designated the CD8 molecule. The CD8 cells are able to recognize when a tissue cell is infected because the tissue cell displays a portion of the infectious agent in a presentation molecule (called MHC I) that is on the surface of the tissue cell. The CD8 T lymphocyte has a molecule on its surface, called the T-cell receptor, which can recognize when a peptide from an infectious agent is being displayed in a MHC I molecule on the tissue cell. When the CD8 lymphocyte binds to the peptide:MHC I complex on the surface of a tissue cell that the lymphocyte has previously been activated to, the CD8 lymphocyte will kill the tissue cell.

delayed hypersensitivity   a localized reaction of CD4 T lymphocytes engaged in an immune response against a foreign antigen displayed on the surface of a cell. The CD4 lymphocytes release cytokines that attract phagocytic cells and contribute to the killing of the infected cell.

dendritic cell   cells that have the capability of presenting antigens to T lymphocytes. The antigens are either ingested into the dendritic cells or synthesized within the dendritic cells. Dendritic cells have a variety of names associated with them, depending on their location. In the skin they are called Langerhan's cells, interstitial dendritic cells in the heart, kidney, intestine, or lung, dendritic cells in the blood, and veiled cells in the afferent lymphatics. Dendritic cells have high concentrations of MHC I and MHC II molecules as well as costimulation molecules on their membranes. Dendritic cells in the spleen or lymph nodes initiate immune responses by interacting with a T cell that has antigen-recognizing receptors for the antigen being displayed on the membrane of the dendritic cell.

effector lymphocyte once a lymphocyte has been activated by an antigen, it is termed an effector lymphocyte. Effector lymphocytes have been activated to carry out process that will rid the body of infectious agents. Before a lymphocyte becomes an effector lymphocyte, it is called a "naive" lymphocyte. An effector lymphocyte that is searching for the antigen to which it is sensitized (activated) but has not found the antigen, is called a "memory" lymphocyte. When the antigen is located on a tissue cell, the memory lymphocyte becomes an "effector" lymphocyte.

hapten a low-molecular-weight chemical that cannot activate an immune reaction unless the hapten is bound to a large protein.

helper lymphocyte a lymphocyte with the CD4 surface marker. The function of help is associated with a CD4 T cell producing soluble cytokines that contribute to antibody production by a B lymphocyte.

humoral immunity plasma (the liquid portion of blood) contains antibodies produced by B lymphocytes. The total amount of antibodies present in plasma that provide protection from infectious agents not located within tissue cells is referred to as "humoral immunity."

hypersensitivity increased sensitivity or responsiveness to an antigen. Only occurs with a second exposure to an antigen after the immune system has been activated by the first exposure. Thus, hypersensitivity is an altered state of responsiveness to an antigen. Immediate hypersensitivity occurs within minutes of reexposure to an antigen and clinically is the allergic reaction. Allergic reactions are mediated by the IgE class of antibody. Delayed hypersensitivity is mediated by CD4 T lymphocytes and does not involve antibodies. Delayed hypersensitivity reactions often take 48–72 hours to become manifest after the T lymphocytes encounter the antigen. Delayed hypersensitivity reactions are produced against intracellular pathogens. Another term used to describe delayed hypersensitivity reactions is "cell mediated immunity."

immune complex the combination of an antigen with antibody that specifically binds to the antigen is called an immune complex. Immune complexes may deposit in tissue and initiate tissue damage.

immune system the immune system has the function of protecting the body from infectious agents (bacteria, viruses, fungi). The immune system consists of soluble substances (antibodies, complement, cytokines) and cells (macrophages, dendritic cells, B lymphocytes, different classes of T lymphocytes). When the various components interact together, the system is capable of contributing to the maintenance of good health.

immunization   deliberately injecting an antigen into an individual (human or animal) for the purpose of producing an immune reaction (antibody or cell mediated) to the antigen.

immunocompetence   the ability to detect that a foreign antigen is present and an immune response to a specific antigen. This involves the synthesis of surface receptors for the antigen and their appearance on the surface of lymphocytes. Each lymphocyte is programmed to recognize and respond to a specific antigen. This occurs before the lymphocyte actually encounters the antigen. Lymphocytes have their first encounter with a specific antigen in the lymph node or spleen.

immunosurveillance   the concept of the immune system looking for cells that have become malignant. It is hypothesized that when the immune system encounters malignant cells, the immune system reacts against these cells and kills them. This is often given as an explanation as to why people do not spontaneously develop malignancies. When the immune system is suppressed, for example to prevent rejection of a tissue transplant, there is an increased risk of developing a malignancy.

inflammation   a response that occurs to rid the body of an infectious agent and that is localized to the site in the body where the infectious agent is found. Inflammation is characterized by pain, heat, redness, and swelling, at the site where the inflammation is occurring. The response consists of altered patterns of blood flow (increased blood flow accounts for the redness), fluid leakage out of small blood vessels (contributing to the swelling), an influx of phagocytic or other immune cells (also contributing to the swelling), and finally removal of the foreign antigen by the infiltrating cells and healing of the damaged tissue. The inflammatory reaction may be acute (occurring without activation of the immune system) or chronic (involving activation of the immune system). The redness and pus (pus is an accumulation of white blood cells in tissue) that occurs at the site of a splinter is an example of inflammation.

leukocyte   the white blood cells are collectively referred to as "leukocytes." Leukocyte is translated as "pale cell." The cells that comprise the leukocytes (white blood cells) are the neutrophils, eosinophils, basophils, monocytes, and lymphocytes.

lymph   during systole (when the heart contracts and sends blood to tissue), plasma passes through the wall of blood capillaries. During diastole (when the heart relaxes), most of the plasma flows back into the vasculature. However, a small amount of plasma does not reenter the vasculature and remains in the extravascular tissue space. If this fluid were not removed, tissue edema (tissue swelling) would result. Within connective tissue there are small capillary tubes, that are closed at one end, and into which the excess plasma flows. The fluid is called "lymph," and the tubes are called the "lymphatic capillaries."

lymphocytes   white blood cells responsible for the immune response. Different types of lymphocytes originate from a common stem cell in the bone marrow.

Lymphocytes that continue their maturation in the bone marrow become "B lymphocytes," which function by producing antibody. Lymphocytes that migrate from the bone marrow to the thymus gland for their maturation, become "T lymphocytes," which function in cell-mediated immunity, which is antibody independent.

MHC I   a molecule on the membrane of all nucleated cells. The major histocompatibility complex (MHC) I molecule presents antigens that are synthesized within the cell that the MHC I molecule is present on. CD8 lymphocytes see antigen bound to MHC I molecules.

MHC II   a molecule on the membrane of all antigen-presenting cells. The MHC II molecule presents antigens that are ingested and then digested by the cell. CD4 lymphocytes see antigen bound to MHC II molecules.

monoclonal   the progeny of a single cell that repeatedly divides is called a clone of cells with each being identical. Monoclonal refers to a single clone of cells.

monoclonal antibody   the descendents of a single B lymphocyte, all of which produce the identical antibody, are monoclonal cells. As each of these B lymphocytes produces the identical antibody molecule, their product is a monoclonal antibody. In vitro cultures of monoclonal B lymphocytes are used to produce large concentrations of a specific antibody.

naive lymphocyte   naive lymphocytes are cells that have not encountered antigen since their exit from the bone marrow and thymus but which have receptors for a specific antigen. Naive cells are not found in tissues; they are found only in the blood and secondary lymphoid tissues. Naive lymphocytes are not actvated at the site of antigen entry into the body, but rather in lymph nodes and spleen.

NK lymphocyte   a lymphocyte that is neither a T cell or a B cell. Natural killer lymphocytes kill tissue cells that are infected by a virus or that display an antigen derived from malignant tissue.

parenchymal tissue   the substance of an organ.

pathogen   an infectious agent that can cause tissue damage and disease. The infectious agent may cause disease by damaging tissue, for example by releasing a toxin that kills tissue cells. An infectious agent may also produce tissue damage by stimulating an immune response that is directed against the infectious agent. In the process of destroying the infectious agent, the immune responses will cause damage to the tissue where the infectious agent is located. An example of this process is viral hepatitis. The virus infects liver cells but does not damage them. A cell mediated immune response against the virus produces killing of the liver cells.

phagocytic cell   white blood cells that can ingest insoluble and soluble materials. Bacteria that are ingested are killed by the phagocytic cell. Neutrophils, monocytes, macrophages, and dendritic cells are examples of phagocytic cells. Some phagocytic cells are antigen presenting cells, but neutrophils are not antigen presenting cells.

phagocytosis   the process of ingestion of insoluble material by a cell.

plasma blood is treated so that it cannot clot. The liquid portion of the blood with all of the cells removed is termed plasma. The liquid portion of clotted blood is called "serum."

primary immune response the immune response which occurs on first expose of the immune system to an antigen. Effector lymphocytes are generated during the primary immune response. The magnitude and duration of a primary immune response is not as great as that of a secondary immune response.

processing of antigen to be presented in the groove of a MHC molecule a large protein molecule must be digested into small peptides of approximately 10–14 amino acids. Ingested antigen is placed into a vacuole in the cytoplasm of the antigen presenting cell into which enzymes are dispensed. Ingested antigen is degraded into small peptides that are placed into the grooves of MHC II molecules for presentation to T lymphocytes. Peptides synthesized within the antigen-presenting cell are placed into the groove of MHC I molecules.

secondary immune response occurs upon a second exposure to the same antigen that elicited the primary immune response. Memory cells which had previously been activated during the primary immune response respond rapidly to the antigen and with greater magnitude than during the primary response. Another name for the secondary immune response is the "anamnestic" response.

serum blood is allowed to clot. The liquid portion lacks cells and also lacks the factors of the coagulation system as they have formed the clot.

specificity in regard to the immune system, indicates that an immune reaction is only directed to the specific antigen that initially activated the particular immune reaction.

T-cell receptor a two-chain polypeptide on the surface of T cells that is capable of binding to a specific antigen. Only those T cells with receptors for a specific antigen can bind to that antigen. The T-cell receptor (TCR) allows the T cell to recognize an antigen.

T lymphocyte a lymphocyte that is formed in the bone marrow that then moves to the thymus gland, where it matures and develops the capability to recognize an antigen. This involves the formation of molecules on the surface of the T lymphocyte that can bind to an antigen. The formation of the antigen-specific surface receptors (called T-cell receptors) is a random process that occurs independently of antigen.

thymus gland the lymphoid organ located just above the heart. Immature T lymphocytes leave the bone marrow and mature in the thymus. T lymphocytes that can react to one's own tissues are eliminated in the thymus.

tolerance the specific absence of an immune response to an antigen. This is usually an active process related to the deletion of antigen-reactive lymphocytes or a mechanism which suppress the ability of the lymphocytes to respond to antigen. Lymphocytes that have receptors for self-antigen (one's own tissue antigens) are eliminated by the tolerance mechanism(s).

white blood cell see leukocyte.

INTRODUCTION

To understand the importance of the immune system for the maintenance of health, it is important to have an understanding of the components and function of the immune system and their role in resistance to infectious diseases or in causing autoimmune diseases or in modifying susceptibility to the onset or progression of a malignant disease. How well or how poorly the immune system works to protect the body from disease is influenced by how individuals respond to stressors in their lives. This occurs because the characteristics of how an individual responds to stressors influences the chemical composition of plasma in which the immune system functions.

We respond to "stress" or "stressors" that are present in our lives with behavioral and physiological responses called the "stress response." Hormones whose concentration is altered by stress or whose synthesis is initiated by stress are classified as "stress hormones." The stress that we respond to may be universal or personal. Having to flee a building that has caught fire is a universal stressor. Everyone is likely to have a physiological response to it. Working in an environment requiring constant supervision may be a stressor to some but not to others. Thus, if an individual does not perceive a particular situation as a stressor, there may be no physiological response to the situation.

If you are not an immunologist, reading this chapter will not make you a card-carrying immunologist. However, this chapter will teach a considerable amount of the essential aspects of basic immunology. After reading it, you will begin to understand how stress-induced modulation of immune system function occurs and how this modulation can affect health. If you are an immunologist, you will develop an appreciation for the influence of our environment on altering the function of the immune system, something that I only began to appreciate when I began my studies of how immune system function is modulated by hormones. Subsequent chapters will expand and clarify the mechanisms and health implications of stressor-induced immune alteration.

DEFINITION OF THE IMMUNE SYSTEM AS A SENSORY ORGAN THAT SURVEYS THE INTERIOR OF THE BODY

The immune system is important for the maintenance of homeostasis within the body. When the internal environment of the body is disturbed by the presence of an infectious agent, the immune system works to eliminate the infectious agent and return the body to the state it was in before the infectious agent was present. In this regard, the immune system patrols the tissues of the body, constantly looking for the presence of substances that are foreign to the body (usually bacteria, viruses, and fungi). In addition, protozoa that are parasitic in humans, and worms, are attacked by the immune system to eliminate them from the body.

When the immune system identifies the presence of an infectious agent, the immune system turns itself on, directs its attention to the infectious material, kills it, and causes it to be removed from the body. A possible scenario suggests that the infectious material presents a "danger signal" to the immune system and that the presence of a dangerous pathogen initiates a response to eliminate the danger. Rather than removing oneself from a dangerous psychological or physical situation, the immune system responds by removing the dangerous situation. To do this, the cells of the immune system must be present throughout the body, especially in areas where infectious agents may gain entrance to the body (skin, gastrointestinal tract, upper and lower respiratory tract).

The immune system is one of the surveillance systems of the body. The immune system is constantly in motion, checking out all parts of the body for the presence of "things" that don't belong there. In this regard, the immune system is similar to other surveillance systems of the body. For example, a particular odor may cause movement toward or away from the smell. Pain indicates that an aversive event is occurring. If heat is applied to an area of the body, the body reacts by moving away from the source of heat, avoiding tissue damage. Indeed, the surveillance properties of the central nervous system (CNS) often allow for the exact localization of a painful (dangerous) stimulus and signal the brain that something is wrong. Thus, there is often conscious perception of potential harm by some of the surveillance systems of the body.

With regard to surveillance by the immune system, there is no conscious perception by the brain that the immune system has identified an aversive (dangerous) event (usually an infectious agent). When the immune system "detects" the "smell" of an infection, it moves toward the infection and eliminates it, usually without our conscious awareness. However, we often experience tiredness, loss of appetite, and fever, as a result of activation of the immune system and the release of cytokines by the activated immune system. The cytokines signal the brain that the immune system is active and influence activities of the brain which then produce effects of tiredness and loss of appetite.

Probably the most dramatic way to describe the importance of the immune system is to describe what happens if an individual has no immune system. The absence of a functional immune system is incompatible with life. Just as the absence of a heart, lungs, or liver is incompatible with life, you cannot live without your immune system. Children born without functioning immune systems will die from overwhelming infections.

YOUR PERSONAL EXPERIENCE WITH IMMUNITY

Rather than beginning a description of the immune system by describing the cells and molecules that produce immune responses, I will first describe one of the primary protective functions of the immune system and provide examples of how stressors can influence this aspect of immune function.

Probably the first experience that one recalls regarding the immune system occurred when one was "immunized" against tetanus. Tetanus is a condition in which there is uncontrolled contraction of the muscles of the body, caused by damage to the nerves that innervate the striated muscles that provide voluntary movements. The damage is caused by a toxin produced by the bacterium *Clostridium tetani.*

Immunization to protect against the development of tetanus involves being injected with the antigen (a material that is foreign to the body and that activates the immune system, which then tries to remove the antigen from the body) tetanus toxoid (tetanus toxoid is tetanus toxin that has been treated so that it cannot bind to nerves but will still elicit an immune response). To be immunized is to be protected. The immunization results in antibody being produced that will bind to the tetanus toxin and prevent it from binding to nerves. Other examples of the immune system being activated to provide protection are immunization against diphtheria, measles, chickenpox, and polio.

The immune system consists of several different parts that must properly interact with each other and with disease-causing infectious agents (bacteria, viruses, fungi, parasites) for protection against infectious diseases to be provided. If there is an imbalance in the function of one of the parts of the immune system, the ability to resist infectious diseases may be compromised or the development of immune reactions that damage tissue may occur (autoimmune disease). The physiological response to a stressor alters the ability of the immune system to function properly.

As will be detailed later, several events must occur before a B lymphocyte is capable of releasing antibody that will combine with the antigen that stimulated the B lymphocyte to produce the antibody. Included in the process of antibody formation to an antigen are:

Cells called "interdigitating dendritic cells" and "follicular dendritic cells"

Lymphocytes called "CD4 T cells"

Soluble substances called "cytokines"

Molecules on lymphocyte and dendritic cell surfaces called "MHC II"

An antigen-recognition molecule on the CD4 T cell called the "T-cell receptor (TCR)"

Costimulation molecules on the T cell called "CD28" and "CD40L"

Costimulation molecules on the dendritic cells called "B7"

It should be obvious from the above list that antibody production is not a simple process. The following examples will show that antibody production does not occur independent of events in an individual's local environment.

EFFECT OF THE NUMBER OF ANIMALS HOUSED IN A CAGE ON ANTIBODY PRODUCTION

Whether one or five mice are housed in a cage would appear to be a benign event that would not be expected to have an impact on how the immune system functions. However, our investigative group and others have shown that housing different numbers of animals in a cage can influence several components of immune system function, including the immune system-dependent susceptibility to infection and possibly the growth of malignant tissue (Andervont, 1944; DeChambre and Gosse, 1973; Plaut et al, 1969; Soave, 1964).

Several studies were conducted in our laboratory that examined immunologic changes that occur when either one or five mice are housed in a cage. The mice were not crowded, had ample room to move around, and had unlimited access to food and water.

Initially, we studied an inbred strain (all animals genetically identical; identical twins) of male mice designated C3H/HeJ. When the mice were approximately 6 weeks of age, they were either housed in cages alone or in cages with four other animals of the same sex.

Our first study involved the injection of the animals with sheep red blood cells (erythrocytes). Sheep erythrocytes were selected as an antigen because antibody production to sheep erythrocytes requires the CD4 T-helper lymphocyte to interact with the antibody-producing B lymphocyte before antibody to the sheep erythrocytes will be produced. Thus, by using sheep erythrocytes as an antigen, we were able to test the functional activity of T-helper lymphocytes and B lymphocytes. In addition, there are assays that allow the actual number of B lymphocytes that are producing antibody to be counted. We found that the number of B lymphocytes in the spleen producing antibody to sheep erythrocytes was significantly lower in C3H/HeJ male mice that were housed five per cage as compared with those housed alone (Rabin et al, 1987).

We then determined whether the T lymphocytes or the B lymphocytes, or both, were functionally altered by the housing conditions. To make this determination, we immunized mice with an antigen that does not require the participation of a CD4 T-helper lymphocyte for antibody production. This is called a T-independent antigen. The antigen used was a carbohydrate that directly interacts with B lymphocytes and causes them to synthesize and release antibody.

When the mice were injected with the carbohydrate antigen, equal numbers of antibody-producing B lymphocytes were produced in the spleen of animals housed either one or five per cage. This indicated that B lymphocyte functional activity was not directly altered by the differential housing conditions. However, when a T-helper lymphocyte was required to facilitate antibody production, less antibody production occurred in the group housed animals. Therefore, the decrease in antibody production in the group housed mice was due to an altered function of the CD4 T-helper lymphocyte population.

To investigate how the function of CD4 T-helper lymphocytes was influenced by housing one or five mice in a cage, we conducted two additional experiments. The first involved stimulation of T lymphocytes with nonspecific mitogenic agents. Nonspecific mitogens will cause lymphocytes to undergo mitosis, regardless of whether the lymphocytes have previously been exposed to the nonspecific mitogen. The nonspecific mitogen that we used was derived from a plant and is called phytohemagglutinin (PHA). PHA will induce T lymphocytes to divide. We found the rate of mitotic division induced in the T lymphocytes to be significantly greater in spleen lymphocytes from individually housed animals in comparison with the group-housed animals. This suggests that the housing environment influenced the functional activity of the T cells.

The second assay of T cell function involved determination of the amount of the cytokine, interleukin-2 (IL-2) that is derived from activated T-helper lymphocytes. IL-2 is essential for the growth of T-helper cells in vitro. The assay measured the amount of IL-2 produced by the T-helper lymphocytes from group-housed and individually housed animals. Significantly more IL-2 was produced by spleen T-helper lymphocytes from individually housed mice than was produced by the group-housed animals. The difference in IL-2 production may account for less antibody production by B lymphocytes (as cytokine produced by T lymphocytes helps B lymphocytes to produce antibody) and the diminished response to mitogenic stimulation of the group housed mice.

Finally, we determined whether there were differences in the production of interleukin-1 (IL-1) between the group and individually housed mice (IL-1 is produced by the macrophage/monocyte and promotes the ability of T lymphocytes to give help to B lymphocytes). We found IL-1 production to be the same in spleen cells of group-housed and individually housed mice. This indicates that the immunologic difference which would explain the difference in the amount of antibody production was at the level of the T helper lymphocyte and involving IL-2 production.

Thus, this relatively simple study shows that the environment in which one resides may influence the function of the immune system. The immune system does not exist in isolation from the events occurring outside the body. It is likely that the outside environment is connected to the environment inside of the body in which the immune system resides, by the brain. As the brain can influence the chemical composition of the body, the environment outside the body can influence how well or poorly the immune system functions. As will be described in Chapter 7, the brain has the capability of modifying how events occurring outside of the body influence the hormonal composition of plasma.

Additional experiments found that:

1. Not every strain of mouse shows an alteration of immune reactivity when different numbers of mice are housed per cage. This suggests that multiple factors will influence how the immune system is altered by the environment that may be related to the genetic background of an animal and activation of areas within the brain by one's environment.

2. In some inbred strains, only male mice show an effect of housing on the immune system. In other strains, mice of both sexes show the effect. This suggests that sex hormones, in some strains of animals, interact with the environment to modify immune alterations.

EFFECT OF SOCIAL RANK ON ANTIBODY PRODUCTION IN MONKEYS

We studied the effect of social rank on antibody production in a group of male cynomolgus monkeys (Cunnick et al, 1991). Monkeys were housed in groups of five in large pens, with access to the outdoors. Control monkeys remained together throughout the course of the study. Experimental animals were reorganized at 4-week intervals, so that each monkey was rehoused with three or four new animals each month. Social rank was determined by observing whether or not a monkey won or lost when fighting with another monkey. The most dominant monkey won all their fights, and the animal that lost all their fights was the least dominant (submissive). All monkeys, regardless of rank, had access to adequate amounts of food. The immune response measured was the amount of antibody produced subsequent to immunization with tetanus toxoid.

For analysis of the data, the monkeys that were ranked numbers 1 and 2 (the dominant monkeys) were grouped together, and the animals ranked 3, 4, and 5 (the subordinate monkeys) were grouped together. Differences in antibody response were not random but were influenced by the social rank of the monkeys. A significant difference in the amount of IgG antibody produced to tetanus was detected between the two groups with the subordinate monkeys producing significantly more antibody. Possibly, the submissive monkey was under the least amount of stress as it knew its place and therefore did not worry about its lowly role (there was enough food and water for all). The dominant monkey had to fight to maintain dominance and was experiencing stress because of this. The stress may have decreased the ability of the dominant monkey to produce antibody. Alternatively, the submissive monkey may have been experiencing more stress than the dominant monkey and the stress response enhanced the antibody response (stress may enhance or suppress immunity; see Chapter 5). Regardless of the actual physiological and biological events that stress induced, at this point in the book the message being put forth is that social situations can influence immune function.

Whether the same hormones that were involved in modifying the antibody response were also involved in contributing to the different behaviors (dominance or submissiveness) of the monkeys is an intriguing question that is present throughout studies of mind–body medicine.

INTERPRETATION OF NORMAL AND ABNORMAL IMMUNE VALUES

A caution that needs to be emphasized in regard to immune function is that the obvious may not be the mechanism that is producing an alteration of the function of the immune system. A clinical example of antibody production being modified by a T cell is found in a disease called "common variable immunodeficiency" (CVI). This is a disease in which an individual grows up healthy and has an immune system that gives no indication of abnormal function. When the individual reaches the second or third decade of life, they begin to develop repeated episodes of infections with bacteria that are normally eliminated through processes that depend on antibody production. For example, they may develop repeated episodes of bacterial pneumonia or bacterial sinusitis or gastrointestinal infections with the protozoan organism *Giardia lamblia.*

When the amount of immunoglobulin present in their serum is measured, it is found to be extremely low. As B lymphocytes are the cells that synthesize and release immunoglobulins, it would be expected that the disease occurs secondarily to a defect in the function of B lymphocytes. However, in many patients with CVI, the B lymphocytes are capable of normal function but are not supplied with the proper stimulatory signals from T lymphocytes that are necessary to begin antibody production. Thus, the disease is actually caused by an abnormality of T lymphocytes.

This is an example of the importance of fully understanding the processes involved in antibody production. An abnormally low concentration of antibody in plasma does not necessarily indicate a defect of B lymphocyte function. It is important to understand the networks that regulate the function of the immune system. As demonstrated above, something that may appear to be benign, such as the number of animals housed in a cage, can influence antibody production.

ANTIGENS ARE SUBSTANCES THAT ACTIVATE AN IMMUNE RESPONSE

An antigen is a substance that elicits or activates an immune response. Once activated, the immune response is directed toward neutralizing or killing the antigen. The immune response may be either cellular or humoral. "Cellular" means that the immune response consists of T lymphocytes directly attacking the antigen. Humoral means that B lymphocytes are releasing antibody into the plasma and tissue fluids (humors) and that the antibodies contribute to elimination of the antigen.

Different types of antigens activate different types of immune responses. For example, bacteria that multiply in extracellular sites of the body will stimulate the production of antibodies by B lymphocytes. The antibodies will participate in killing and removal of the bacteria from the body. A virus that multiplies within a tissue is inaccessible to antibodies and therefore stimulates a different type of immune response. Viruses activate T lymphocytes to either directly attack and kill the infected cell or to focus an inflammatory response of phagocytic cells and tissue killing cytotoxic CD8 lymphocytes at the location of the infected cell, which will kill the infected cell.

Polysaccharide antigens do not stimulate cell-mediated immunity. Polysaccharides bind to receptors on B lymphocytes and stimulate the B lymphocyte to synthesize antibody to the polysaccharide. Polysaccharide antigens are not taken up by APCs such as dendritic cells and are not presented to CD4 T lymphocytes in major histocompatibility complex (MHC) molecules (concepts that will be explained later in this chapter). Therefore, polysaccharide antigens are unable to induce interaction between B lymphocytes and CD4 lymphocytes. As the T-cell B-cell interaction is required as part of the process that causes B lymphocytes to produce different classes of immunoglobulin (eg, IgG, IgA, IgE), polysaccharide antigens stimulate B lymphocytes to produce the IgM class of antibody molecules.

Protein antigens are taken up and processed by the APCs. T lymphocytes interact with the antigen that has been taken up and processed by the APCs. Through specific T-cell interactions with the APC and T-cell interactions with B cells, either cell-mediated immunity or production of antibody of different classes occurs.

Another type of antigen is termed the "superantigen." Although not actually functioning as an antigen, these substances have a profound effect on the immune system. Superantigens are soluble substances (termed "exotoxins") secreted by several types of bacteria. The superantigen binds to the outside portion of the T-cell receptor (TCR) (not the part of the TCR that binds to the antigenic peptide). As the binding does not depend on antigen–antibody specificity, a superantigen may bind to 30% of all T cells. The superantigen bound to a TCR also binds to the outside portion of the MHC molecule on APCs (not the part of the MHC that binds the antigenic peptide). The result of this bridging of T cells with APCs is that as many as 30% of T lymphocytes will be bound to APCs. This interaction stimulates a massive release of cytokines from the APC, often in concentrations that can have negative effects on health. A clinical example of this interaction is the "toxic shock syndrome," which occurs in association with bacterial infection and produces profound hypotension, sloughing of skin, failure of kidney and pulmonary function, and possibly death.

COMPONENTS OF THE IMMUNE SYSTEM

Where are the cellular components of the immune system formed, and where is the immune response initiated?

Lymphoid tissues are divided into two classes, the "primary lymphoid tissues," consisting of the bone marrow and thymus, and the "secondary lymphoid tissues," the spleen, lymph nodes, and lymphoid tissues of the gastrointestinal tract and pulmonary system. Lymphocytes are produced in the bone marrow, where an initial determination is made as to whether they will become T or B lymphocytes. The lymphocytes become activated to antigen in the secondary lymphoid tissues, not in the primary lymphoid tissues. The bone marrow is where white blood cells originate.

There are immature cells in the bone marrow, termed "stem cells," that have the potential of becoming one of several types of white blood cells (if blood is collected and prevented from clotting and allow to settle in a tube, the red blood cells will fall to the bottom, and a white layer of cells will lie on top of the red cells. The cells which form this white colored layer are commonly called "white blood cells"). The maturation of the cells of the marrow is under the influence of hormonal factors called "colony-stimulating factors." These soluble substances act upon immature cells in the marrow and induce them to mature to become either a granulocyte (of which there are several types; the neutrophil, the eosinophil, and the basophil), a monocyte, a lymphocyte, or a megakaryocyte.

To identify the granulocyte (also called polymorphonuclear leukocytes because of the variable shape of their nucleus) class of white blood cells, a drop of blood is placed on a microscope slide, spread into a single cell layer, and dried. A stain is then applied to the blood smear. The stain contains two dyes: methylene blue (blue color) and eosin (red color). The granules in basophils pick up the blue dye. Because the blue dye has a basic pH value, the blue-stained cells are called "basophils." Granules of eosinophils take up the red (eosin) dye. The granules of the cells called neutrophils take up both dyes and stain pale pink or purple. In each type of granulocyte, the nuclei stain dark purple and the cytoplasm gray to blue.

Lymphocytes and monocytes have a round nucleus and are not granular. These cells are collectively called "mononuclear cells." As monocytes are phagocytic cells, they are frequently called "mononuclear phagocytes." A list of white blood cells and a brief comment of their functions follows.

Neutrophil. These cells are granular leukocytes possessing a nucleus with three to five lobes. The granules in their cytoplasm contain enzymes that can digest bacteria. Neutrophils are involved in ingestion (phagocytosis) of solid particles such as bacteria. Neutrophils have the properties of being attracted to areas where they are needed by the mechanism of chemotaxis and the capability, via receptors for complement and antibodies, of binding foreign particles (eg, bacteria) to their surface so that the particles can be ingested and killed. Antibodies produced by the immune system participate by helping neutrophils ingest bacteria. Neutrophils do not present antigen to lymphocytes as part of the process by which an immune reaction is initiated (Fig. 2.1).

Eosinophil. These cells help protect against infections with some worms by releasing proteins that are toxic to the worms. They migrate to sites of allergic reactions that lead to damage of normal tissue (Fig. 2.2).

Basophil. Basophils arise from the bone marrow and circulate in the blood. They have granules containing histamine and surface receptors for the Fc portion of the IgE antibody molecule. Basophils usually do not enter tissue. A cell with a similar morphology is the mast cell. Mast cells also have histamine-containing granules and surface receptors for IgE. Mast cells do not circulate. Chemical factors released from mast cells mediate many allergic reactions (Fig. 2.3).

Monocyte. This cell ingests foreign materials that get into the body. When the monocyte enters tissue, it enlarges in size and is called a macrophage. They express

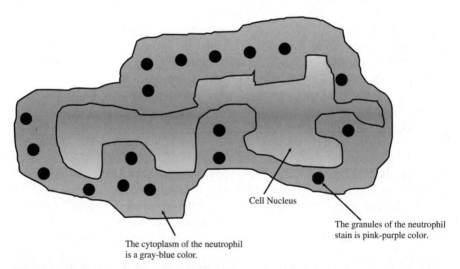

Cell Nucleus

The granules of the neutrophil stain is pink-purple color.

The cytoplasm of the neutrophil is a gray-blue color.

FIG. 2.1 *Lysosomal granules within the cytoplasm contain enzymes that will digest substances that the cell ingests. Phagocytosed substances are placed into vacuoles called "phagosomes". When the lysosomal granule fuses with the phagosomes, the lysosomal enzymes are released to digest the contents of the phagosome. The vacuole is then called a phagolysosome.*

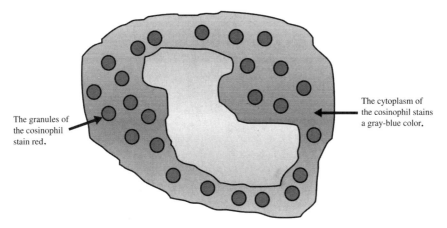

The granules of the cosinophil stain red.

The cytoplasm of the cosinophil stains a gray-blue color.

FIG. 2.2 *The granules in eosinophils are stained by the red dye "eosin." There is a protein in the granules that is toxic for microorganisms and tissue cells. The protein is released from the granules and will damage tissue at sites where the eosinophils accumulate.*

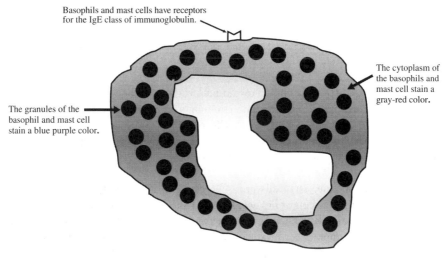

Basophils and mast cells have receptors for the IgE class of immunoglobulin.

The granules of the basophil and mast cell stain a blue purple color.

The cytoplasm of the basophils and mast cell stain a gray-red color.

FIG. 2.3 *The granules in basophils and mast cells (which stain with a blue dye having a basic pH) contain preformed chemical mediators of allergic reactions. The primary mediator is histamine which is released from the granules when the IgE immunoglobulin molecules on the cell membrane bind to the antigen to which they have specificity.*

class I and class II MHC molecules. Infectious agents that are ingested by monocytes and macrophages are often killed when the monocyte or macrophage is activated by a T lymphocyte. The T lymphocyte recognizes a portion of the infectious agent in MHC II molecules on the membrane of the monocyte or macrophage (Fig. 2.4).

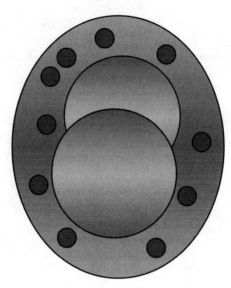

FIG. 2.4 *The monocyte will ingest microorganisms and kill them. Cytokines released from CD4 lymphocytes enhance the ability of monocyte (and macrophages) to kill ingested bacteria. The nucleus of the monocyte has a folded appearance.*

Lymphocyte. There are several types of lymphocytes, each with a different function (Fig. 2.5).

T Lymphocytes. These lymphocytes do not produce antibody. They are active in immune reactions termed "cell-mediated immunity." There are several different populations of T lymphocytes. T lymphocytes bearing the CD4 identification marker can be subcategorized into two classes: Th1 and Th2. The two different classes produce different cytokines and have different functional properties.

1. As a general rule, Th1 cells are effective against intercellular pathogens by being the effector cell of delayed hypersensitivity reactions and by producing cytokines which activate macrophages and cytotoxic CD8 lymphocytes. They also help B lymphocytes produce the classes of antibody that activate the complement system. Thus, they promote immune responses where phagocytosis of foreign material is important. Cytokines produced by Th1 cells are interferon-γ (IFN-γ), IL-2, and tumor necrosis factor-β (TNF-β).

2. As a general rule, Th2 cells are important in inducing B cells to produce IgE, IgA, and the noncomplement activating IgG4 class of antibodies. Cytokines produced by Th2 cells inhibit macrophage function. Th2 cells tend to be associated with phagocytic cell-independent reactions such as allergic reactions and the antibody that is secreted onto the mucosal surface of the body. Th2 cells produce IL-4, -5, -6, -10, and -13.

B lymphocytes. These lymphocytes produce antibody.

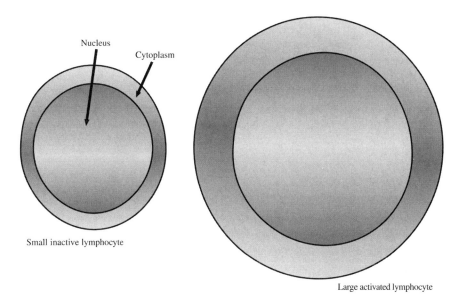

Nucleus

Cytoplasm

Small inactive lymphocyte

Large activated lymphocyte

FIG. 2.5   There are several different functional types of lymphocytes that all look alike under a microscope. However, they have different molecules on their surface that are used to tell them apart. Small sized lymphocytes are usually inactive (not having been activated to an antigen or being memory cells after having interacted with an antigen). Large lymphocytes, with large nucleus, usually are in the process of reacting to an antigen.

NK Lymphocytes. These lymphocytes are not T or B cells. They contain granules in their cytoplasm and have the capability of killing tissue cells that have been infected by a virus or that may be malignant.

Dendritic cell. The dendritic cell is found in secondary lymphoid organs, the skin, and all tissues of the body (Fig. 2.6). Technically, it is not a white blood cell. However, it is pictured and described here because of its importance to the immune system. Dendritic cells have high concentrations of MHC I and MHC II molecules, as well as costimulation molecules on their membranes. Thus, they are very efficient at activating a primary immune response. Dendritic cells in the spleen or lymph nodes initiate immune responses by interacting with a T cell that have antigen-recognizing receptors for the antigen being displayed on the membrane of the dendritic cell.

B Lymphocytes in the Marrow

In the marrow, newly formed B lymphocytes may be tolerized (inactivated or killed) if they have receptors for antigens that are constituents of the individual in whom the B lymphocytes are being formed (referred to as "self-antigens"). The receptor on the B lymphocyte that binds to an antigen is the antibody that the B lymphocyte will produce. Of the B lymphocytes that are not tolerized in the marrow, most die within a few days after leaving the marrow, unless they encounter antigen. The bone marrow

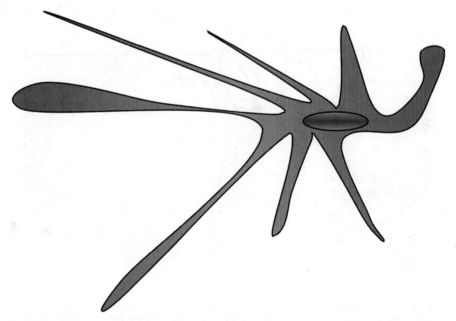

FIG. 2.6   *Dendritic cells have long filamentous processes which encounter foreign antigen.*

FACTOID: The production of cells from the bone marrow is influenced by the production of soluble factors, commonly referred to as "colony-stimulating factors." The source of the factors are fibroblasts that form the stroma (support meshwork) of the marrow and by T lymphocytes. Stress has been reported to alter the growth of bone marrow derived cells. The bone marrow of male C3H/HeJ mice housed either one or five per cage was studied for the ability to generate localized colonies of stem cells in an agar matrix (Salvin et al, 1990). Each colony that forms when bone marrow cells are suspended in a semisolid agar placed into petri dishes is derived from a single precursor cell in the marrow. Marrow obtained from mice house individually produced 1.6 times the number of colonies as cells from the marrow of mice housed five per cage. Lymphocytes of mice housed individually produced twice the amount of factors as did lymphocytes of mice housed five per cage.

In another study, the stress of physical restraint enhanced both the number of colony forming bone marrow cells and the production of colony-stimulating factors in experimental mice (Goldberg et al, 1991).

At least one factor, IL-3, is derived from T cells. Studies of the alteration of bone marrow growth promoting cytokine production by stressors will contribute to our understanding of the regulation of hematopoiesis.

is constantly producing lymphocytes which would accumulate in excessive amounts unless there is a mechanism to remove lymphocytes that are not being utilized. Thus, in order to survive, lymphocytes must interact with an antigen.

The maturation of B lymphocytes in the bone marrow proceeds through a series of steps characterized by (1) the random and non-antigen-dependent rearrangement of immunoglobulin genes, and, (2) by the production of enzymes and proteins that are required for the expression of the immunoglobulin molecule on the membrane of the B lymphocyte.

The stages of B-lymphocyte maturation are designated as:

Progenitor B lymphocyte—At this stage, the variable portion of the immunoglobulin heavy chain gene is rearranging. This occurs independently of antigen (Fig 2.7a).

Pre-B lymphocyte—These cells have μ heavy chains in the cytoplasm. μ heavy chains are synthesized by the B lymphocyte as part of the maturation process and independently of antigen or help from a T lymphocyte (Fig. 2.7b).

Immature B lymphocyte—These cells have intact IgM molecules inserted into the cell membrane. The IgM is not secreted from the lymphocyte but remains inserted into the membrane. At this stage of maturation the B lymphocyte can bind to the antigen that the IgM molecule has specificity for. This will initiate a series of events that will result in tolerance (Fig 2.7c).

Mature B lymphocyte—IgM, IgG, IgA, or IgE, are present on the B-cell membrane. As the expression of IgG, IgA, or IgE requires the input of cytokines from a T lymphocyte, this stage indicates that the B cell has interacted with the antigen that its surface-bound immunoglobulin has specificity for, and, in addition, with an activated T cell that interacted with an antigenic peptide in a MHC II molecule on the B cell.

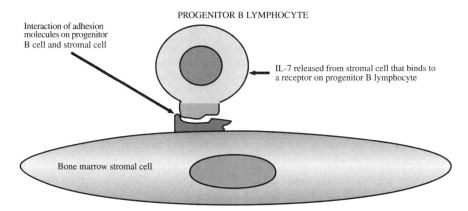

FIG. 2.7a *At the progenitor stage, the B lymphocyte adheres to adhesion molecules on the bone marrow stromal cells and binds IL-7 that is produced by the stromal cells. The immunoglobulin heavy chain genes in the progenitor B cell begin to rearrange the variable portion of the molecule. No immunoglobulin is synthesized at this stage of development.*

PRE B LYMPHOCTE

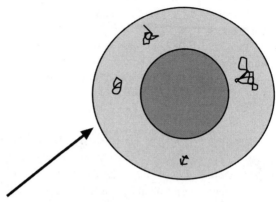

Rearranged μ heavy chain and light chain are
present in the cytoplasm

FIG. 2.7b   *Small pre-B lymphocytes arise as larger progenitor B cells divide. The pre-B lymphocyte contains rearranged μ heavy chains in the cytoplasm and light chains begin to undergo arrangement.*

IMMATURE B LYMPHOCYTE

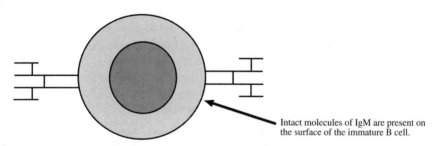

Intact molecules of IgM are present on
the surface of the immature B cell.

FIG. 2.7c   *Intact molecules of IgM are expressed on the cell membrane. At this stage of maturation the B lymphocyte is capable of recognizing antigen. If the antigen to which the IgM can bind is present in the bone marrow environment, the B cell will die or become functionally inactivated.*

Plasma cell—This cell is the end stage of maturation of the B lymphocyte. It synthesizes and releases the largest amount of immunoglobulin of any of the B cells. It has a distinct morphology and is rich in endoplasmic reticulum (where protein is synthesized within the cytoplasm of a cell). Even though the plasma cell releases large amounts of immunoglobulin, they do not have membrane bound immunoglobulin molecules as do the B lymphocytes. The plasma cell also lacks surface MHC molecules (Fig. 2.7d).

MATURE B LYMPHOCYTE

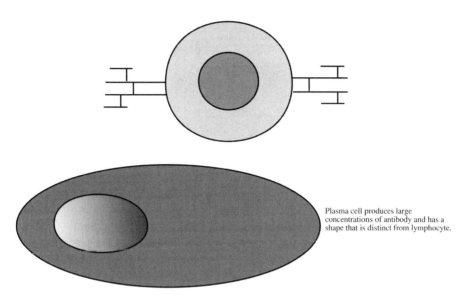

Plasma cell produces large
concentrations of antibody and has a
shape that is distinct from lymphocyte.

FIG. 2.7d   At this stage of maturation the B lymphocytes have IgM on their membrane and leave the bone marrow. The cells can be activated to secrete antibody to the antigen that fits into the rearranged variable region of the immunoglobulin molecule. Cytokines, which are released from CD4 T lymphocytes that interact with the B lymphocyte, induce the B lymphocyte to produce the IgG, IgA, or IgE classes of antibody molecules. Some mature B lymphocytes will become plasma cells and produce large amounts of antibody for several weeks, before dying. Many of the plasma cells producing antibody are located in the bone marrow.

Thymus Gland

The thymus gland is responsible for the maturation of lymphocytes that originate in the bone marrow and which will become functional T lymphocytes. It is likely that T lymphocytes that leave the bone marrow and enter the thymus do so because there is an adhesion molecule on the lymphocytes which binds to a receptor on the arterial or venous capillaries in the thymus (adhesion molecules cause the binding or sticking of a cell to another cell or of a cell to extracellular structures such as collagen). When this occurs the immature T lymphocytes will move across capillaries into the thymus parenchyma.

The thymus consists of two lobes, each wrapped in a capsule that sends membranous projections (septae) into the thymus dividing it into numerous small lobules (compartments). Each lobule consists of an outer portion called the "cortex" and an inner portion called the "medulla." Blood vessels migrate out of the septae and course through the outer (cortex) portion of the thymic lobules. A separate blood supply is present in the inner portion (medulla) of the thymus. Lymphatic vessels are found at the junction of the cortex and medulla (corticomedullary junction) and in the area adjacent to the blood vessels in the medulla. The lymphatics drain to lymph nodes and remove mature lymphocytes from the thymus.

The lobules of the thymus are filled with a meshwork of epithelial cells, macrophages, and dendritic cells. The remaining space is filled with lymphocytes. When the immature T cells enter the thymus they lack the CD4 and CD8 markers. However, both markers appear on the T cells once they are in the thymus and the cells undergo cell division. Most of these double positive cells will die with a small proportion (approximately 5%) surviving and leaving the thymus as single positive cells with either the CD4 (helper) or CD8 (cytotoxic) marker.

The T cells mature in the cortex of the thymus and leave the thymus through lymphatics that are at the corticomedullary junction and the medulla. The cells that leave the thymus have the capability of reacting to antigens that are foreign to the body. As will be described, an interaction between the thymic lymphocytes and antigen being presented by the epithelial cells, macrophages, and dendritic cells, determines whether the immature T lymphocytes will die in the thymus or leave the thymus as functional T cells.

The thymus participates in the elimination of immature bone marrow-derived T lymphocytes that (1) have a receptor for "self-antigens" that are constituents of the individual, or (2) are functionally useless.

During the maturation of T lymphocytes in the thymus, a receptor that binds to antigenic peptides presented in MHC molecules is generated on the T cell surface (the T-cell receptor [TCR]). The TCR is generated independently of an interaction with antigen. As formation of the TCR is a totally random process, some of the TCR that are produced will have the capability of binding to self antigen.

When immature T lymphocytes are in the thymus gland, a selection process takes place that evaluates the TCR on each of the immature T cells. Within the lobules of the thymus there are APCs, which have MHC I and MHC II (see Fig. 2.15) molecules on their surface. The MHC molecules are occupied with peptides derived from self-antigens. Assuming that the inside of the body is free of infectious agents, the only antigens present in the body will be self-antigens.

The TCR of the immature T cells can bind to the MHC molecules expressing self-antigens (which are the predominant antigens present in the fetus and throughout life); one of three events may occur:

Positive selection—During the random formation of the TCR, a configuration may have been generated that will fit into the peptide binding groove of the MHC molecule presenting the antigenic peptide, but the TCR does not have a shape that will bind tightly to the self peptide in the MHC molecule. At this stage of maturation, the immature T cell has both the CD4 and CD8 molecules on its surface. If the T cell has bound onto a MHC I molecule on an APC in the thymus, the CD8 molecule will bind to the CD8 receptor on MHC I. Synthesis of CD4 will cease. The binding of the CD8 molecule to its receptor on the MHC I molecule and, the TCR fitting into the MHC molecule but not binding tightly to the peptide in the molecule, will positively select the T cell for survival. The CD8 cell leaves the thymus and is considered naive until it binds to an APC in a lymph node or the spleen that contains the peptide to which the TCR can bind in a MHC I molecule. The formation of mature CD4 cells follows the same pattern except that the peptide is presented in a MHC II molecule (Fig. 2.8).

Negative selection of autoreactive cells—If the TCR binds tightly to the peptide in the MHC molecule, the CD4 or CD8 molecule will also bind to its receptor (depending on whether the cell is binding to a peptide presented in a MHC I or MHC II molecule). The combination of a tight binding of the TCR and the CD molecule binding to its receptor will result in T-cell death by apoptosis. Apoptosis is death of a cell that occurs when a trigger mechanism instructs the cell to kill itself. The tight binding of the TCR indicates that the T cell is binding to a self antigens and is an autoreactive T cell. To lessen the possibility of developing autoimmune diseases, autoreactive T lymphocytes are eliminated in the thymus (Fig. 2.9).

Negative selection of useless cells—During the random formation of the TCR, a configuration may have been generated that will not fit into the particular

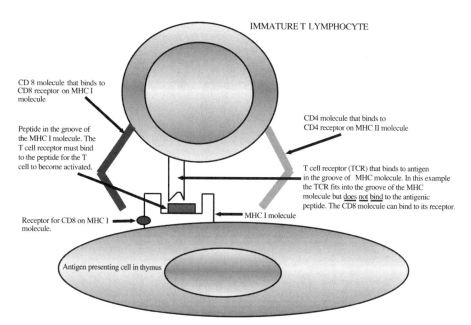

FIG. 2.8 *Note that the TCR and the peptide have different shapes. However the TCR can fit into the groove of the MHC molecule. When this occurs the CD8 molecule will bind to the CD8 receptor. This combination of events (the TCR fitting into the groove which allows the CD8 molecule to get enough to bind to its receptor) provides the immature lymphocyte with 1 signal indicating that the T cell will be able to recognize peptides in MHC molecules. This becomes a useful T lymphocyte which stops production of the CD4 molecule and leaves the thymus as a naive lymphocyte.*

shape of the MHC molecule presenting the antigenic peptide. In this case, the T lymphocyte would not be useful, as the TCR could not approach and bind to a foreign peptide. In the thymus, these immature T cells cannot recognize a peptide in a MHC molecule, and their CD molecule cannot bind to its receptor. These immature T lymphocytes die by apoptosis (Fig. 2.10).

Approximately 5% of all the immature T cells that enter the thymus leave as mature T cells.

The epithelial cells of the thymus produce hormones, called "thymic hormones." These thymus-derived hormones act on the immature T cells in the thymus and help them to mature into T cells that can become functional effector cells. The concentration of thymic hormones in the blood begins to decrease at approximately 60 years of age. A question of concern to immunology research will be whether individuals who experience high levels of stressors during their lifetime are more likely to undergo earlier decreases in the ability of the thymus to promote maturation of T lymphocytes in comparison with individuals who experience lower life time levels of stress.

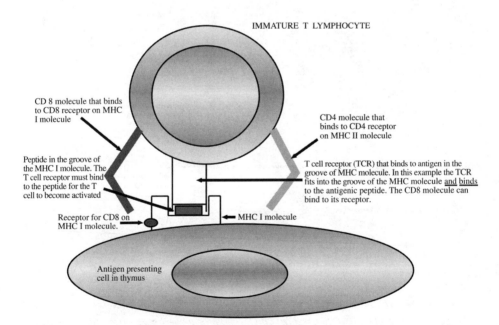

FIG. 2.9   *Note that the TCR and the peptide have the same shape. The TCR binds to the peptide in the groove and the CD8 molecule will bind to the CD8 receptor. This combination of events (the TCR binding to the peptide in the groove which allows the CD8 molecule to get close enough to bind to its receptor) provides the immature lymphocyte with two signals indicating that the T cell will be able to recognize self peptides in MHC molecules. This represents a T lymphocyte with autoreactive capabilities. This lymphocyte dies in the thymus gland.*

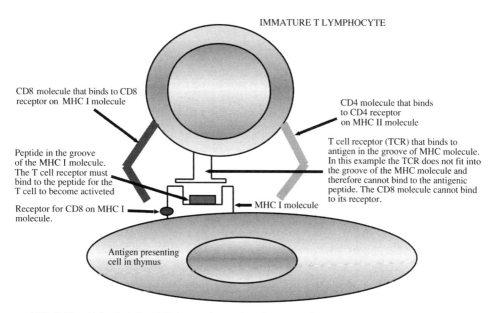

IMMATURE T LYMPHOCYTE

CD8 molecule that binds to CD8 receptor on MHC I molecule

CD4 molecule that binds to CD4 receptor on MHC II molecule

T cell receptor (TCR) that binds to antigen in the groove of MHC molecule. In this example the TCR does not fit into the groove of the MHC molecule and therefore cannot bind to the antigenic peptide. The CD8 molecule cannot bind to its receptor.

Peptide in the groove of the MHC I molecule. The T cell receptor must bind to the peptide for the T cell to become activeted

Receptor for CD8 on MHC I molecule.

MHC I molecule

Antigen presenting cell in thymus

FIG. 2.10   Note that the TCR has a shape that does not allow it to fit into the MHC groove. Therefore, the CD8 molecule will be unable to bind to the CD8 receptor. This combination of events (the TCR not fitting into the groove and the CD8 molecule not binding to its receptor) provides the immature lymphocyte with 0 signals. This represents a T lymphocyte that will be unable to recognize peptides in MHC molecules. This lymphocyte is useless, and it dies in the thymus gland.

Glucocorticoids produced by the adrenal gland in response to stressors have the capability of decreasing the size of the thymus gland (Damjanov and J. Linder, 1990). Do individuals with high levels of stress in their lives have a more rapid decline of immune function as they age than do individuals with low levels of life stressors?

A determination of the amount of thymosin α_1, one of the hormones produced by thymic epithelial cells, found that the stress associated with separation from their peers reduced the amount of measurable hormone in the blood of young squirrel monkeys (Coe and Hall, 1996). If the amount of thymic hormone being produced by the thymus gland is important for the maintenance of T-lymphocyte function, factors such as stress, which lead to a decrease in the ability of the thymus to produce such factors, may accelerate the decrease of immune function found as individuals age.

It is difficult to relate a specific amount of thymic hormone to the function of the cell mediated immune system and T-cell-mediated regulation of antibody production. This is partially due to the lack of an in-depth understanding of how the different thymic hormones integrate their function. Regardless, thymic hormones are important for a properly functioning immune system. Children who are born without a thymus (a disease called "thymic alymphoplasia" or "DiGeorge syndrome") have little if any T-cell activity.

The autoimmune disease insulin-dependent diabetes has a peak age of onset at puberty, which is when the thymus begins to decrease in size (Nystrom et al, 1992). As individuals age the amount of thymic hormones in blood decreases along with a decrease in the activity of their T-lymphocyte function (Hadden, 1992). As stressors are associated with an increase in the concentration of glucocorticoids, the sequelae of the effect on the thymus, immune function, and health are obvious concerns for the psychoneuroimmunologist.

There are studies that have used hormonal or nutritional factors to restore decreased thymic function in older experimental animals. These studies have found that aspects of decreased thymic function can be restored and that there is an accompanying increase in immune function in aged animals. For example, zinc supplementation will reverse decreased thymic hormone production in older animals, restore the histology of the thymus to that found in younger animals, and produce an increase in the function of lymphocytes (Dardenne et al, 1993; Mocchegiani and Fabris,1995; Mocchegiani et al, 1995b; Saha et al, 1995).

Providing exogenous melatonin, a product of the pineal gland, or actual transplantation of the pineal gland from young into older animals, has been shown capable of altering some of the histological and functional changes present in the thymus of older animals (Maestroni, 1993; Mocchegiani et al, 1994a,b; Persengiev et al, 1991; Pierpaoli, 1993; Pierpaoli and Regelson, 1994; Poon et al, 1994; Provinciali et al, 1996). Associated with the functional and histologic changes in the thymus is an increase of the function of lymphoid cells of the older animals.

There is also a nerve supply to the thymus, consisting of both sympathetic and parasympathetic nerve fibers (further described in Chapter 3). In rats there is a dense innervation of sympathetic nerve fibers at the corticomedullary junction, while in humans the medulla may have more sympathetic innervation. The sympathetic and parasympathetic nervous systems have been shown to influence T-cell maturation and emigration from the thymus. The role of the thymic innervation in modifying thymic hormone production has not been defined. The thymus gland increases in size from birth to puberty and then slowly undergoes involution, but it is often still functionally active, producing thymic hormones, into the seventh decade of life.

OVERVIEW OF ANTIBODY FORMATION

Before describing the various types of cells and how they function in producing an immune response, I will provide an overview of the cellular interactions that occur after the injection of antigen, which elicits a specific antibody response. This introduction will help in understanding the significance of each type of immune cell.

1. A specific immune response to a protein antigen first involves the protein being ingested by a dendritic cell. Dendritic cells are located in various tissues

of the body, including the skin. If an antigen (eg, an infectious agent) enters the body through a break in the skin or an injury, it is ingested by dendritic cells. After ingestion, the protein is digested in vacuoles to small peptides (short lengths of amino acids) as the dendritic cell moves from the skin to the para-cortical region of the lymph node that is draining the tissue site where the dendritic cell is located. The digested protein is then bound into a groove on a major histocompatibility complex molecule (MHC) that displays the protein on the surface of the dendritic cell (Fig. 2.11).

2. The dendritic cell localizes in the paracortical region of the lymph node. The paracortical region also contains "naive" CD4 T lymphocytes, ie, lymphocytes that have not interacted with an antigen but that have matured in the thymus and rearranged their TCRs so that they recognize an antigenic peptide bound into the MHC molecule. If the TCR of a CD4 T lymphocyte sees a peptide that it recognizes, the CD4 T lymphocyte becomes active and divides and releases soluble factors called cytokines, which help maintain activation of the CD4 lymphocyte but which will also help the CD4 lymphocyte induce a B lymphocyte to produce antibody. The activated CD4 cell may move from the paracortical region to the follicle (the B lymphocyte area) of the lymph node (Fig. 2.12).

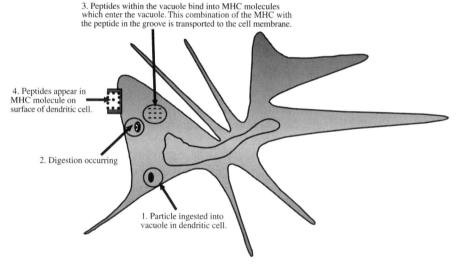

3. Peptides within the vacuole bind into MHC molecules which enter the vacuole. This combination of the MHC with the peptide in the groove is transported to the cell membrane.

4. Peptides appear in MHC molecule on surface of dendritic cell.

2. Digestion occurring

1. Particle ingested into vacuole in dendritic cell.

FIG. 2.11 *Dendritic cell ingests antigen, degrades the antigen into small peptides, and places the peptides into the groove of MHC molecules. A single dendritic cell may have tens of thousands of MHC molecules on its surface, each with a different peptide in it. The dendritic cell migrates from the site, where it ingests the antigen to the T-cell areas of lymph nodes. This is where the dendritic cell presents antigen to naive T lymphocytes. In the spleen, the dendritic cell ingests and processes antigen that passes in the blood stream, through the spleen. The dendritic cells move from the marginal zones of the spleen to the periarteriolar lymphocyte sheath, where they interact with naive T cells.*

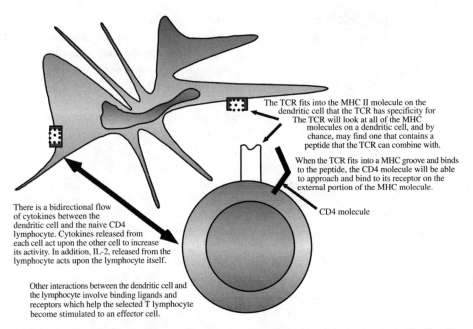

The TCR fits into the MHC II molecule on the dendritic cell that the TCR has specificity for The TCR will look at all of the MHC molecules on a dendritic cell, and by chance, may find one that contains a peptide that the TCR can combine with.

When the TCR fits into a MHC groove and binds to the peptide, the CD4 molecule will be able to approach and bind to its receptor on the external portion of the MHC molecule.

CD4 molecule

There is a bidirectional flow of cytokines between the dendritic cell and the naive CD4 lymphocyte. Cytokines released from each cell act upon the other cell to increase its activity. In addition, IL-2, released from the lymphocyte acts upon the lymphocyte itself.

Other interactions between the dendritic cell and the lymphocyte involve binding ligands and receptors which help the selected T lymphocyte become stimulated to an effector cell.

FIG. 2.12 *Once a CD4 lymphocyte has been activated the lymphocyte can go to the B cell containing follicles of the node or spleen and provide help to a B lymphocyte for antibody synthesis. Or the T cell may leave the lymphatic tissue and travel through the tissues of the body looking to attack the antigen that the T cell is activated against.*

3. Simultaneously with the antigen being processed and presented to CD4 lymphocytes, the intact antigen passes through lymphatic vessels to the draining lymph node. In the node, the antigen is recognized by naive B lymphocytes, which have a protein on their surface (the immunoglobulin molecule) that is capable of recognizing foreign protein in an intact form. After the antigen binds to the immunoglobulin molecule on the B lymphocyte, it is ingested by the B lymphocyte and is then digested; the peptides are presented on the surface of the B lymphocyte in the same type of molecule (MHC II molecules) that the dendritic cell used to present the peptides to CD4 lymphocytes. Naive B lymphocytes that have processed antigen react with activated T cells in the paracortical area of the node or in the follicles. If the reaction is in the paracortical area the cells then move into the follicles for expansion and antibody production.

4. The CD4 lymphocyte that recognized the peptide on dendritic cells will also recognize the peptide when presented by B lymphocytes. However, now there is a difference. The CD4 cell had been activated and is capable of producing cytokines that will stimulate antibody production by the B lymphocyte. The activated CD4 cell, reacting with the MHC–peptide complex on B lymphocytes will induce the B lymphocyte to become activated, to proliferate, and to release antibody against the protein. This is called "T-cell help" (Fig. 2.13).

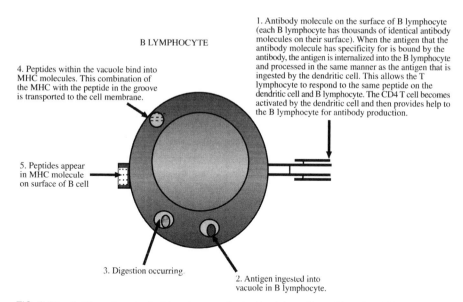

B LYMPHOCYTE

1. Antibody molecule on the surface of B lymphocyte (each B lymphocyte has thousands of identical antibody molecules on their surface). When the antigen that the antibody molecule has specificity for is bound by the antibody, the antigen is internalized into the B lymphocyte and processed in the same manner as the antigen that is ingested by the dendritic cell. This allows the T lymphocyte to respond to the same peptide on the dendritic cell and B lymphocyte. The CD4 T cell becomes activated by the dendritic cell and then provides help to the B lymphocyte for antibody production.

4. Peptides within the vacuole bind into MHC molecules. This combination of the MHC with the peptide in the groove is transported to the cell membrane.

5. Peptides appear in MHC molecule on surface of B cell

3. Digestion occurring.

2. Antigen ingested into vacuole in B lymphocyte.

FIG. 2.13 *A T lymphocyte that has been activated by interacting with a dendritic cell that is displaying the antigenic peptide that the TCR reacts with will move to the B-cell-rich follicle and bind to an MHC molecule on the B-cell membrane that is displaying the same peptide. Cytokines released from the T lymphocyte will cause the B lympocyte to produce either IgG, IgA, or IgE antibody molecules.*

5. B lymphocytes have a surface marker named CD40. The ligand (what CD40 binds to) for CD40, on the surface of activated helper CD4 cells, is termed CD40L (CD40 ligand). CD40L is transiently present on activated CD4 cells. It appears on T cells after the TCR binds to an antigen. The CD40 : CD40L interaction is termed "costimulation." The interaction between the CD40 and the CD40L ensures that only the B lymphocyte that is interacting with the T cell will be activated. Other B cells in the area may be bathed in cytokines, but they will not have a costimulatory molecule being activated and therefore, they will not synthesize and release antibody.

6. The B-cell-rich follicles (saclike accumulations of B cells) contain follicular dendritic cells (FDC) that trap antigen in the form of immune complexes (antigen bound to its specific antibody). Once a B cell is activated to produce antibody, the antigen bound to the cell membrane of the FDC selects (binds) those B cells that produce antibody of the highest affinity for survival. B cells that produce antibody of low affinity will die. Antibody that binds tightly to an antigen will be more useful than antibody that does not bind tightly (Fig. 2.14).

7. In addition to helping B lymphocytes produce antibody, the activated CD4 lymphocyte may leave the lymph node, migrate through tissue, and look at the surface of tissue cells for the presence of a peptide in a MHC II molecule that the TCR can bind to. The CD4 cell may then initiate a process that will kill the cell which is displaying the peptide on its surface. If the CD4 cell attracts other

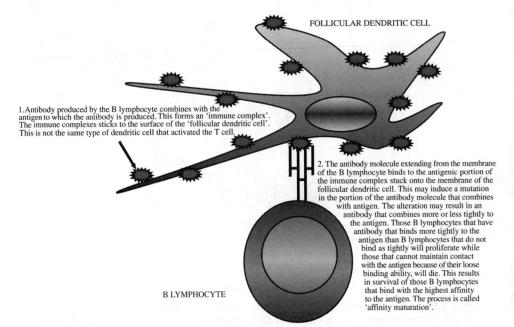

FOLLICULAR DENDRITIC CELL

1. Antibody produced by the B lymphocyte combines with the antigen to which the antibody is produced. This forms an 'immune complex'. The immune complexes sticks to the surface of the 'follicular dendritic cell'. This is not the same type of dendritic cell that activated the T cell.

2. The antibody molecule extending from the membrane of the B lymphocyte binds to the antigenic portion of the immune complex stuck onto the membrane of the follicular dendritic cell. This may induce a mutation in the portion of the antibody molecule that combines with antigen. The alteration may result in an antibody that combines more or less tightly to the antigen. Those B lymphocytes that have antibody that binds more tightly to the antigen than B lymphocytes that do not bind as tightly will proliferate while those that cannot maintain contact with the antigen because of their loose binding ability, will die. This results in survival of those B lymphocytes that bind with the highest affinity to the antigen. The process is called 'affinity maturation'.

B LYMPHOCYTE

FIG. 2.14 Antibody production is maintained by the B lymphocyte binding to specific antigen held on the surface of follicular dendritic cells.

cells to help in this process (cells such as polymorphonuclear leukocytes, eosinophils, and monocytes) the reaction is called a "delayed hypersensitivity reaction." If the T cell, by itself, kills the cell displaying the peptide, the reaction is called "cytotoxicity." Cytotoxicity is mediated by activated CD8 lymphocytes.

B lymphocytes are present in all tissues of the body. They are probably exposed to numerous cytokines that are present in plasma and extracellular fluids. If activation of B lymphocytes occurs subsequent to exposure to signals from the nonspecific cytokines, all B lymphocytes would be activated, all the time. However, as polyclonal activation usually does not occur, it is clear that a specificity factor must be in place. Indeed, it has been found that resting B lymphocytes cannot be induced to grow and differentiate to thymus dependent antigens by exposure of the lymphocytes to cytokines. This indicates that the selection process for determining which B lymphocyte will be activated, must first involve the binding of an antigen to the immunoglobulin receptor on the B lymphocyte and then costimulatory activation by the appropriate T cell.

Stressors can alter the function of most of the components of the immune response (APCs, MHC molecules, T lymphocytes, B lymphocytes, cytokines). These alterations will be described in Chapter 4.

Antigen-Presenting Cells

A critical component of the initiation of an immune response is a requirement for protein antigen to be processed byAPCs. Once the protein antigen is processed by APCs, T and B lymphocytes can become activated. The antigen presenting cells are the dendritic cells (probably the most important antigen presenting cell because of a high concentration of costimulatory molecules on its surface) macrophages and B lymphocytes.

APCs other than B lymphocytes do not specifically recognize antigen but are capable of ingesting and digesting antigen and presenting it in a form in MHC molecules that can activate T lymphocytes. The APCs are constantly ingesting proteins which are in their microenvironment (the fluid surrounding the APCs). Most of the time, the proteins will consist of one's own proteins (these are self-antigens). The APCs ingest these self-antigens and process them for presentation to naive T cells. However, because self-reactive T lymphocytes are eliminated in the thymus, autoimmune reactions usually do not occur.

Dendritic cells are found in a variety of tissues and have different names depending on the site of localization:

Veiled cells in afferent lymphatics (these are dendritic cells that have left the anatomic region, where they have ingested foreign antigen and are moving to the draining lymph node)

Interdigitating dendritic cells in thymus

Interstitial dendritic cells in heart, kidney, intestine, lung

Langerhans cells in skin and mucous membranes

If a foreign antigen, such as a bacteria, gains entrance to the body and is processed by the dendritic APCs, the sequence of events will ensue as outlined above. The dendritic cell will leave the site where it processed the antigen, for example the skin, and will enter the lymphatic capillaries and join the lymph fluid as it passes to the lymph node draining the anatomical region.

B lymphocytes that are also APCs recognize antigen by means of antibody specific for the antigen and which is on the surface of the B lymphocyte. Thus, B lymphocytes can only present the antigen to which they make antibody. Once they process the antigen and display it on their surface in a MHC II molecule, the B lymphocyte can interact with an activated T cell and be stimulated to release antibody.

All the potential portals of entry of infectious agents, such as the lungs and gastrointestinal tract, have their own collections of APCs to facilitate antigen processing and immune activation.

Major Histocompatibility Complex Molecules

The term major histocompatibility complex (MHC) is derived from the initial identification of molecules on the surface of tissue cells that were found to be important in stimulating the immune reaction that produced rejection of transplanted tissue. Thus, these molecules were called major (because they were important), histocompatibility

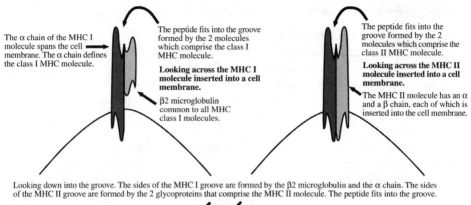

The α chain of the MHC I molecule spans the cell membrane. The α chain defines the class I MHC molecule.

The peptide fits into the groove formed by the 2 molecules which comprise the class I MHC molecule.

Looking across the MHC I molecule inserted into a cell membrane.

β2 microglobulin common to all MHC class I molecules.

The peptide fits into the groove formed by the 2 molecules which comprise the class II MHC molecule.

Looking across the MHC II molecule inserted into a cell membrane.

The MHC II molecule has an α and a β chain, each of which is inserted into the cell membrane.

Looking down into the groove. The sides of the MHC I groove are formed by the β2 microglobulin and the α chain. The sides of the MHC II groove are formed by the 2 glycoproteins that comprise the MHC II molecule. The peptide fits into the groove.

FIG. 2.15   *MHC class I and MHC class II molecules.*

(because they were involved in determining if transplanted tissue would be compatible when taken from an organ donor and given to an organ recipient), complex (because there are many different molecules which are coded for by several genetic loci (location on a chromosome) with multiple alleles (alternate choices of a gene from the total population).

In addition to their role in organ transplantation, the MHC molecules are important as they are located on cells which present antigens to lymphocytes as part of the process of a lymphocyte being converted from a naive state (before being activated to an antigen) to an effector state (after interaction with an antigen and ready to react against infectious agents). There are two major groupings of MHC molecules, designated "MHC I" and "MHC II."

MHC I molecules present antigens to the CD8 class of T lymphocytes (cytotoxic lymphocytes), and MHC II molecules present antigens to the CD4 class of T lymphocytes (helper and mediators of cell-mediated immunity). MHC molecules contain a groove in the portion of the molecule which is oriented away from the surface of the APC. The groove contains a peptide of approximately 10–14 amino acids derived from an antigen that is either a component of self (autologous antigen) or from a foreign material. The groove presents the antigenic peptide to predetermined T lymphocytes that react with the peptide through their TCR. MHC I molecules present antigenic peptides that are synthesized within a cell (usually derived from viruses) and MHC II molecules present antigenic peptides derived from the degradation of antigens, such as bacteria or large proteins, that are ingested into a APC. Every MHC molecule must have a peptide in its groove, or the MHC molecule will not move from the cytoplasm of the APC to the cell membrane of the APC.

HLA MOLECULES

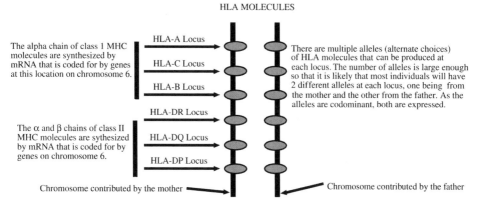

The alpha chain of class 1 MHC molecules are synthesized by mRNA that is coded for by genes at this location on chromosome 6.

HLA-A Locus

HLA-C Locus

HLA-B Locus

HLA-DR Locus

The α and β chains of class II MHC molecules are sythesized by mRNA that is coded for by genes on chromosome 6.

HLA-DQ Locus

HLA-DP Locus

There are multiple alleles (alternate choices) of HLA molecules that can be produced at each locus. The number of alleles is large enough so that it is likely that most individuals will have 2 different alleles at each locus, one being from the mother and the other from the father. As the alleles are codominant, both are expressed.

Chromosome contributed by the mother

Chromosome contributed by the father

FIG. 2.16   *The HLA molecules that appear on the surface of tissue cells and that present anti-genic peptides to the TCR of T lymphocytes, are coded for by genes on the number 6 chromosome. Proteins coded for by genes from both chromosomes are synthesized. Therefore, each cell has two molecules of HLA-A, one from each parent. There are several thousand of each of the HLA-A molecules on the surface of a cell. There are a total of 12 different HLA molecules that are present on a cell membrane, six from each parent (HLA-A, B, C, DR, DP, DQ). The different HLA alleles are assigned numbers. For example, some of the alleles at the HLA-A locus have been assigned numbers 1, 2, 3, 9, 11, 24, 26. Thus, HLA-A1 refers to a MHC class I molecules that can be identified as being the A1 molecules. As both alleles are present on a cell the complete HLA identification of an individual may be: HLA-A1, A3, C1, C2, B7, B8, DR1, DR3, DP1, DP2, DQ2, DQ3.*

As the inside of the body is usually free of infectious agents, most MHC molecules will contain peptides derived from our own proteins (the "self-antigens"). During the development and maturation of T and B lymphocytes, all the lymphocytes that develop receptors than can recognize self-antigens (immunoglobulin on B lymphocytes and the TCR on T lymphocytes) should be eliminated by the process of tolerization. Thus, the remaining lymphocytes that can recognize foreign antigens must search throughout the body looking for foreign peptides in MHC molecules. This is an extremely active process, with T lymphocytes rolling over APC and sampling the peptide in the MHC groove. If the TCR does not fit onto the peptide, the T lymphocyte keeps on rolling. If the TCR fits onto the peptide, adhesion molecules stop the rolling of the T lymphocyte and initiate its conversion from a naive to an effector T lymphocyte.

In humans the MHC molecules are part of the human leukocyte antigen (HLA) system. Class I HLA genes code for the MHC I molecules and class II HLA genes code for MHC II molecules. For class I molecules, there are three loci (locations on chromosome number 6 where the genes for MHC I are located): HLA-A, HLA-B, and HLA-C. For class II molecules, there are three loci: HLA-DR, HLA-DP, and HLA-DQ. The class I and class II molecules are polymorphic (many possible genes at each locus) at each of the loci. Therefore, there are many different proteins that can be synthesized within the human population. For example, there are more than 20 alleles at the HLA-A locus and 40 at the HLA-B locus (Figs. 2.15 and 2.16).

T Lymphocytes

Progenitor T lymphocytes from the bone marrow migrate to the thymus, where they accomplish most of their differentiation. There are three stages to thymic differentiation. The maturation consists of rearrangements in the genome that produces the two polypeptide chains that make up the TCR (the TCR is what binds to the antigen that is presented bound to the MHC molecule by the APC). There are four possible polypeptide chains for the TCR, termed α, β, γ, and δ. On functional T cells, the TCR consists of either dimers of the alpha and beta chains (the predominant type of T cell), or the γ and δ chains.

During early maturation, the TCR genes begin to rearrange. The T cells begin to express the surface markers CD1, CD2, CD4, CD5, CD8. The CD nomenclature is a standardized system that is used to designate a specific substance which is present on the surface of a cell. Many of the CD markers have been well characterized both as to the cells they are present on and as to what they do on that cell. For example, all T lymphocytes have CD3 on their surface. Some T lymphocytes also have CD4 and are termed CD4+; others are CD8+. Regardless of whether they have CD4 or CD8, they also have CD3. The CD3 participates in signaling the T cell that the TCR has bound an antigenic peptide.

Thus, several different CD markers are present on the surface of the same cell. CD markers are commonly detected by reacting the cells with an antibody that is specific for the CD marker. Thus, to determine if a cell is CD3+, the cells would be incubated with an antibody that is reactive to CD3. To detect whether or not the antibody bound to the cells, the anitbody has a dye attached to it. If the color product of the dye is visualized on the cell, it would be known to be CD3+. A common procedure to detect CD markers on lymphocytes is termed "flow cytometry" (see Fig. 2.41). The two major populations of T lymphocytes in the peripheral blood are CD3+ CD4+ CD8- and the CD3+ CD4- CD8+ cells.

CD4 T Lymphocytes. Effector CD4 T lymphocytes are capable of binding to an antigen presented in MHC class II molecules on the surface of a tissue cell and then releasing soluble factors (called cytokines), which attract inflammatory cells (neutrophils, eosinophils, monocytes, and macrophages) to the tissue site where the CD4 lymphocyte has bound. The inflammatory cells release enzymes to kill infectious agents in tissue. The phagocytic cells then ingest the killed or damaged tissue. Cytokines released from effector CD4 T lymphocytes will activate a macrophage that has ingested an infectious agent to kill the infectious agent (Fig. 2.17).

The CD4 lymphocyte population has two functional components: Th1 cells and Th2 cells. Both populations have important functional differences. When an activated Th1 lymphocyte binds to the MHC II molecules of a B lymphocyte that has processed an antigen, the Th1 cell releases cytokines that cause the B lymphocyte to release the IgG1, IgG2, and IgG3 classes of immunoglobulin. These immunoglobulin classes participate in the removal of bacteria from the body by enhancing the ability of the bacteria to be ingested by neutrophils. The process is called "opsonization." In addition, the Th1 cells are responsible for reactions called "cell-mediated immunity" or "delayed hypersensitivity," which produces an inflammatory response at the site of an infection as a means of removing the infectious agent.

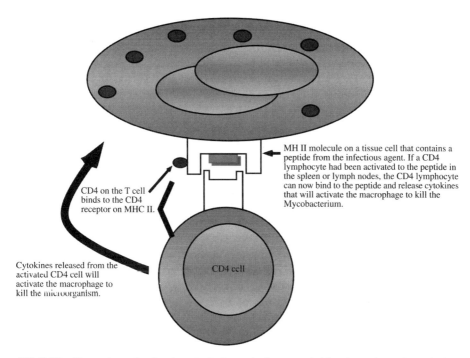

MH II molecule on a tissue cell that contains a peptide from the infectious agent. If a CD4 lymphocyte had been activated to the peptide in the spleen or lymph nodes, the CD4 lymphocyte can now bind to the peptide and release cytokines that will activate the macrophage to kill the Mycobacterium.

CD4 on the T cell binds to the CD4 receptor on MHC II.

Cytokines released from the activated CD4 cell will activate the macrophage to kill the microorganism.

CD4 cell

FIG. 2.17 *Macrophage that has ingested a bacteria, for example* Mycobacterium tuberculosis.

Th2 cells produce different cytokines than the Th1 cells. The Th2-derived cytokines stimulate B lymphocytes to produce the IgA, IgE, and IgG4 classes of immunoglobulin. Th2 cells do not participate in cell mediated immune reactions.

There is a down-regulating interaction between Th1 and Th2 cells. Cytokines released by either Th1 or Th2 cells will decrease the activity of the other cell population. Thus, increased activity of one of the cell populations is associated with decreased activity of the other population.

Several factors may participate in directing a CD4 cell to the Th1 or Th2 pathway, although the precise mechanism is still under study:

1. The local cytokine environment that is present when the T cell interacts with an APC (eg, IL-12 released from macrophages that ingest an antigen promotes the development of Th1 cells; IL-4 in the microenvironment where the CD4 T lymphocyte is interacting with the APC promotes the development of Th2 cells)

2. The density of the peptide being presented to the CD4 T cell in MHC molecules on the surface of the APC with a higher density of peptide associated with development of the Th1 cells

3. The strength of binding of the TCR with the peptide in the MHC molecule on the APC with tighter binding being associated with development of Th1 cells

4. The density and types of costimulatory molecules on the APC

5. The types and concentration of hormones that are present when the T cell interacts with an APC

FACTOID: The balance of activity between the CD4 Th1 and CD4 Th2 populations of lymphocytes is important to the overall function of the immune system and the onset or exacerbation of immunologically mediated disease. Cytokines produced by the Th1 or Th2 cell populations will modify the function of the other population. High levels of Th1 activity are associated with cell mediated immune activity (resistance to viral infections, fungal infections, and intracellular bacterial infections) and decrease the function of the Th2 lymphocyte population. High levels of Th2 function will promote the production of the IgE, and IgA classes of antibody (associated with resistance to parasitic disease, an increased clinical development of allergic disease, and increased resistance to infections on the mucosal surfaces of the body) while decreasing Th1 function.

A predominance of Th1 function has been associated with progression of autoimmune disease, and increased resistance to fungal infection (Charlton and Lafferty, 1995; Crucian et al, 1996; Kallmann et al, 1997; Kobrynski et al, 1996; Kroemer et al, 1996; Nicholson and Kuchroo, 1996; Olsson, 1995; Vandenbark et al, 1996). Thus, environmental factors which influence the balance between Th1 and Th2 may modify the course of immune-mediated disease.

An inverse relationship has been reported between whether an individual has a positive delayed hypersensitivity skin-test response to tuberculin and also has asthma. A positive delayed hypersensitivity skin test response is an indicator of a functioning Th1 CD4 population of lymphocytes. IgE production is regulated by cytokines produced by Th2 lymphocytes, in particular IL-4. As cytokines released from Th1 cells are capable of decreasing the function of Th2 cells, it can be hypothesized that those subjects who have good Th1 lymphocyte function will be producing cytokines that decrease the ability of Th2 cells to stimulate IgE antibody production by B lymphocytes. It would be anticipated that such individuals would have less IgE-mediated disease, such as asthma (Shirakawa et al, 1997). On the other hand, individuals who produce more IgE, and may be considered more likely to develop allergic disease, would have more Th2 lymphocyte function and a lower function of the Th1 population. Indeed, an inverse correlation between the plasma concentration of IgE antibody and the amount of induration (swelling) of the tuberculin delayed hypersensitivity skin test was found. This interesting observation will most likely stimulate considerable research interest to clarify whether the hypothesis of the relationship between activation of Th1 responses by infectious agents, or possibly vaccination, can suppress the development of allergic diseases. Careful attention will have to be directed to parameters that predispose to allergic disease as the effect of tuberculin immunization may not be present in subjects with a strong genetic predisposition to the development of allergy (Alm et al, 1997). Possibly, a strong genetic predisposition will overcome the influence of a deliberate alteration of the balance between Th1 and Th2 cells.

However, the relationship of positive Th1 cell mediated skin reactivity and a decreased allergic predisposition may increase a predisposition to other medical problems. For example, one of the ways that worms are removed from the body is by an IgE-mediated response to antigens of the worm. IgE is involved with histamine release and histamine produces a contraction of smooth muscle cells. If a worm clamps its mouth onto intestinal tissue and some of the antigens of the worm bind to IgE on the surface of histamine containing mast cells in the mucosa of the intestine, the histamine that is released may cause the worm to open its mouth and be discharged from the body. If procedures are developed to decrease allergic diseases through immunization to increase Th1 lymphocyte activity, the possible resultant decrease of IgE antibody may increase the susceptibility to worm infections.

The balance between Th1 and Th2 is altered by stress. Studies in experimental animals indicate that catecholamines do not affect the function of Th1 and Th2 cells equally. Chemical sympathectomy (the use of chemicals to remove the ability of nerves to release catecholamines) of mice suggest that catecholamines may shift the balance between Th1 and Th2 cells with catecholamines decreasing Th1 activity (Kruszewska et al, 1995). Indeed, high-affinity β-adrenergic receptors are found on mouse Th1 lymphocytes but not on mouse Th2 lymphocytes (Sanders et al, 1994). We have found, in humans, that exercise alters the production of cytokines by Th1 cells with an increase of the Th1 cytokines but no alteration of Th2 cytokines (Moyna, 1996).

A study of cytokines produced by Th1 and Th2 lymphocytes in humans undergoing the stress of surgery for cholecystectomy (gallbladder removal), has been reported. Some subjects had conventional surgery involving an incision into the peritoneal cavity, manipulation of organs, and suturing of the incision site and the skin, while others had a less traumatic and painful procedure with the gallbladder being removed through a laproscopic procedure (Decker et al, 1996). The cytokines produced by Th1 and Th2 cells were measured before surgery and for 48 hours afterward. Conventional surgery significantly increased cytokine production by Th2 cells (measured by IL-4 production) more than laparoscopic surgery (although both types of surgery increased IL-4 production). Cytokine production by Th1 cells (measured by IFN-γ production) was decreased to a greater degree by conventional than by laparoscopic surgery.

Thus, exercise and the stress of surgery produce different alterations of Th1 and Th2 function. It is likely that the differences are related to the specific hormonal response and the quantity of the various stress hormones produced. The ultimate effect of stress hormones on any particular cell will be the summation of the various effects of each hormone (described in Chapter 5). In this regard there is an indication, from studies in mice, that glucocorticoids may contribute to the development of a predominantly Th2 response (Daynes and Araneo, 1989). If glucocorticoids are elevated as a result of a stressor, and the glucocorticoid elevation decreases the ability of Th1 cells to produce cytokines, there may be unopposed activation of the Th2 cell population. This observation also suggests that circadian rhythm may influence the characteristics of an immune response as the concentrations of various hormones differ during the light and dark phases of a day. The characteristics of an immune response occurring during daylight may differ from the characteristics of an immune response occurring during the dark cycle.

The importance of the balance between Th1 and Th2 cells on resistance to infectious and malignant disease is becoming increasingly recognized. As the hormonal environment that is present during the development of an immune response may contribute to the characteristics of the response, the influence of stressors on the hormonal milieu in which the immune response develops, will have to be clearly and completely understood.

CD8 T Lymphocytes. This class of T lymphocytes is capable of binding to an antigen being presented in MHC class I molecules on the surface of a tissue cell and then killing the tissue cell. These are commonly called "cytotoxic" lymphocytes.

CD8 lymphocytes have the capability of binding to a foreign antigenic peptide in the groove of a class I MHC molecule and of releasing an enzyme that will kill the cell displaying the foreign peptide. The influence of hormones that are increased in concentration by stress on the functional activity of the CD8 cells is an important and needed area of investigation. As CD8 cells are important for the elimination of virus-infected cells, a decrease in their activity may contribute to an increased susceptibility to viral infection. CD8 activation and killing of target cells are illustrated in Figures 2.18 and 2.19.

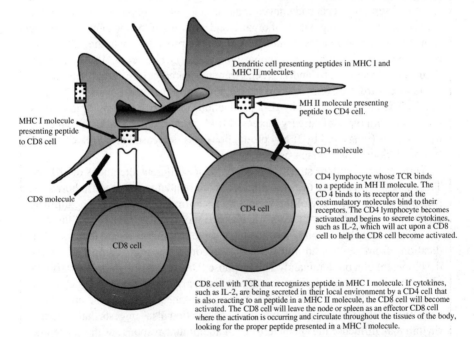

FIG. 2.18 *The activation of a CD8 lymphocyte requires both a CD4 and CD8 lymphocyte to react with antigenic peptides on a dendritic cell. The CD4 and CD8 cells must be in proximity to each other to allow the cytokines produced by the CD4 lymphocyte to promote activation of the CD8 cell.*

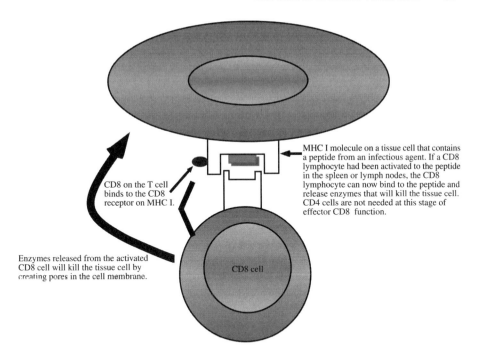

FIG. 2.19 *A CD8 lymphocyte that has been activated can exert its cytotoxic activity on an infected cell without help from a CD4 lymphocyte.*

FACTOID: In several studies of humans, in which subjects were exposed to an acute laboratory stressor, the number of CD8 cells circulating in the blood increased significantly (Herbert et al, 1994; Manuck et al, 1991; Naliboff et al, 1991). However, these were short-term studies and only quantitated the numbers of CD8 cells, providing no information about their function. The acute stress to medical students of taking an examination has been reported to decrease or have no effect on the numbers of CD8 lymphocytes (Kiecolt-Glaser et al, 1985, 1986). Thus, an acute stressor devised and delivered in a laboratory setting may not replicate the quantitative alteration of CD8 cells induced by an acute stressor associated with a life event. Chronic life event stressors have been reported either to increase the number of CD8 cells present in blood (Herbert and Cohen, 1993); produce no change (Kiecolt-Glaser et al, 1987, 1991); or decrease of CD8 (McKinnon et al, 1989; Spratt and Denney, 1991) numbers.

The reason for the differences in acute laboratory vs. acute naturalistic vs. chronic stressors on CD8 numbers in blood can be due to several factors. The data may reflect differences in technical procedures between laboratories that precluded the ability to duplicate the findings of different research groups. The assessment of acute or chronic stress may have differed between different research groups. Coping skills may have differed between subjects in different environments. Obviously, the reason for the discrepancies cannot be determined, nor

can the health implications of alterations of CD8 numbers by stress be determined. However, the data do indicate that careful attention to laboratory techniques, the coping skills of the experimental subjects, and the careful assessment
of stressors that an individual is experiencing, are essential components of psychoneuroimmunology research.

The differences may also reflect different concentrations of stress hormones
induced by acute or chronic stressors, different hormones being produced, or alterations in the number of receptors for stress hormones on cells of the immune
system.

T-Cell Receptors

A lymphocyte can only recognize an antigen for which the lymphocyte has a receptor. The receptors are the eyes of the lymphocyte. Thus, for T lymphocytes to be able
to identify millions of different foreign antigens, there must be millions of T lymphocytes, each bearing a different receptor for foreign antigen. Each T lymphocyte

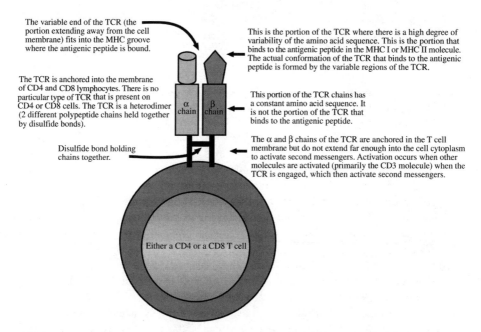

The variable end of the TCR (the
portion extending away from the cell
membrane) fits into the MHC groove
where the antigenic peptide is bound.

This is the portion of the TCR where there is a high degree of
variability of the amino acid sequence. This is the portion that
binds to the antigenic peptide in the MHC I or MHC II molecule.
The actual conformation of the TCR that binds to the antigenic
peptide is formed by the variable regions of the TCR.

The TCR is anchored into the membrane
of CD4 and CD8 lymphocytes. There is no
particular type of TCR that is present on
CD4 or CD8 cells. The TCR is a heterodimer
(2 different polypeptide chains held together
by disulfide bonds).

This portion of the TCR chains has
a constant amino acid sequence. It
is not the portion of the TCR that
binds to the antigenic peptide.

α chain   β chain

The α and β chains of the TCR are anchored in the T cell
membrane but do not extend far enough into the cell cytoplasm
to activate second messengers. Activation occurs when other
molecules are activated (primarily the CD3 molecule) when the
TCR is engaged, which then activate second messengers.

Disulfide bond holding
chains together.

Either a CD4 or a CD8 T cell

FIG. 2.20   *Each T cell has many (thousands) of TCRs protruding from the cell membrane. All
the TCR on a single T cell are identical. As the T cell rolls over dendritic cells or tissue cells, the
TCR sample the peptide in the MHC molecules that the TCR encounter. As long as one of the
TCR does not bind to a peptide, the T cell keeps rolling. Once a TCR binds to its appropriate
peptide the T cell stops rolling and the CD4 or CD8 molecule bind to their receptor. This
strengthens the binding between the T cell and the target cell. Other adhesion molecules are
then engaged to hold the T cell to allow secondary messengers to become activated which then
activate the T cell to become an effector cell.*

only has a receptor for a single antigen. The receptors on T lymphocytes that recognize antigen are called TCRs.

The TCR has a variable portion that is the region that combines with the antigenic peptide in the MHC. The rearrangement of the variable region genes is a totally random process which occurs independently of antigen. The combination of gene segments that is available for formation of the variable region of the TCR, and the combination of two chains forming the antigen receptor site, results in the possibility of producing approximately 10^{15} TCR.

Of course, not all these T cells will leave the thymus gland. Only those T cells that do not contain an autoreactive TCR and that have a TCR that can bind a peptide in a MHC will leave the thymus (Fig. 2.20).

NAIVE AND EFFECTOR CD4 CELLS DIFFER IN THEIR REQUIREMENTS FOR ACTIVATION

Regulation of the activity of effector CD4 T lymphocytes differs from the activation of naive T cells. By definition, naive CD4 cells have not encountered antigen since their exit from the thymus. Before encountering the antigenic peptide that their TCR binds to, they are lacking effector function. Naive CD4 cells become activated when they recognize antigen bound into class II MHC molecules on APC that express costimulatory molecules. These interactions induce the responding CD4 cells to secrete IL-2, which in turn drives their proliferation and eventually their differentiation into effector CD4 cells.

Several costimulatory pathways have been identified that regulate (promote or inhibit) the T-cell response by providing signals that interact with the signals received as a consequence of TCR antigen recognition. These include the interaction of CD28 on the T cell with ligands of the B7 family on the APC. The response of naive T cells is also dependent on the strength of TCR-mediated signals, which are optimum only at high densities of MHC-peptide presentation on APC.

Costimulation is a signaling pathway separate from TCR-mediated signaling. Costimulation involves induction of intracellular signals that are not activated through TCR binding to the MHC II molecule. Costimulation molecules may also increase signaling by mediating tight adhesion between CD4 cells and APCs.

Once effector CD4 cells are generated, the next step in the immune response is the elicitation of effector cell function. After activation, effector cells circulate through the tissues of the body and localize to sites of infection. They enter tissues by attaching and passing between the endothelial cells lining blood vessels.

Effector function by CD4 cells involves recognition of peptides from pathogens presented in MHC II molecules of macrophages or tissue cells. Effector populations are much less dependent on costimulation molecules than are naive cells. CD4 effector cells, unlike naive cells, proliferate and produce their respective cytokines in response to a strong TCR signal alone. Thus, an activated CD4 cell that is present in tissue at a site where a pathogen has been processed by a macrophage (which has fewer costimulatory molecules than dendritic cells) or a tissue cell, may interact with a specific MHC-peptide and release cytokines that mediate an inflammatory response.

TABLE 2.1   Surface Marker Differences Between Naive and Memory Lymphocytes

Surface Marker	Naive Lymphocyte	Memory Lymphocyte
CD45R	Hi	Lo
CD44	Lo	Hi
L-selectin	Hi	Lo

Naive and memory lymphocytes have different circulation patterns. Naive lymphocytes pass into the node through high endothelial cells lining postcapillary venules (HEV). Effector/memory lymphocytes migrate into parenchymal tissue through flat endothelium lining blood vessels and pass into the afferent lymphatics for passage back to the blood. Thus, the tissues of the body are constantly being surveyed by effector/memory lymphocytes that are looking for the antigen to which they were sensitized.

Naive CD4 lymphocytes that have been activated in the spleen or lymph nodes to a foreign antigenic peptide are termed "effector/memory" lymphocytes. These CD4 cells have the capability of reacting to the MHC presentation of the foreign peptide on the membrane of macrophages or tissue cells; while the activated cells are circulating and searching for the peptide, they are "memory" cells. When they find the peptide and participate in an immune response (eg, a delayed hypersensitivity type of reaction) they are called "effector" cells.

The surface markers of memory cells differ from the surface markers of naive cells, a few examples of which are shown above for T lymphocytes. There are other surface differences on T cells in addition to those presented in Table 2.1.

Finding differences between the surface characteristics of naive and memory lymphocytes is compatible with some of the functional aspects of naive and memory cells differing. Not only do the markers on their surface make the cells look different, they also behave differently.

NATURAL KILLER LYMPHOCYTES

Natural killer (NK) lymphocytes lack the surface markers and functional aspects of T and B lymphocytes. They have no memory and do not react to an antigen upon a second exposure to it any differently than they did the first time they encountered the antigen. The NK cell does not have a receptor for antigen but rather has a molecule on its membrane that binds to a configuration on the outside of the MHC I molecule. As long as a self-peptide is in the MHC I groove, the NK cell receptor can bind to the outside of the MHC I. However, when the groove is occupied by a foreign antigen derived from a virus or possibly a tumor specific antigen, or the concentration of MHC I molecules are decreased on a cell, the NK receptor cannot bind to the MHC I.

The altered binding of the NK receptor to MHC I has significant functional significance as the NK cell receptor is an inhibitory molecule that prevents the release of a lytic enzyme from the NK cell. NK cells are constantly rolling over the surface membrane of tissue cells while a surface receptor on the NK cell called "NKR-P1" binds to carbohydrate ligands on the cell surface. The binding of the NKR-P1 receptor to its ligand activates the NK cell to release enzymes to kill the target cell. However, as long as the MHC I binding receptor on the NK cell is bound, the release of enzymes from the NK cell is inhibited. If a viral infection decreases MHC I production and placement on the cell membrane, or interferes with the binding of the NK inhibitory receptor, the NK cell will release enzymes that kill the target cell (Fig. 2.21).

There is a subset of NK cells that has a receptor for the Fc portion of an immunoglobulin molecule. When an antibody binds to a tissue antigen, the Fc part of the antibody molecule is exposed and may bind to the Fc receptor on this subset of NK cells. When this occurs the NK cell releases an enzyme that kills the tissue cell. The phenomenon is termed antibody-dependent cellular cytotoxicity (ADCC). Its contribution to producing damage to tissue is uncertain (Fig. 2.22).

Many studies find a decrease of NK cell function in association with stressors. However, some studies of the effect of acute stress on the function of the immune system find an increase of NK cell numbers and function that occurs simultaneously with a decrease of T-lymphocyte function (Naliboff et al, 1991; Tonnesen et al, 1987). When a stressor-induced increase of NK function occurs, it may represent a homeostatic mechanism which provides the body with a mechanism of resistance to viral infections during a time that immune function is compromised. However, as stress is

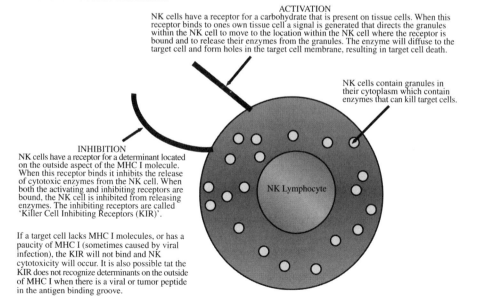

NK cells have receptors that regulate both activation and inhibition of NK cell function.

ACTIVATION
NK cells have a receptor for a carbohydrate that is present on tissue cells. When this receptor binds to ones own tissue cell a signal is generated that directs the granules within the NK cell to move to the location within the NK cell where the receptor is bound and to release their enzymes from the granules. The enzyme will diffuse to the target cell and form holes in the target cell membrane, resulting in target cell death.

NK cells contain granules in their cytoplasm which contain enzymes that can kill target cells.

INHIBITION
NK cells have a receptor for a determinant located on the outside aspect of the MHC I molecule. When this receptor binds it inhibits the release of cytotoxic enzymes from the NK cell. When both the activating and inhibiting receptors are bound, the NK cell is inhibited from releasing enzymes. The inhibiting receptors are called 'Killer Cell Inhibiting Receptors (KIR)'.

If a target cell lacks MHC I molecules, or has a paucity of MHC I (sometimes caused by viral infection), the KIR will not bind and NK cytotoxicity will occur. It is also possible tat the KIR does not recognize determinants on the outside of MHC I when there is a viral or tumor peptide in the antigen binding groove.

NK Lymphocyte

FIG. 2.21 *NK lymphocytes react against cells which have been infected by a virus or which have become malignant and present a nonself antigen in their MHC I molecules. The NK cell recognizes that the MHC I contains nonself and exerts a cytotoxic activity against the target cell.*

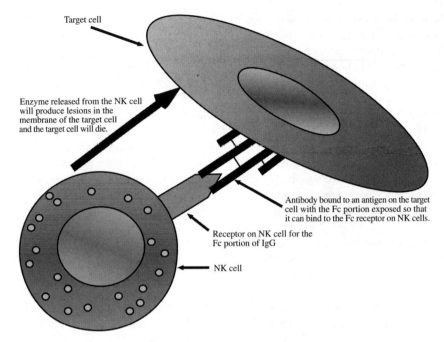

Target cell

Enzyme released from the NK cell
will produce lesions in the
membrane of the target cell
and the target cell will die.

Antibody bound to an antigen on the target
cell with the Fc portion exposed so that
it can bind to the Fc receptor on NK cells.

Receptor on NK cell for the
Fc portion of IgG

NK cell

FIG. 2.22   Antibody-dependent cellular cytotoxicity (ADCC).

associated with an increased susceptibility to infection, it is likely that the mechanism of increased NK function does not totally compensate for the decreased immunity (Cohen et al, 1991). Yet, without an increase in NK function, it is possible that
much more severe viral diseases would occur.

In addition, during stress there is a decrease of IFN-α and IFN-β production (Kita
et al, 1989; Sonnenfeld et al, 1988). Interferon alpha and beta induce cells to increase
their expression of class I MHC molecules. A stressor-induced decrease of interferon
production and MHC I expression may increase the ability of NK cells to kill virally
infected tissue cells (by decreasing the inhibitory signals to NK cells). Thus, although
stress decreases specific immune reactions, it may enhance the protective effects of
NK resistance to viral infection.

MAST CELLS

Mast cells (Fig. 2.3) are derived from bone marrow hematopoietic progenitors and
mature in all vascularized peripheral tissues. Mast cells are especially numerous in
the skin and in the gastrointestinal and respiratory tracts. In these locations they are
often close to blood vessels and nerves. Some of the mediators of allergic reactions
are preformed in cytoplasmic granules of mast cells: histamine, heparin, neutral pro-

teases and acid hydrolases. Other mediators are generated upon stimulation of the mast cells; these include platelet activating factor and products of arachidonate metabolism (eg, prostaglandin and leukotrien). Mast cell function in allergic diseases or parasite infections occurs upon activation of the cells through Fc receptors that bind IgE. The cells also can be activated to release mediators by complement degradation products (C3a and C5a) and neuropeptides.

B LYMPHOCYTES

B lymphocytes produce the various classes of immunoglobulin molecules. The B lymphocytes mature in the bone marrow where, under ideal circumstances, all autoreactive B lymphocytes are eliminated. However, that this does not occur is apparent, as many individuals produce autoantibodies that react to self-antigens. It is important to note that the presence of an autoantibody does not indicate the presence of an autoimmune disease. Autoimmune disease is only present when their is tissue damage or physiological abnormalities induced by the autoreactive antibody.

During maturation, each B lymphocyte undergoes a process of random rearrangement of the variable portion of the immunoglobulin molecule (the portion that combines with antigen). The rearrangement is not antigen driven and results in approximately 10^9 different specificities of antibody molecules capable of binding to antigen.

ANTIBODY

All serum proteins can be divided into one of five subgroups termed albumin, α_1-globulin, α_2-globulin, β-globulin, and γ-globulin. The proteins produced by B lymphocytes are γ-globulins. All antibody molecules are γ-globulins. The terms γ-globulins, immunoglobulin, and antibody are often used interchangeably.

Purpose of Antibody Molecules

Humans and animals are constantly being exposed to infectious agents such as bacteria, viruses, fungi, and parasites. Many of these pathogens (agents that can produce pathological [harmful] damage to the body) can produce lethal infections or problems caused by their toxins (eg, tetanus). The production of antibody that will react with the specific infectious agent will prevent disease. Antibodies can only bind to infectious agents in an extracellular location. Infectious agents that are intracellular are attacked by T-cell-mediated immunity.

The Basic Antibody Molecule

All antibody has a basic structure which consists of four separate protein chains and carbohydrate which is bound to the protein. The protein chains are bound together by interchain disulfide bonds and have loops formed by intrachain disulfide bonds.

The four protein chains are oriented in a specific arrangement with two lower-molecular-weight chains (22,000 daltons (L chains)) overlying a portion of the 2 higher molecular weight chains (53,000 daltons [H chains]). The end of the antibody molecule where the L and H chains are overlapping is where the antigen binds. The opposite end, where the H chains are extended, is where the antibody molecule attaches to cells such as mast cells, polymorphonuclear leukocytes, or macrophages, and where activation of substances that mediate inflammation occurs. The basic structure of the antibody molecule is shown in Figure 2.23.

It can be deduced that the portion of the antibody molecule that combines with antigen must have a structure that depends on the antigen for which the antibody has specificity. Thus, the terminal end of the Fab portions are termed the variable portion of the immunoglobulin molecule. The remaining portions of the H and L chains are termed constant regions. There are three constant domains for the H chain and one for the L chain.

The immunoglobulin classes are IgG, IgA, IgM, IgD, and IgE. The constant region is the same for all immunoglobulins within a given class; indeed, it is the constant region that provides a means of differentiating one class of immunoglobulin

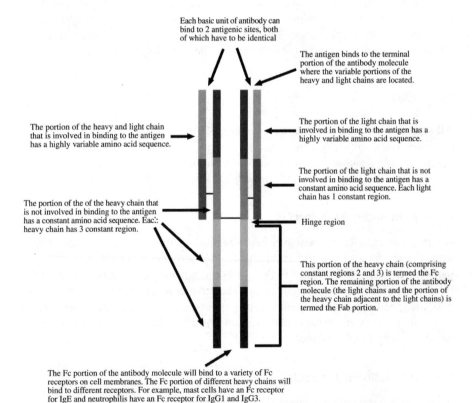

Each basic unit of antibody can bind to 2 antigenic sites, both of which have to be identical

The antigen binds to the terminal portion of the antibody molecule where the variable portions of the heavy and light chains are located.

The portion of the heavy and light chain that is involved in binding to the antigen has a highly variable amino acid sequence.

The portion of the light chain that is involved in binding to the antigen has a highly variable amino acid sequence.

The portion of the light chain that is not involved in binding to the antigen has a constant amino acid sequence. Each light chain has 1 constant region.

The portion of the of the heavy chain that is not involved in binding to the antigen has a constant amino acid sequence. Each heavy chain has 3 constant region.

Hinge region

This portion of the heavy chain (comprising constant regions 2 and 3) is termed the Fc region. The remaining portion of the antibody molecule (the light chains and the portion of the heavy chain adjacent to the light chains) is termed the Fab portion.

The Fc portion of the antibody molecule will bind to a variety of Fc receptors on cell membranes. The Fc portion of different heavy chains will bind to different receptors. For example, mast cells have an Fc receptor for IgE and neutrophilis have an Fc receptor for IgG1 and IgG3.

FIG. 2.23 *Basic structure of the immunoglobulin molecule.*

from another. Thus, all immunoglobulin molecules that are of the IgG class have identical aspects to their constant regions that allow them to be identified as IgG. Similarly IgA, IgM, IgD, and IgE have identical characteristics to their constant regions.

Not every part of the variable region is as variable as every other part of the variable region. The variable end of the H and L chains begins at the amino-(N-)terminal end of the chain. The first 110 amino acids are involved in the variable portion of the H and L chains. The amino acids at positions 30–34, 48–56, and 94–99 are much more variable than the amino acids at the other positions. The highly variable regions are termed the hypervariable regions and the amino acids between the hypervariable regions are termed the framework regions. The intrachain disulfide bonds bring the hypervariable regions together to form the actual site that combines with the antigen.

Another aspect of the immunoglobulin molecule is termed the hinge region. The hinge region is located between the first (CH1) and second (CH2) constant regions of the H chain. This region allows the two Fab portions to have mobility, so that the two portions that combine with antigen can move. The primary shape of the immunoglobulin molecule is that of a "Y" with flexibility of the two arms given by the hinge region.

Classes of Immunoglobulin

There are five classes of immunoglobulin: IgG, IgA, IgM, IgD, and IgE. Each class of immunoglobulin has its own characteristic and identifiable heavy chain. It is the heavy chain that allows for the identification of each class as the light chains are common to all classes (there are only two classes of light chains: κ and λ). The term applied to the class differentiation of immunoglobulin is "isotype." Thus, there are five isotypes of immunoglobulin: IgG, IgA, IgM, IgD, and IgE (Table 2.2).

The molecular weight of the light chain is approximately 22,000 daltons. There are only two classes of L chains and they are termed κ and λ. The two L chains that comprise a single basic immunoglobulin unit are both κ or both λ. Thus each immunoglobulin class (IgG, IgA, IgM, IgD, IgE) is composed of κ-containing molecules and λ-containing molecules. The difference between kappa and lambda is due to different amino acid sequences. The basic structure of each immunoglobulin isotype is shown in Figure 2.24.

TABLE 2.2   Heavy Chain Designation for each Isotype

Isotype	Heavy Chain
IgG	γ
IgA	α
IgM	μ
IgD	δ
IgE	ε

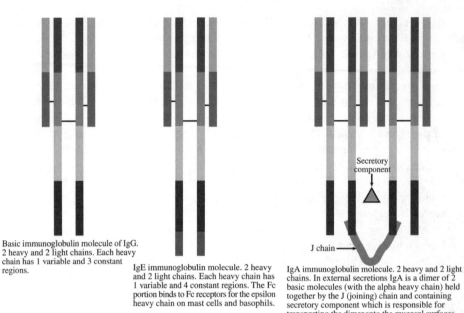

Basic immunoglobulin molecule of IgG. 2 heavy and 2 light chains. Each heavy chain has 1 variable and 3 constant regions.

IgE immunoglobulin molecule. 2 heavy and 2 light chains. Each heavy chain has 1 variable and 4 constant regions. The Fc portion binds to Fc receptors for the epsilon heavy chain on mast cells and basophils.

IgA immunoglobulin molecule. 2 heavy and 2 light chains. In external secretions IgA is a dimer of 2 basic molecules (with the alpha heavy chain) held together by the J (joining) chain and containing secretory component which is responsible for transporting the dimer onto the mucosal surfaces.

FIG. 2.24   *Basic structure of the immunoglobulin isotypes.*

Assuming that IgG represents the basic subtype of two light chains bound to two heavy chains, the following characteristics of the different isotypes are noted:

1. IgM is composed of five basic subunits.
2. The H chain of IgE and IgM has four constant domains.
3. Serum IgA is composed of two basic subunits, held together by a joining J chain.
4. The IgA in external secretions is composed of two basic subunits, held together by a J chain and an additional component termed "secretory component."

Hinge region—The place where the Fc and Fab regions join together, which is where the arms of the Ig molecule move

Secretory component—a protein derived from epithelial cells that binds to dimeric IgA (two basic molecules of IgA bound together) and transports the immunoglobulin across the mucous membrane

Joining chain (J chain)—a polypeptide that links the monomeric immunoglobulin units that form secretory IgA (two IgA monomeric units bound together by J chain and containing secretory component) or secreted IgM (five IgM monomeric units with J chain)

Some of the properties of the various immunoglobulin classes are presented in Table 2.3.

Immunoglobulin Subclasses

The IgG, IgA, and IgM classes of immunoglobulin also contain subclasses. There are four subclasses of IgG: two of IgA and two of IgM. The subclasses have different amino acid sequences on the constant region of the H chain. The four subclasses of IgG have different biological properties, as shown in Table 2.4.

Physiological Functions

IgG. This class of immunoglobulin is effective in neutralizing toxins (eg, tetanus or diphtheria toxin) that are produced by microorganisms. The IgG1 and IgG3 subclasses are able to activate the complement system and adhere to phagocytic cells and are therefore effective in providing protection against many microorganisms by

TABLE 2.3   Properties of Immunoglobulin

	IgG	IgA	IgM	IgD	IgE
Serum concentration (g/dl)	1.2	0.3	0.12	0.03	0.0005
Molecular weight ($\times 10^5$)	1.6	1.8[a]	9.0	1.8	1.9
Serum half-life (days)	23	6	5	3	2

[a]IgA found in external secretions of the body (tears, saliva, colostrum, gastrointestinal fluid, bronchial fluid) is a dimer of two molecules of IgA held together by a joining (J) chain with secretory component.

TABLE 2.4   Subclasses of IgG

	IgG1	IgG2	IgG3	IgG4
Serum concentration (% of total IgG)	70	20	7	3
Half-life (days)	23	23	7	23
Relative ability to activate the complement system	3+	1+	4+	+
Relative ability to adhere to phagocytic cells and enhance phagocytosis	3+	1+	4+	+

participating in the removal of infectious agents. IgG2 activates complement poorly and IgG4 does not activate complement. At birth, the fetus is protected from infection by maternal IgG, which has crossed the placenta.

IgA. IgA is found in serum and in the eternal secretions of the body. In serum, IgA primarily exists as the monomeric unit, with approximately 15% of the IgA being dimers (two basic units). In the external secretions (sweat, colostrum, tears, saliva, gastrointestinal tract, bronchi) IgA is a dimer of two basic units held together by a joining chain and containing a polypeptide component termed secretory component. The function of IgA in serum is not well understood. The major interest in IgA is due to its role as a protective substance in the external secretions. Secretory IgA may interfere with the ability of microorganisms to adhere to the mucosal surfaces of the body and to penetrate tissue. Secretory component is synthesized in the epithelial cells which line the mucosal surfaces. The IgA that appears in the external secretions is produced locally by plasma cells underlying the epithelium. The locally produced IgA forms a dimer that binds to secretory component precursor on the surface of the epithelial cells on mucosal surfaces. The complex is endocytosed by the epithelial cell and the endocytic vacuole releases the complex on the mucosal surface, where the secretory component precursor is cleaved to form secretory component (see Fig. 2.34).

IgM. IgM is the largest immunoglobulin, consisting of five of the basic units. As such, it is more efficient as a protective agent against infectious agents. The reason for its efficiency is that one molecule of IgM can initiate activation of the complement system (the major mediator of inflammation). Complement activation by IgG requires two molecules of IgG that are close enough together on a membrane to allow the first component of complement to attach to the two IgG molecules. This requires approximately 800 molecules of IgG to be present on a red blood cell.

IgD. Most of the IgD class of immunoglobulin is found on the surface of immature B lymphocytes. The serum concentration of IgD is very low. The role of IgD on the cell surface is not well defined.

IgE. Small amounts of IgE are found in serum. IgE in serum does not have a biological function. Most IgE, and the IgE that is responsible for producing the clinical symptoms of allergy, is bound to the surface of tissue mast cells. Degranulation of mast cells occurs when two molecules of IgE that are reactive to the same antigen locate next to each other on the surface of the mast cell, and both bind to the same molecule of antigen (see Fig. 2.35). The products that are released from the mast cell are responsible for producing the changes in tissue which are referred to as allergy.

Antibody Maturation

Heavy Chain Class Switching. After a lymphocyte interacts with an antigen, the variable region stays the same, but the constant region may change. The initial isotype of immunoglobulin produced is IgM, but activation of B lymphocytes and T-cell help causes class switching to IgG, IgA, or IgE. Class switching changes the functional characteristics of the antibody, while retaining the antigenic specificity. The class switch is caused by a B-cell-specific switch recombination. The C μ gene H chain genes are deleted, and a C_H gene for γ, α, or ε heavy chain is brought to the V region and expressed with it.

Selection of the isotype of immunoglobulin that will be produced by a B cell depends on the types of cytokines produced by the T cell providing help to the B cell. Different cytokines will induce specific class switches, but varying concentrations of the same cytokine may induce a different class switch. Also combinations of cytokines may induce different class switches than either individual cytokine.

Somatic Hypermutation. The affinity of IgG and IgM antibody for binding to T-cell-dependent antigen increases as the antibody response continues. This occurs because the variable genes in a mature B lymphocyte can mutate. This increases the binding ability of the surface immunoglobulin receptors for its specific antigen.

This hypermutation occurs in B cells in germinal centers. Antigen bound to the surface of follicular dendritic cells in the germinal center is the likely inducer of the hypermutation process and cytokines released from T cells may participate in inducing this process.

Once the B lymphocyte, which is activated in the follicle and which divide to form a germinal center begin to release antibody to the antigen, the antigen present in the germinal center will bind the antibody. This forms an immune complex that will be a combination of antigen and its specific antibody. Once the antibody binds to the antigen, the Fc portion of the antibody molecule is exposed and this will attach to a receptor on the dendritic cells in the follicle. The immune complex will then localize the antigen at the follicular dendritic cell surface. These are not the same dendritic cells that were involved with presenting the antigen to the T cell in the paracortical area of the node (see Fig. 2.14).

CYTOKINES

Cytokines are usually designated as IL followed by a number (eg, IL-2). There are numerous cytokines. These low-molecular-weight substances are produced by a cell and have three types of properties: autocrine (act on the cell that produces them), paracrine (act on cells near the cell that produces them), and endocrine (act on cells distant from the cell that produces them). Cytokines are usually produced after a cell receives an activation signal. They mediate their effects after binding to receptors on cell surfaces. They are involved in cell growth, inflammation, immunity, cell differentiation, hormone production.

Cytokines are produced by different cell types, including monocytes, lymphocytes, mast cells, astrocytes, mesangial cells, endothelial cells, and fibroblasts. Cytokine production is induced by infectious agents such as bacteria, viruses, fungi, and parasites. Cytokines have redundancy and ambiguity in that different cytokines have very similar actions and individual cytokines have different activities on different cells. Some of the properties of cytokines are presented in Table 2.5.

Some cytokines enhance the innate defense mechanisms of the body by conferring resistance to viral infections, increasing the lytic potential of NK cells and increasing expression of MHC molecules. IL-1 is produced by mononuclear phagocytes and astrocytes in the brain and has a very wide range of biological activities. In vivo, IL-1 induces hypotension, fever, weight loss, slow-wave sleep, and increased synthesis of proteins called "acute-phase proteins" that enhance the inflammatory response. Chemotactic cytokines such as IL-8 act primarily on neutrophils and function as mediators of acute inflammation. Chemotactic cytokines stimulate the directed migration of leukocytes that attach to cytokine-activated vascular endothelium through induced adhesion molecules.

Cytokines, produced by activated Th1 and Th2 CD4 lymphocytes regulate the growth and differentiation of T and B lymphocytes. IL-2 is the major autocrine (act on the cell that produces it) and paracrine (act on cells adjacent to cells producing it)

TABLE 2.5   Properties of Cytokines

Property	Description
Ambiguity	Individual cytokines act on many different cell types.
Redundancy	Different cytokines have similar actions.
Synergism and antagonism	Exposure of cells to two cytokines can produce qualitatively different responses than when the cells are exposed to either alone.
Cytokine cascade	One cytokine may increase (or decrease) the production of another.
Receptor binding	Cytokines initiate their action by binding to specific receptors on the surface of target cells.
Receptor transmodulation	One cytokine may increase or decrease the expression of receptors for another.

growth factor for T lymphocytes. IL-2 also stimulates the growth and function of NK cells and B lymphocytes. IL-4, produced by Th2 lymphocytes, is an important regulator of allergic reactions as it stimulates the switching of B lymphocytes to IgE production. It also stimulates growth of mast cells

IFN-γ is produced by Th1 helper CD4$^+$ T cells. Its production is enhanced by IL-2 and IL-12. IFN-γ is a powerful activator of macrophages and induces killing of bacteria the macrophages have ingested. It increases both MHC class I and class II expression on cells. Lymphotoxin (TNF-β) and TNF-α are produced by activated Th1 cells and promote killing of intracellular bacteria and may cause apoptosis of tissue cells.

IL-10 is produced by the Th2 subset of T lymphocytes. One of its major activities is to inhibit cytokine production by macrophages. IL-5 produced by Th2 cells stimulates growth and differentiation of eosinophils. IL-12 produced by activated monocytes and B cells is a very potent NK cell stimulator, inducing transcription of IFN-γ by NK cells. It enhances the cytolytic activity of NK cells.

Several cytokines stimulate the growth and differentiation of bone marrow progenitor cells. Cytokines that stimulate growth and differentiation of bone marrow progenitor cells are termed colony-stimulating factors (CSFs). The names given to CSFs reflect the types of colonies that they stimulate when bone marrow cells are cultured in agar.

IL-3 is produced by Th1 and Th2 lymphocytes and promotes the growth of immature progenitors to cells that differentiate into mature cells. IL-7 is secreted by bone marrow stromal cells and acts on immature lymphoid progenitor cells committed to the B-cell lineage.

Some lymphocyte-derived cytokines have been shown to bind to receptors within the central nervous system (CNS) and to activate the hypothalamic–pituitary–adrenal (HPA) axis and the sympathetic nervous system. Cytokines that are locally synthesized within the CNS may also be involved in the HPA axis, sympathetic nervous system activation, and the alteration of behavior. These characteristics of cytokines are reviewed in Chapter 3.

Mononuclear phagocytes are common to the immune system and the CNS. Mononuclear phagocytic cells produce IL-1, IL-6, TNF, and TGF, These cytokines are involved in the regulation of the inflammatory response. As early participants in the response of the immune system, their interaction with the CNS may serve to signal the CNS that an infectious agent or other antigen is being processed by the immune system. This suggests that these particular cytokines may have a major role in communication between the immune system and CNS.

Our studies, as well as those of others, have shown that in response to stressors, cytokines are produced by non-immune cells and thus, may (1) participate in stressor-induced activation of the HPA axis and the sympathetic nervous system, and (2) induce functional alterations of the immune system. As cytokine production occurs in response to both exogenous stress and immune challenge, it is possible that cytokine production occurs in response to stimuli that threaten the integrity of the organism.

Chemokines

Chemokines are a family of low-molecular-weight chemoattractant molecules that mediate inflammation. Chemokines induce target cell-specific directional migration of leukocytes (lymphocytes, monocytes, and neutrophils) within tissue sites of inflammation. Chemokines act in conjunction with adhesion molecules to give specificity to the cell composition of inflammatory infiltrates. The leukocyte composition at an inflammatory focus is determined, in large part, by the spectrum of chemokines produced at the site.

COMPLEMENT

During the late 1800s, it was noticed that the killing of bacteria by serum required a heat-stable and a heat-labile substance. The heat-stable substance was identified as antibody and the heat-labile substance was termed "complement" because it complemented the action of antibody on bacteria. Today we know that complement is not a single substance but consists of at least 20 different proteins, which are termed the "complement components."

Most of the proteins are in an inactive form, but when the first protein with the capability of initiating activation of the next protein becomes activated, a cascade of complement activation ensues. Activation of the complement system is important in mediating inflammatory reactions, bacterial killing, the enhancement of phagocytosis, and the destruction of cells by producing holes in cell membranes.

There are two pathways of complement activation. The first to be discovered is termed the "classic" activation pathway and is initiated by immunoglobulin binding to antigen. The other pathway is termed the "alternative pathway," which is activated by repeating polysaccharide or other polymeric structures on tissue cells or bacteria. The classic and the alternative complement pathways converge into a common track termed the "lytic" pathway. As several of the complement components are enzymes which, when activated, have the potential of causing tissue damage, a system of regulatory proteins has evolved to prevent complement activation from damaging one's own tissue.

The complement system has powerful cytolytic activity against which an individual's own cells must be protected. Several proteins have evolved to control the extent of complement activation in fluid and on the surfaces of ones own cells. The proteins that inhibit complement activation limit the generation of complement fragments such as C4b and C3b and render the generated fragments inactive, thereby reducing the extent of cellular damage.

Several of the complement components are present in serum in inactive forms. After they are activated, they are split into fragments, usually designated by the suffixes "a" (smaller fragment released into body fluid) and "b" (larger membrane-bound fragment). For example, the C3 component, when activated, splits into C3a and C3b. The C3b fragments are further degraded into "c" (which is released into body fluids) and "d" (which remains membrane bound). However, the C2 component does not follow this rule as C2a is bound and C2b released.

Several biological activities that result from complement activation:

Lysis. Holes are punched into the membranes of cells which have activated complement on their surfaces. This will lead to cell death.

Phagocytosis. Phagocytic cells (polymorphonuclear leukocytes and macrophages have a receptor on their membrane for a component of complement called "C3b." C3b attaches to the membrane of cells where complement is activated (for example, if an antibody binds to a bacteria and activates complement, the complement will adhere to the membrane of the bacteria and C3b will be attached to the bacteria). The C3b also binds to a receptor on the membrane of phagocytic cells and this induces the phagocytic cell to ingest the bacteria.

Chemotaxis. Activation of the complement system results in the cleavage of small peptides from some of the protein molecules that are part of the complement system. These small peptides have the biological function of attracting inflammatory cells to the location at which the complement is being activated.

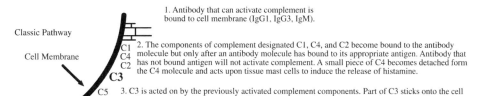

Classic Pathway

Cell Membrane

1. Antibody that can activate complement is bound to cell membrane (IgG1, IgG3, IgM).

C1
C4
C2
C3

2. The components of complement designated C1, C4, and C2 become bound to the antibody molecule but only after an antibody molecule has bound to its appropriate antigen. Antibody that has not bound antigen will not activate complement. A small piece of C4 becomes detached form the C4 molecule and acts upon tissue mast cells to induce the release of histamine.

C5
C6
C7
C8
C9

3. C3 is acted on by the previously activated complement components. Part of C3 sticks onto the cell membrane and a small piece (called C3a) becomes detached and acts upon tissue mast cells to induce the release of histamine and also attracts neutrophils to the location where the C3a is being generated. The C3 on the cell membrane enhances the ability of neutrophils to ingest the particle that the C3 is located on.

4. The terminal complement components, C5-C9, become activated once C3 is activated on the cell membrane. A piece of C5, called C5a, is split off and contributes to causing the release of histamine from mast cells, and also attracts neutrophils to the location where the C3a is being generated. C7-C9 will produce a hole in the cell membrane which leads to death of the cell.

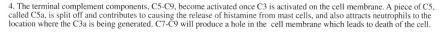

Alternate Pathway

C3

1. C3 complement is continuously activated by the alternate pathways and deposits on cell membranes. On human and animal tissue cells, the C3 is immediately inactivated, preventing damage to tissue. However, inactivation of C3 deposited on the membranes of microorganisms does not occur. Therefore, there is rapid activation of the alternate pathway without having to wait for the production of antibody. Thus, the alternate pathway provides a rapic defense against infectious agents.

C5
C6
C7
C8
C9

2. The terminal complement components, C5-C9, become activated once C3 is activated on the cell membrane. A piece of C5, called C5a, is split off and contributes to causing the release of histamine from mast cells, and also attracts neutrophils to the location where the C3a is being generated. C7-C9 will produce a hole in the cell membrane which leads to death of the cell. This is identical in both pathways.

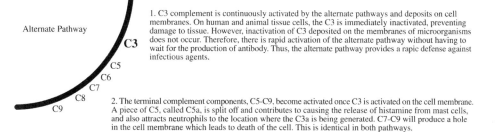

FIG. 2.25 *There are two pathways for complement activation. The classic pathway, depicted above, is initiated when an antibody IgG1, IgG3, or IgM class binds to an antigen. The alternate pathway is constantly active and places C3 onto cell membranes. However, when this occurs on human tissue cells, a rapid inactivation of the C3 occurs. This prevents complement mediated damage to human tissues. Many microorganisms will bind C3 through the alternate pathway. The microorganisms are unable to inactivate the C3. Therefore, inflammatory cells are attracted to the microorganism to ingest and kill it.*

FACTOID: The total activity of the complement system can be measured by determining the ability of complement in a defined volume of serum to lyse (destroy) red blood cells that are coated with antibody. The assay is called the CH50 test and defines the amount of serum required to lyse 50% of a specified number of red blood cells. In rats, chronic stress has been reported to be able to decrease the amount of CH50 complement (Ayensu et al, 1995). Whether this is a specific response to chronic stress or associated with a generalized decrease of protein synthesis caused by stress or decreased nutrition, is unclear. An important consideration relates to how low serum complement levels must go before there are biological consequences (an increased risk of infection). It is unlikely that the hormonal response induced by stress would be capable of lowering complement levels sufficiently to increase the risk of infectious diseases.

INNATE DEFENSE AGAINST INFECTIOUS DISEASES

An innate defense system is essential to the maintenance of health. The innate defenses differ from the immune defenses in that the innate system does not remember that it has previously seen an infectious agent and it is fully developed without the body having had prior experience with the infectious agent. Therefore, the innate system always reacts against the infectious agent as if it were the first time the agent was present in the body and the innate defense system rapidly responds to the presence of an infectious agent.

If all we could rely on was the immune system, we would likely die of infections before the immune system is turned on, as it may take 4–5 days for the immune response to become activated. The innate defense system against infectious organisms is activated very quickly, often within minutes. Both white blood cells and soluble substances in plasma are involved in the innate defense system.

Innate defense mechanisms have the following characteristics:

Rapid action

No learning ability—do not respond any quicker a second time

No specificity—cannot distinguish between infectious agents

The white blood cells that participate in "innate" defenses are called "inflammatory cells." The inflammatory cells are primarily the neutrophils, monocytes, and macrophages. All are cells that can ingest and digest foreign material or tissue cells that have been damaged. In addition, the NK cell is part of the innate defense system.

The attraction of inflammatory cells of the innate defense system to the site of an infectious agent is mediated by chemokines that are released at the site of the infectious agent. When an infection is present, it is likely that cells, which are at the site of the infectious agent, can release soluble substances which attract inflammatory cells.

FACTOID: Neutrophils are important cells for the elimination of bacteria that will cause pyogenic infections (infections that cause the accumulation of pus). In humans, reports suggest that stress is associated with an increased risk of infection with gram-positive bacteria (gram-positive bacteria are associated with the accumulation of pus in tissue) (Meyer and Haggerty, 1962; Peterson et al, 1991). If stress increases susceptibility to gram-positive bacterial infection, an associated alteration of neutrophil function may be present. Indeed, there are reports of stressor-induced alteration of neutrophil function in humans.

Neutrophil phagocytic activity was decreased by 2 days of the combination of the lack of sleep and psychological stressors in humans (Palmblad et al, 1976). In rats, exposure to 3 hours of footshock stress increased phagocytic activity and 18 hours of restraint stress increased macrophage phagocytosis (Harmsen and Turney, 1985; Zwilling et al, 1992). Superoxide production which contributes to the killing of ingested bacteria increases in neutrophils in humans in association with surgical stress (Yokota et al, 1993). In humans, running until a state of exhaustion, produces an enhancement of the ability of neutrophils to ingest and kill *Candida* fungi (Rodriguez et al, 1991).

We found that after 3 consecutive days of a 1-hour session of a footshock stress, neutrophil function in regard to both phagocytic ability and killing were altered, however, in opposite directions. Phagocytosis increased and killing ability decreased (Shurin et al, 1994).

Inflammation requires that neutrophils relocate from the vascular system into tissue. The neutrophil population of leukocytes is important for the ingestion and killing of bacteria in tissue. Neutrophils roll along the endothelial cells lining blood vessels (the rolling is caused by a weak adhesion interaction between surface molecules (called "selectins") on the neutrophil and the endothelial cells) and the movement is caused by the flow of blood. However, when the neutrophils encounter endothelial cells that have increased their expression of adhesion molecules (this is caused by an event occurring in the tissue underlying the endothelial cells, usually the presence of an infectious agent) the neutrophils will stop rolling and firmly adhere to the endothelial cells.

If neutrophils are released from their location along the endothelial cells into the bloodstream, their will be fewer neutrophils rolling along the endothelial cells which are available to migrate into sites of tissue inflammation. Catecholamines, which are increased in plasma by stress, have been found to decrease the adherence of neutrophils to endothelial cells (Benschop et al, 1996). Thus, stress may decrease the ability of the innate defense system to develop a localized inflammatory response that will remove bacteria from tissue that they have invaded.

For a normal inflammatory response to occur, neutrophils must migrate from their point of adherence on endothelial cells to the tissue site where they are needed. Studies done in patients experiencing the anticipatory stress of surgery were found to have neutrophils that had a decreased ability to migrate toward a chemotactic stimulus (a chemical stimulus which attracts the cells) (Fricchione et al, 1996). This is similar to an observation we made many years ago. Our laboratory used to perform a test called the "leukocyte inhibition factor" assay. The test uses neutrophils collected from a normal individual and measures their migration, through agar, to a stimulus provided by cytokines released from the lymphocytes of a subject whose ability to produce chemotactic factors was being determined. Whenever the donor of the normal neutrophils was nervous about having their blood drawn the test did not work because the neutrophils would not migrate.

INFLAMMATION

Although white blood cells circulate in the blood, they are frequently needed in tissue as part of the response to the presence of infection. The migration of white blood cells to tissue and their accumulation in tissue is the inflammatory response. The inflammatory response is the process of cells and soluble substances that are involved with attracting and activating the cells accumulating at the site of an infectious agent.

In a healthy person, the response to infectious agents or tissue injury is rapid and efficient and will frequently lead to resolution (resolution means that the eliciting agent is removed) before the immune system is activated (this is called "acute inflammation"). In an individual with an overwhelming infection or who is chronically ill with an impaired acute inflammatory response, the immune system becomes activated and participates in the inflammatory response (this is called chronic "inflammation").

Characteristics of Inflammation

Redness (erythema)—caused by vasodilation

Swelling (edema)—caused by leakage of fluids from enlarged and more permeable blood vessels

Fever—(a) local warmth caused by increased blood flow; (b) systemic fever caused by release of IL-1 from macrophages acting in the brain

Pain—results from heat and swelling acting on local nerves

There are two phases to inflammation: (1) the inflammatory phase, and (2) the reparative phase. The inflammatory phase destroys or walls off the invading agent and removes dead cells and debris. Successful repair returns the tissue to its original state and function. If the inflammatory reaction has been extensive, the tissue may be replaced by a fibrotic scar.

The process of inflammation can be initiated within minutes of entry of a bacterium into the body (initiation of a primary immune response may require days. Thus, it should be obvious that the acute inflammatory response is a major factor in preventing many infectious diseases—if we had to wait for the immune system to become activated serious diseases could result from the tissue damage produced by infectious agents and the soluble toxins that they release).

White blood cells normally marginate along the lining of blood vessels by adhering to the endothelial cell surface through interactions of adhesion molecules on the white blood cell and endothelial cell surfaces. When a stimulus (such as the presence of an infectious agent) elicits the production of proinflammatory molecules (proinflammatory molecules are produced before there is evidence of inflammation and are responsible for bringing about the inflammatory response), polymorphonuclear leukocytes adhere to the endothelial cells in the local tissue. This causes the polys to stop flowing past the site. The cells then pass between the endothelial cells and through the vascular basement membrane. Polys go through first (0–24 hours) and then monocytes accumulate (24–48 hours). This may be related to different chemotactic stimuli being produced, the cells responsiveness to chemotactic stimuli, or the disappearance of the polys after initially accumulating in tissue.

The relevant endothelial molecules for adhesion are expressed at a greater density by venules than by capillaries explaining the preference for attachment of cells to

---

FACTOID: There are two aspects to tissue inflammation. One is the removal of an infectious agent from the tissue and the other is healing of the inflammatory site with return of the tissue to its original architecture and function. Healing requires the removal of damaged tissue, usually done by macrophages, and growth of new tissue. The production of tissue growth factors may contribute to the repair process. The interaction on cell growth of hormones that are elevated during stress, such as catecholamines, and growth-promoting factors, needs to be determined. One such interaction has been reported to augment the growth of non-myocyte cells, in vitro, of neonatal rat hearts (Long et al, 1993). Growth-promoting interactions between growth factors involved in the regeneration of liver cells and norepinephrine have also been observed (Michalopoulos and DeFrances, 1997). Thus, it is possible that stress is associated with a positive effect on tissue repair.

However, an experimental study of wound healing in individuals experiencing the stress of caring for a relative who has Alzheimer's disease reports an inhibition of tissue repair by stress. A small biopsy of skin was removed from the arm of the experimental subjects and control individuals. Healing required approximately nine more days in the individuals with higher levels of stress than in the controls (Kiecolt-Glaser et al, 1995). Thus, in addition to altering the accumulation of inflammatory cells at a site of infection, stress may also alter the repair process. This area of research needs considerable attention to determine the conditions under which the hormonal response to stress either promotes or interferes with wound healing and tissue repair. Uneventful or eventful recovery of patients from surgical procedures may be better understood if the influence of stress hormones on wound healing were clarified.

venules. Cytokines can cause a gradual and sustained increase in adhesion molecules on endothelial cells. IL-1 and TNF cause increases in adhesion molecules for granulocytes and lymphocytes, while IFN-γ or IL-4 can cause a selective increase in adhesion molecules for T lymphocytes. Since different inflammatory stimuli elicit different patterns of cytokine production, the nature of the inflammatory agent may contribute to determining the pattern of leukocyte adhesion.

The time-dependent variations in the patterns of cytokine-induced expression of leukocyte adhesion molecules on endothelial cells may underlie the sequential recruitment of neutrophils followed by lymphocytes seen in various inflammatory processes. However, it should be remembered that the combination of cytokines can alter the time dependent patterns of adhesion molecule expression that is observed in vitro when only a single cytokine is being studied.

The basal level of adhesion is inadequate to sustain attachment of lymphocytes to the surface of endothelial cells in the face of shear forces applied by flowing blood.

The cells of chronic inflammation are lymphocytes, macrophages, and plasma cells. The cells of chronic inflammation are collectively termed "mononuclear cells." Lymphocytes are the immune specific effector cells of delayed hypersensitivity reactions. They react with antigen to release soluble factors which mediate the delayed hypersensitivity response and have properties of mediating an inflammatory response (attract macrophages, increase vascular permeability, kill target cells). The finding of cells and processes which are associated with immune reactions (delayed hypersensitivity) in chronic inflammation, suggests that chronic inflammation occurs when the agent that elicited the acute inflammatory response is not removed by the acute process with the resultant activation of the immune system.

ADHESION MOLECULES

Cell adhesion molecules (CAM) are appendages on the surface of cells and are used by cells to grip onto each other or onto connective tissue fibers. CAM help cells haul themselves by one another. CAM enable white blood cells to travel to injured tissues or to tissues that are infected with microorganisms.

The inflammatory process involves cell adhesion events. White blood cells must be able to move about in the intravascular space but they must also be able to adhere to endothelial cells which are lining the blood vessels at sites where an inflammatory process is required. Such interactions between lymphocytes and postcapillary venule endothelial cells are constantly occurring in lymph nodes as part of the mechanism by which lymphocytes migrate from the circulation to lymph nodes.

Leukocyte emigration from the blood stream into tissue involves a coordinated series of complex events. The presence of an infectious agent or tissue damage sends signals to the adjacent endothelial cells, which causes these cells to become "activated." The activation is expressed by an increase of adhesion molecules on the endothelial cell membrane. The rolling leukocytes stick at the specific location on the endothelium which has expressed an increased concentration of adhesion molecules which arise due to signals generated by the inflammatory process in the tissue.

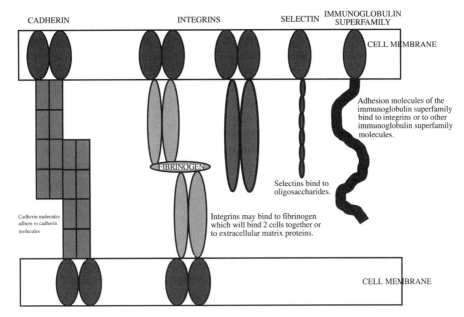

FIG. 2.26 *The basic structure of the four different types of cell adhesion molecules.*

There are four major types of CAM, which are classified on the basis of their structure. Figure 2.26 illustrates the characteristics of CAM.

1. *Cadhedrin*—penetrates the cell membrane and helps hold cells together.
2. *Integrins*—heterodimers whose two chains contribute to binding. Many integrins bind to proteins in the extracellular matrix. Integrins are involved in cell–cell and cell–matrix adhesion functions. A feature of integrins is that they extend into the cytoplasmic side of the plasma membrane and interact with components of the cytoskeleton. This allows them to link the extracellular environment to the cytoskeleton. Subfamilies of integrins include:

   VLA proteins—integrins of the VLA family are expressed on different types of white blood cells (eg, T cells have VLA-4, VLA-5, and VLA-6; B cells have VLA-2, VLA-3, and VLA-4). VLA-4 binds to a ligand on endothelial cells called VCAM-1, which is activated by cytokines (VCAM-1 is a member of the immunoglobulin superfamily class of cell adhesion molecules). VLA proteins appear to be inactive on resting lymphocytes and become active on stimulated lymphocytes.

   Leukocyte adhesion molecules—LFA-1, which is present on all leukocytes, binds to ICAM-1 (ICAM-1 is a member of the immunoglobulin superfamily class of cell adhesion molecules). LFA-1 becomes activated on T lymphocytes after the T cell receptor binds a peptide in the MHC molecule. The binding of LFA-1 to ICAM-1 provides strength for the adhesion of T cells to target cells.

3. *Selectins*—Selectins emerge from the cells outer membrane as a single protein string with a zig-zag appearance. Selectins protrude from the endothelial cells lining blood vessels and slow the rolling of white blood cells (like a shag carpet slowing the rolling of a ball). There are three members of this group of adhesion molecules:

> *L-selectin* is present on naive lymphocytes and allows the lymphocytes to attach to a ligand on high endothelial venule cells in secondary lymph nodes.
>
> *E-selectin:* found on cytokine-activated endothelial cells and binds to sugars on monocytes and polymorphonuclear leukocytes. This interaction may be associated with the accumulation of inflammatory cells in tissue.
>
> *P-selectin:* found on the surface of activated platelets and participate in platelet adherence to monocytes and polymorphonuclear leukocytes.

4. *Immunoglobulin superfamily*—mediate cell–cell adhesion. Immunoglobulin superfamily adhesion molecules on a cell may bind to integrins on another cell or to immunoglobulin superfamily adhesion molecules on another cell.

Function of Adhesion Molecules

Rolling. Selectins cause the white blood cell to slow down and to roll along the blood vessel wall. The weak binding and transient contact of the selectins allows the white cells to roll. If the blood vessel has dilated, the blood flow along the wall is slower than in a narrow blood vessel, and there is more chance for interaction between the white cell and the endothelial cells. Dilation occurs during inflammation.

Activation. Once the white cell has slowed down, it can sense the presence of chemical attractants which may be produced by clotted blood, infiltrating leukocytes, endothelial cells, damaged tissues, or infectious agents. These chemoattractants can initiate changes in the white cells which lead to their activation and sticking to the endothelial cells. Locally derived chemoattractants cause changes in the presence of adhesion molecules on endothelial cells and on white blood cells which cause a conformational change in integrins which produces an increase in leukocyte integrin affinity for immunoglobulin-like adhesion receptor ligands on endothelial cells.

Firm adhesion. Transendothelial migration: Subendothelial migration—The integrin receptor on the white blood cell latches onto an immunoglobulin-like adhesion receptor on endothelial cells. Binding of the integrin to ICAM-1 causes the white blood cell to flatten against the vessel wall and locate a gap between the endothelial cells. The white blood cell then squeezes through the space between the endothelial cells into the tissue. When in tissue the white cell will move in the direction of increasing concentration of a chemoattractant. Chemoattractants not only activate integrin adhesiveness, they also give direction to the migration of leukocytes. When the white cells get to where they are needed the polymorphonuclear cells will ingest and kill bacteria.

FACTOID: T lymphocytes that are in the circulation and that have not been activated to the antigen for which their TCR has specificity, are termed "naive" T lymphocytes. The naive T cells are unable to migrate from the bloodstream to the tissues and organs of the body. However, the naive T lymphocytes are capable of entering lymph nodes by adherence to and migration through the high endothelial venule cells that are present on the postcapillary venules of the nodes.

An alteration in the pattern of trafficking of the naive lymphocyte population may influence the number of naive cells available to interact with antigen presenting dendritic cells in lymph nodes. If the lymphocytes do not adhere to the high endothelial venule cells when they pass through the nodes, their capability of entering the node would be decreased.

Once activated and now referred to as "effector/memory" cells, lymphocytes no longer migrate into lymph nodes through the high endothelial venule cells, but rather migrate into tissue through the flat endothelial cells that form the lining of blood vessels. Once in tissue, the effector/memory lymphocytes search for the MHC presentation of antigen to which they have been activated as a part of their surveillance function of eliminating antigen from tissue. Thus, alterations of lymphocyte trafficking may influence both the activation of lymphocytes in nodes and the presence of lymphocytes in organs and tissue.

Stress hormones have been found capable of altering the adhesive properties of leukocytes. Injection of catecholamines into humans produces an increase in the number of lymphocytes present in the blood (Schedlowski et al, 1993). Catecholamines have been found to decrease the interaction between human lymphocytes and endothelial cells cultured from umbilical cords that have been treated with IL-1 to activate their adhesion molecules (Carlson et al, 1996).

A factor that must be considered in studies of stress hormones and alteration of immune function is whether the stress is acute or chronic. Differences in the alterations of the number of circulating lymphocytes may occur as a result of the duration of the stressor. For example, in subjects who have heart failure with a chronic elevation of plasma catecholamine levels, there is a decrease in the number of lymphocytes in the blood (Maisel et al, 1990), while acute stress may increase lymphocytes in blood (Herbert and Cohen, 1993).

In rats, the number of lymphocytes present in blood decreases during stress and the decrease has been shown to be mediated by corticosterone binding to the type II adrenal steroid receptor (Dhabhar et al, 1996). Whether hormones other than glucocorticoids and catecholamines can influence the number of lymphocytes bound to endothelial cells, and the strength of binding to the endothelial cells, remains to be determined.

The reason that the number of lymphocytes is altered when blood is collected for counting lymphocytes, is important. If the lymphocyte count is reduced because the cells are induced to adhere more tightly to endothelial cells, an enhanced ability to migrate into tissue may be expected. However, if stress hormones cause the lymphocytes to be sequestered, for example, in the spleen, the number of lymphocytes available to provide protective functions would be decreased.

With regard to lymphocytes entering an area of inflammation, lymphocyte VLA-4 binds to VCAM-1, an adhesion molecule on the surface of endothelial cells induced by inflammatory mediators. This may differ from the selectin-ligand interactions that are used by neutrophils to enter sites of inflammation. With lymphocytes, capture, rolling adhesion and tight adhesion may all be mediated by VLA-4. This contrasts with neutrophil capture, rolling and tight adhesion, where capture and rolling adhesion is mediated by selectins, while tight adhesion is mediated by integrins.

THE IMMUNE SYSTEM AS A DEFENSE AGAINST INFECTIOUS AGENTS

Infectious agents multiply outside the cells of the body (many bacteria localize in the extracellular spaces of the body) or within cells of the body (eg, viruses). Different types of immune reactions are needed to rid the body of extracellular and intracellular infections. Antibody is the primary immune defense against extracellular infections and T lymphocytes are the primary defense against intracellular infectious agents.

The substance that initiates an immune response is the antigen. When an antigen is injected into a subject (human or animal) and an immune response occurs, it is called active immunization. The first time the immune system reacts to an antigen is called a "primary response," and the second time it is called a "secondary" or

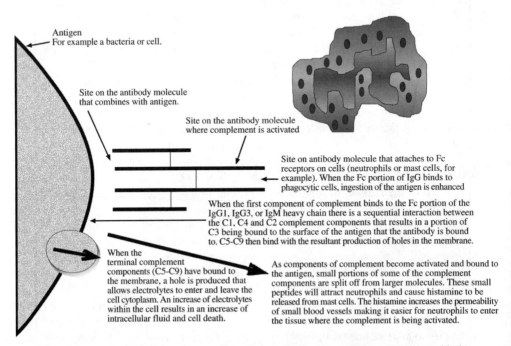

FIG. 2.27 *Antibody binding to its specific antigen activates the complement system with the subsequent alteration of vascular permeability, the attraction of phagocytic cells, and removal of the antigen.*

"anamnestic response." When the antigen is injected a second time, the immune response occurs more rapidly and is quantitatively greater than after the first exposure to antigen. Figures 2.27 and 2.28 illustrate some of the pathways that the immune system uses to resist infectious diseases.

Many bacteria produce toxins. The toxins will attach to receptors on tissue cells and interfere with cell function. Antibodies that are produced to a toxin will bind to the toxin and "neutralize" the toxin so that it cannot disrupt cell function. Immunization with tetanus toxoid is done to produce an antibody that will neutralize the tetanus toxin before the toxin attaches to a receptor on a cell.

Viral inactivation occurs in a similar manner to toxin neutralization. Viruses bind to specific receptors on cell surfaces. They then enter the cell and replicate. If an antibody is present that binds to the surface of a virus, the virus may be unable to bind to and infect a tissue cell (Fig. 2.29).

When a pathogen is within a tissue cell, it cannot be bound to an antibody. Antibody molecules are too large to penetrate a cells membrane. Intracellular infectious agents are attacked by the component of the immune system termed "cell-mediated immunity." Cell-mediated immunity works by killing the tissue cell in which the pathogen resides. If, as a result of the cell dying, the pathogen is released to an extracellular location, the pathogen may then be eliminated by antibody.

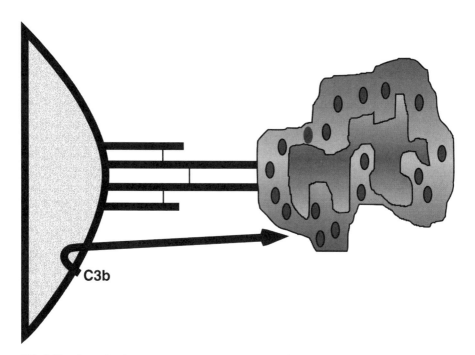

FIG. 2.28 *Opsonization occurs when antibody and the C3b component of complement bind to the surface of an antigen. Phagocytic cells have receptors for C3b and the Fc fragment of IgG1, IgG3, and IgM. The adherence of these molecules to their receptors on the surface of phagocytic cells enhances their ingestion. The process is opsonization.*

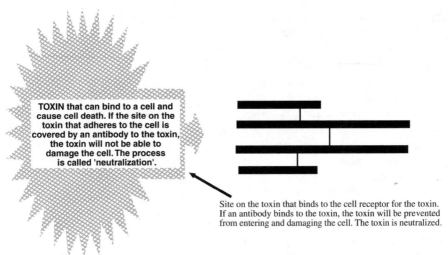

TOXIN that can bind to a cell and cause cell death. If the site on the toxin that adheres to the cell is covered by an antibody to the toxin, the toxin will not be able to damage the cell. The process is called 'neutralization'.

Site on the toxin that binds to the cell receptor for the toxin. If an antibody binds to the toxin, the toxin will be prevented from entering and damaging the cell. The toxin is neutralized.

A similar process occurs with viral neutralization. A virus has to bind to a receptor on a cell as part of the process of the virus entering the cell. If the site on the virus that binds to the receptor is covered by an antibody, the virus will be unable to adhere to its receptor and will not be able to infect a cell. The process is referred to as 'viral neutralization'.

FIG. 2.29   Neutralization of a toxin or of the ability of a virus to bind to a receptor on a cell oc-curs when specific antibody binds to the toxin or virus.

Cell-mediated immunity depends on an infected cell providing an indication to T lymphocytes that indicate that the cell is infected. This is done by a small piece (actually peptides of the infectious agent of about 12–14 amino acids) being displayed on the surface of the tissue cell. The peptides are displayed in peptide presentation molecules that are termed "MHC molecules."

FACTOID: There are studies that suggest that stress (most likely the hormonal response induced by stress) can influence the ability of antigen-processing cells to ingest foreign antigen. The ability of antigen presenting cells to present antigen is critical to the development of the immune response to protein antigen. Several factors are associated with the APC's ability to present antigen, including the number of MHC molecules on the APC, the presence of costimulatory molecules, and the production of cytokines.

The number of mice housed in a cage was found to effect the ability of APC to activate an immune response (Grewal et al, 1997). Mice were housed in groups of six or individually and immunized to hen lysozyme antigen. The response of lymphocytes to mitogenic stimulation in vitro to the immunizing antigen was determined. The group-housed mice had lower proliferative responses than the individually housed mice. APC were isolated from the spleens of the mice and used to present antigen to lymphocytes from immunized mice. APC from group-housed mice had a decreased ability to present antigen in comparison to the APC from individually housed mice. Thus, housing density altered the function of APC.

There are studies which suggest that the expression of MHC molecules on the surface of APC is influenced by the hormones produced in response to stress

(Sonnenfeld et al, 1992). Rats were exposed to a 1 hour session of intermittent footshock and the spleen cells evaluated for the presence of MHC II. A decrease in the number of spleen cells expressing MHC II was found. A similar finding has been reported using peritoneal macrophages of mice that were stressed by restraint (Zwilling et al, 1990). Modification of MHC II expression may alter the ability of the immune response to become properly activated by reducing the number of presentation molecules for antigenic peptides.

FACTOID: The influence of stress-induced hormones on the production of T lymphocytes and the maturation of T lymphocytes with a wide variety of T-cell receptors has not been adequately studied. Stress hormones may affect the development of T lymphocytes from bone marrow precursor cells or may influence the maturation of T lymphocytes in the thymus gland. Indeed, the thymus gland is susceptible to the influence of glucocorticoid hormones (which increase in concentration during stress) which cause the thymus gland to decrease in mass.

FACTOID: Studies of the effect of stress hormones on the development and function of costimulation molecules are needed.

FACTOID: Many studies, in humans and experimental animals, have found that stress hormones alter the activity of the CD4$^+$ T-lymphocyte population. Thus, if an immune response is occurring at a time when stress hormones are increased, it is possible that there will be a decreased function of the T-cell immune system, which would increase susceptibility to viral and protozoan infections and an altered ability to produce antibodies to antigens. In addition, a decrease in the function of cell-mediated immunity may result in activation of a latent virus infection. Latent viral infections occur following an active virus infection when the virus remains within a cell but is not actively replicating. It is likely that an active cell-mediated immune response keeps the virus in a latent state.

ANATOMY OF LYMPHOID TISSUE

The following section will summarize the anatomy of the secondary lymphoid tissues. As these are the locations in which immune system activation occurs, they are locations where neuropeptides and other hormones can influence immune system activation. Chapters 3 and 4 will prove additional information regarding how activation of the immune system in the secondary lymphoid tissues may be modified by stress.

Lymph Nodes

Lymph nodes are organized accumulations of lymphocytes, and dendritic cells, surrounded by a capsule and having a blood supply, supporting connective tissue fibers, and the flow of lymph through it.

The lymphatic capillaries form a dense network within all tissues. The capillaries merge together to eventually form two large "lymphatic vessels" that empty back into the blood stream and return the plasma (which is called "lymphatic fluid" when in the lymphatic system) to the blood. There are two places that the lymphatic fluid returns to the bloodstream:

> *Right lymphatic duct*—drains the upper right part of the body and empties into the right subclavian vein
>
> *Thoracic duct*—drains the rest of the body and drains into the left subclavian vein

Along the path that the lymphatic vessels take to the subclavian veins are accumulations of lymphocytes that form into nodules called "lymph nodes." The lymph nodes are located along the pathway of flow of lymph fluid from the periphery to the vasculature.

There are several lymph nodes located along the lymphatic vessels so that the fluid passes through a sequence of nodes as it moves from the periphery to the vasculature. As the lymph fluid passes through the lymph nodes, it accumulates lymphocytes from the nodes and, eventually, the lymphocytes are passed into the bloodstream at the subclavian arteries.

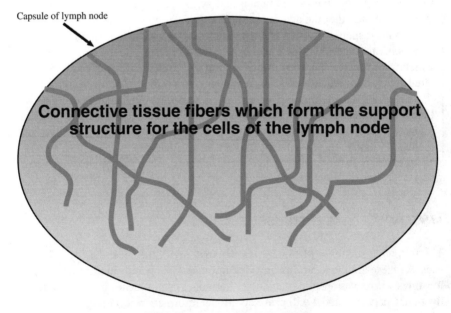

FIG. 2.30   *Connective tissue fibers.*

Each lymph node, which is approximately the shape of a kidney bean, is covered by a capsule. Connective tissue projects off of the capsule into the interior of the node and forms a three-dimensional support meshwork inside the node (Fig. 2.30).

Lymphatics that bring lymph fluid to the node pass through the capsule and discharge their contents into the node. Just beneath the capsule the lymph node is not very dense and their are spaces called sinuses into which the lymph fluid and cells are discharged from the lymphatic vessel (Fig. 2.31).

Just below the sinuses is the parenchyma (the functional part) of the node. The parenchyma can be divided into two parts; the outer part which is called the cortex and the inner part called the medulla (Fig. 2.32).

The outer part of the cortex contains lymphoid follicles which are sacs of B lymphocytes. The follicles can be either primary or secondary (primary have mostly small dark staining lymphocytes and secondary are larger with less darkly staining lymphoyctes in the center indicating that the lymphoyctes are activated. The secondary follicles are also called "germinal centers"). In between the follicles (the interfollicular area) is a diffuse array of T lymphocytes and dendritic cells and just below the follicles is a diffuse band of T lymphocytes and dendritic cells in an area called the paracortex.

The medulla is below the paracortex and is divided into segments by connective tissue. Each segment is called a "medullary cord." Lymphocytes draining from the node and plasma cells (mature antibody-producing lymphocytes) are found in the medullary cords. The plasma cells may be leaving the node to localize in the bone marrow, where they will release specific antibody molecules (Fig. 2.33).

A single artery supplies blood to the node. The artery enters the node at the hilus and sends branches along the connective tissue that form the medullary cords.

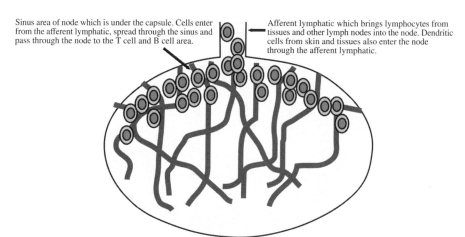

Sinus area of node which is under the capsule. Cells enter from the afferent lymphatic, spread through the sinus and pass through the node to the T cell and B cell area.

Afferent lymphatic which brings lymphocytes from tissues and other lymph nodes into the node. Dendritic cells from skin and tissues also enter the node through the afferent lymphatic.

The lymphocyte which enter the node from tissue are called 'effector' or 'memory' lymphocytes. They had previously been activated in the spleen or lymph nodes and entered tissue through blood vessels. In tissue, their TCR look at the peptides in MHC molecules on tissue cells and macrophages. If they do not find their appropriate peptide they enter lymphatic vessels, pass through lymph nodes to the thoracic duct, and recirculate.

FIG. 2.31

Cortex where the B lymphocytes aggregate into round balls called 'follicles'. The interfollicular spaces between the follicles are filled with T lymphocytes and dendritic cells.

Parafollicular area where naive T lymphocytes and dendritic cells interact. T lymphocytes become activated to an antigenic peptide to which their TCR has specificity.

Sinus where cells enter the node from the afferent lymphatic

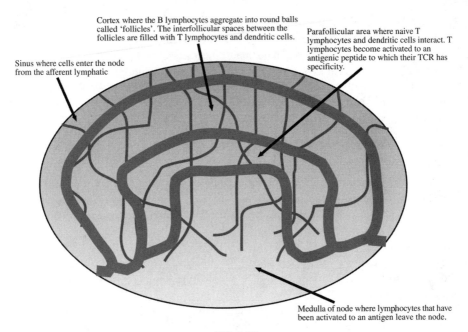

Medulla of node where lymphocytes that have been activated to an antigen leave the node.

FIG. 2.32

Secondary lymphoid follicle with large dividing B lymphocytes. This indicates that the B lymphocytes have been activated by an antigen and the appropriate CD4 helper lymphocyte.

Primary lymphoid follicle consisting of naive B lymphocytes and follicular dendritic cells. The B lymphocytes are small as they have not been activated.

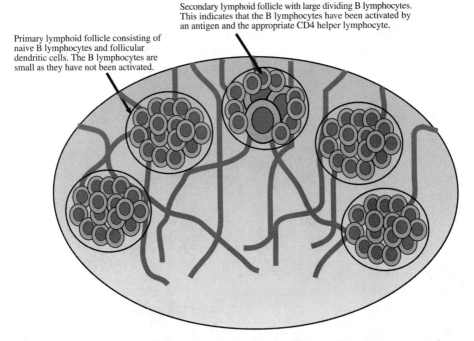

FIG. 2.33   Paracortex where naive T lymphocytes interact with dendritic cells that carry antigen to the node and present the antigen in MHC molecules. Once activated the T lymphocytes move to the follicle to interact with a B lymphocyte that is presenting the same antigenic peptide in MHC molecules.

The arteries branch and decrease in size as they become capillaries that enter the follicles.

The endothelial cells that line the postcapillary venules have a unique shape that is much higher than are other endothelial cells. These are called high endothelial venule cells (HEV). HEV are found in all secondary lymphoid tissue other than the spleen. HEV are involved in the passage of both T and B naive lymphocytes from the blood to the nodes. HEV cells have adhesion molecules that bind to receptors on naive, but not activated lymphocytes. High concentrations of cytokines may induce flat endothelial cells to become HEV as HEV are also found in chronically inflamed nonlymphoid tissue and may support lymphocyte migration at these sites. The venules leave the follicles and then pass as veins back through the cortex and medulla and leave the node at the hilus. When afferent lymph flow to the node is interrupted, the HEV convert to flat endothelial cells. Lymphocyte sticking to HEV occurs within milliseconds.

Approximately 14,000 lymphocytes extravasate from blood into a single lymph node every second, approximately 5×10^7/hour or 1.2×10^9/day/node. These are primarily naive, which have an adhesion molecule that binds to a receptor that is present on the high endothelial cells.

Spleen

The spleen is the largest lymphoid organ. There are no afferent lymphatics to the spleen, only a blood supply as the spleen is inserted into the blood circulation. The spleen filters blood and removes antigens and old or damaged erythrocytes. The spleen is covered with a capsule that sends projections into the spleen, dividing it into segments. Each of the projections of the capsule sends out additional projections which form a meshwork within the spleen. The spaces formed by the meshwork are filled with cells.

A single artery splits into six branches as it enters the spleen and then each branches further. Each arterial branch becomes covered with a mass of lymphocytes which are called the periarteriolar lymphocyte sheath (PALS). As the artery is in the center of the lymphoid tissue, it is called the *central artery*. The portion of the PALS nearest the artery is rich in T lymphocytes and the outer portion of the PALS is a mixture of T and B lymphocytes. As in the lymph nodes, accumulations of B lymphocytes are grouped into follicles.

Both primary and secondary follicles (containing germinal centers of activated B lymphocytes) are present in the PALS. A spleen may contain 10,000–20,000 follicles. The PALS is referred to as the "white pulp."

The central arteries send off perpendicular branches that open into spaces called the "marginal sinus." The marginal sinuses contain dendritic cells, macrophages, T and B lymphocytes. Surrounding the marginal sinus is the "marginal zone" that covers the PALS. At its termination, the central artery discharges into a venous sinus or ends in a space between the venous sinuses called a "splenic cord." The venous sinuses are lined by endothelial cells. The splenic cords consist of erythrocytes, macrophages, monocytes, and lymphocytes. Cells pass between the sinuses and cords. The cords and sinuses are called the "red pulp" because of the large amount of erythrocytes. The venous sinuses coalesce and form veins that leave the spleen at the hilus.

Although there are no afferent lymphatics to the spleen, there are efferent lymphatics which leave the spleen. They originate as closed ended tubes in the follicles of the PALS, merge together, and drain as a single lymphatic to a lymph node located in the hilus of the spleen.

Antigen that is in the blood stream will pass into the spleen, where it is ingested by dendritic cells in the marginal zone and venous sinuses. The dendritic cells move to the PALS of the white pulp. In the PALS, the dendritic cells interact with naive T cells, which then move to the B-cell follicles. Antibody production is initiated and the antibody-producing B lymphocytes leave the spleen by moving to the red pulp or marginal sinuses, or through the lymphatic. Activated T lymphocytes probably migrate to the venous sinus and then to the circulation. Other lymphocyte aggregations in the body include the following.

Diffuse Lymphoid Tissue

The connective and parenchymal tissue of the body contain large numbers of effector/memory lymphocytes in its meshwork. Where these accumulations are particularly dense, they are referred to as diffuse lymphoid tissue. The lungs, gastrointestinal tract, and skin, are areas particularly rich in such lymphocyte accumulations. It make sense for lymphocytes to be in these locations, as they are areas where it is most likely that foreign antigens will gain access to the body.

Solitary Lymphoid Follicles

B and T lymphocytes that aggregate into a dense sphere containing dendritic cells mixed with the B lymphocytes surrounded by T lymphocytes are called "solitary lymphoid follicles." They do not occur in fixed sites but are transiently present. They occur in the same tissue locations as the diffuse lymphoid tissue. Their presence may indicate an active immune response occurring within the tissue.

Aggregated Lymphoid Follicles

Accumulation of several solitary lymphoid follicles. Examples are the "tonsils" found at the posterior part of the nasopharynx; bronchiole-associated lymphoid tissue (BALT) found in the lungs; Peyer's patches, which are aggregated lymphoid follicles in the wall of the small intestine; and the appendix.

Mucosal Associated Lymphoid Tissue

MALT protects the mucosal surfaces of the body and provides immunity to the respiratory tract (BALT) and the gastrointestinal tract (gut-associated lymphoid tissue; GALT; Peyer's patches).

These are the areas of the body that receive the highest volume of exposure to foreign antigens (food, microorganisms, environmental pollutents, parasites, allergens).

The mucosal immune system can produce cell-mediated immune reactions and a specialized antibody mediated immunity that consists of "secretory IgA." This is IgA antibody that is synthesized by B lymphocytes in submucosal sites and transported across the epithelium to the lumen. Secretory IgA binds to pathogens and prevents them from adhering to the mucosal surface.

The MALT is found below all mucosal surfaces and has a greater mass of lymphocytes than all of the other lymphoid tissues in the body combined. The MALT is dispersed in the mucosa at some sites and at others it is organized into lymphoid follicles.

Once an antigen reaches the mucosal surface it must cross the epithelium. There are specialized cells in the gastrointestinal and respiratory tracts, called "M cells," that assist in this process. These cells have a folded membrane or are flattened (the adjacent cells of the gastrointestinal or respiratory tract are columnar). They endocytose (take into a vacuole) soluble and particulate antigen and transport the antigen to the submucosal side of the M cell, where it is released. The M cell cannot present antigen to lymphocytes, they are only involved with transporting the antigen across the mucosa.

On the side of the M cell that is opposite to the lumen of the gut or respiratory tract there are dendritic cells that are in contact with the M cell. The dendritic cells take up the antigen and migrate to follicles or present the antigen to T cells at the submucosal site. The antigen is also taken up by B cells, so that both humoral and cellular immune responses occur.

Once a B lymphocyte has reacted with an antigen and received the necessary help to begin to produce antibody they leave the MALT in efferent lymphatics (the MALT has no afferent lymphatics) and go the the mesenteric lymph nodes where they mature to plasma cells or become B memory cells. The cells then leave the node through the efferent lymphatic, enter the thoracic duct, go to the bloodstream, and then through a specific adhesion system reenter the mucosal tissue. It is possible that B lymphocytes derived from mucosal sites produce all classes of immunoglobulin and that only the cells that produce IgA go back to the mucosal sites, but this has not been determined. Regardless of the mechanism, the predominant class of immunoglobulin produced in mucosal sites is IgA.

The predominant secretory immunoglobulin is IgA. Secretory IgA (sIgA) is resistant to digestion by intestinal enzymes. The secretory immunoglobulins prevent microorganisms, antigens, and toxins from gaining entry to the body. As sIgA lacks the ability to activate the complement system, it cannot elicit an inflammatory response, and therefore works by excluding harmful substances from the body.

Approximately 80% of all immunoglobulin-producing B lymphocytes are in the mucosa. More sIgA is passed into the intestinal lumen than the total amount of IgG produced/day (30 mg/kg).

If a pathogen, or other antigen, crosses the mucosal surface, a backup protective mechanism is in place. There is IgG antibody present to combine with the foreign material (approximately 50% of IgG is extravascular) provided the immune system had previously been activated to produce IgG antibodies (Fig. 2.34).

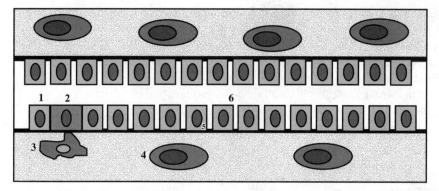

FIG. 2.34 *Steps involved in the production of IgA on the mucosal surfaces of the body using the gastrointestinal tract as an example: 1, Antigen enters the lumen of the intestine after being ingested. 2, The antigen binds to the surface of a transport cell, called the M cell, and is moved across the M cell. 3, The antigen is passed by the M cell to a dendritic cell. The dendritic cell carries the antigen to secondary lymphoid tissue where activation of IgA producing B lymphocytes occurs. The B cells generate plasma cells that migrate to the wall of the intestine. 4, The plasma cells release IgA which forms dimers held together by the J chain. 5, The IgA binds to the membrane of mucosal epithelial cells and is transported through the epithelial cell where it binds to "secretory component" which transports the IgA onto the mucosa of the intestine. 6, The secretory IgA will bind to antigen in the lumen of the intestine and prevent the antigen from crossing the intestine and entering the body.*

SUMMARY OF ACTIVATION OF AN IMMUNE RESPONSE

It is possible to look at the development of an effective immune response as a fairly rigid sequence of events that occur after the introduction of an antigen into the body. Indeed, the various steps which occur do follow a fixed sequence with more than a single activity occurring at the same time. At each step of the process, there are multiple influences that can direct the immune response to a different functional endpoint. It is likely that different hormones, or concentrations of hormones present due to an individuals emotional environment, contribute to the characteristics of the final immune response.

The basic steps that occur subsequent to the introduction of a foreign protein antigen into the body are:

1. The protein must be ingested and digested by a cell termed an "antigen processing cell (APC)". These cells which become involved in activating a specific immune response do not recognize foreignness. Rather, they ingest all proteins by phagocytosis or pinocytosis. Included are populations of cells that are dendritic cells, macrophages, and monocytes. This usually occurs in tissue such as the skin or in the internal organs of the body. If the antigen is in the blood stream, this process takes place in the spleen. The dendritic cell is the most important APC for initiation of the primary immune response.

2. The APC will move from tissue to a draining lymph node. If the APC is in the spleen it will remain in the spleen. Peptides derived from the ingested protein are displayed on the surface of the APC in a presentation molecule called a major histocompatibility complex (MHC) protein of which there are two types: MHC I and MHC II. MHC I molecules are usually associated with presenting peptides derived from antigens which are synthesized within a cell, for example, peptides derived from viruses. MHC II molecules are usually associated with presenting peptides derived from antigens that have been ingested into the APC (bacteria or soluble proteins).

3. A naive CD4 positive (CD4+) T lymphocyte that can recognize the peptide will bind to the peptide displayed in a MHC II molecule. This occurs in a lymph node or in the spleen. Only those T cells that have antigen recognizing receptors, called "T cell receptors (TCR)" that are specific for a particular peptide, will bind to the peptide.

4. The T cell that has bound to the peptide will receive an additional signal, called a costimulation signal, that will activate the T cell to become a T lymphocyte that can do something (the T lymphocyte will be called an "effector lymphocyte"). The number of costimulation molecules on the APC have not been fully characterized. Some costimulation molecules may activate the T lymphocyte, while other costimulation molecules may decrease T-lymphocyte activity.

5. The effector T lymphocyte (either the CD4 or CD8) can leave the lymph node or the spleen and search throughout the tissues of the body for the antigen that caused the T lymphocyte to become activated. If the T lymphocyte finds its activating antigen, the T lymphocyte will participate in the killing of the cell where the antigen resides, or activating the cell (if it is a macrophage) to kill the bacteria. Tissue cells that are infected by a virus are killed by cytotoxic T lymphocytes (CD8 lymphocytes). Infectious agents such as those that cause some fungal infections are eliminated by helper/inducer T lymphocytes (CD4 lymphocytes) that focus inflammatory cells at the site of the foreign organism.

Alternatively, the T lymphocyte may move to an area of the lymph node or spleen where B lymphocytes have accumulated (called "primary follicles"). At these sites, the CD4+ T lymphocyte will interact with a particular B lymphocyte and determine the class of immunoglobulin that the B cell will produce.

IMMUNOPATHOLOGICAL MECHANISMS OF DISEASE

The immune system can bring about the removal of injurious infectious agents and their products. During the course of these events, often producing tissue inflammation, there may be some damage to the host tissue. However, this is outweighed by the potential damage, perhaps even leading to death, that could ensue if the immune response did not exist. However, the same protective responses when produced against harmless, noninvasive elements that form part of the normal environment (eg, pollen from plants) or even against self-antigens or infectious agents, which by themselves do not damage tissue, can lead to tissue inflammation, and hence actually cause disease.

The immune-mediated mechanisms of resistance to foreign antigens uses a variety of effector molecules. The reactions are frequently referred to as hypersensitivity reactions as an indicator of the heightened immune reactivity associated with these reactions. There is clear evidence for at least four types of hypersensitivity reactions:

Type 1: Immediate hypersensitivity reactions—(Reactions that involve the IgE class of immunoglobulin).

Type 2: Antibody-mediated (non-IgE) reactions—(Reactions in which an antibody binds to a tissue and either mediates killing, removal, or functional alteration. These reactions may be complement dependent or complement independent).

Type 3: Immune complex reactions—(Antigen and antibody combine and become fixed in tissue where they mediate a complement-dependent reaction).

Type 4: Cell-mediated hypersensitivity reactions—Delayed hypersensitivity reactions (antibody-independent reactions involving Th1 CD4 T lymphocytes that participate in an inflammatory response); and Cytotoxic cellular reactions (Antibody-independent reactions involving CD8 lymphocytes that participate in a cell-mediated cytotoxic response).

On occasion, the hypersensitivity mechanisms may mediate an attack on an individuals tissue with a resultant damage to the tissue. When disease of self tissue occurs, it is frequently referred to as an autoimmune disease process.

Type 1 Reactions

Not every individual who is exposed to an allergen becomes allergic. Allergic conditions, such as asthma, can be induced by exercise. Thus, the primary defect that leads to the development of allergy is not fully resolved and the interaction of immunological, genetic, and other physiological factors must be considered as important in the causation of allergy.

Mechanism of IgE-Mediated Effect on Mast Cells and Basophils. IgE binds to tissue mast cells. There are approximately 40,000–80,000 Fc receptors for IgE/mast cell. The binding of IgE to mast cells has no effect on the cells. However, when the antibody interacts with specific antigen, a programmed sequence of events starts.

The antigen must be multivalent and binds by 1 epitope to one IgE molecule and by another epitope to an adjacent molecule of IgE. This cross-linking causes an aggregation of Fc receptors. Changes occur in the cytoplasmic cytoskeleton to which the receptors are attached and a signal is given that leads to release of the contents of the granules of the basophils and mast cells. The granules fuse with the plasma membrane and degranulation occurs. In addition to degranulation, there is increased synthesis and release of prostaglandins and leukotrienes (Fig. 2.35).

Mast cell with histamine being released from intracytoplasmic granules.

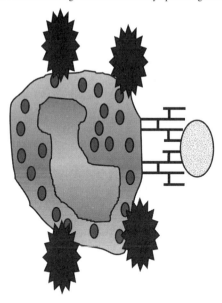

FIG. 2.35 *Molecule of antigen that has been bound by two molecules of IgE which are next to each other on the membrane of the mast cell. When this occurs the contents of the cytoplasmic granules are released. If two molecules of IgE that are reactive to the same antigen molecule are not adjacent to each other, degranulation will not occur. Thus, in those individuals who are synthesizing large amounts of an IgE antibody with specificity for the same antigen, the chance of binding two adjacent IgE molecules that react to the same antigen is increased.*

Soluble Mediators Released by Basophils and Mast Cells. The mediators of type I immediate hypersensitivity reactions stored in the granules are:

Histamine: Increases vascular permeability and causes smooth muscle contraction

Serotonin: Increases vascular permeability and causes smooth muscle contraction

Proteases: Degrade blood vessel basement membranes; activates the third component of complement so that C3a is formed which produces degranulation of mast cells

Mediators Synthesized After the IgE on Mast Cells Bind Antigen.

Leukotrienes: Increase vascular permeability; contract pulmonary smooth muscle

Prostaglandins: Inhibit effects of heparin on smooth muscle cells and vascular endothelial cells; increase platelet aggregation

Bradykinin: Increase vascular permeability and smooth muscle contraction

Platelet activating factor: Promote platelet aggregation and degranulation; contraction of pulmonary smooth muscle

Release of the various mediators produces smooth muscle contraction, vascular leakage, hypotension, mucous secretion, wheal and flare (swelling and redness of skin), itching, and pain. These events occur within minutes of a second exposure to the antigen (the first exposure initiates IgE synthesis), and by 60 minutes they are over. This is termed the immediate hypersensitivity reaction which is followed in 2–8 hours by a late-phase response that lasts for 1–2 days. The late-phase response is an inflammatory reaction mediated by synthesized mediators and consists of lymphocytes, neutrophils, eosinophils, monocytes, and a few basophils. The late-phase reaction results in a localized burning sensation, tenderness, erythema, and induration.

Leukotrienes are not formed until the mast cell degranulates. Therefore, it takes a longer time for the biologic effect of the leukotrienes to occur. The effects of leukotrienes last longer than those induced by histamine. The leukotrienes are more potent in their effects than is histamine. In patients with asthma leukotrienes are associated with prolonged bronchoconstriction and mucous accumulation.

Both the immediate and late phases of the type 1 response are influenced by the autonomic nervous system. Both afferent (sensory) and efferent neurons (ending in smooth muscle, blood vessels, glands) are involved. Afferent neurons can be stimulated by heat, pressure, or chemicals and result in efferent neuron stimulation. In tissue the sympathetic efferent neurons release neuropeptides such as Substance P, vasoactive intestinal peptide (VIP), norepinephrine, and the parasympathetic neurons release acetylcholine. The neuropeptides bind to receptors on mast cells, smooth muscle cells, endothelial cells, and goblet cells and produce changes associated with an allergic reaction.

Type 2 Reactions

Definition-Cytotoxic reactions which involve the combination of IgG or IgM antibodies with accessible antigens on cell surfaces. The antigen may be a natural constituent of the cell surface or may be adsorbed onto the cell surface. The interaction of antigen and antibody may activate the complement system and cause death or lysis of the target cell, or, result in adherence of antibody-coated cells to phagocytic cells and phagocytosis of the antibody coated cell (see Figs. 2.26 and 2.27).

Antibodies directed to cell surface antigens do not necessarily destroy the cell. Sometimes antibodies to cell surface receptors may alter the physiology of the cell. Examples are myasthenia gravis (an antibody to the acetylcholine receptor at the neuromuscular junction of striated muscle causes removal of the receptor and interferes with transmission of the signal that initiates contraction of striated muscle) and Graves' disease (an antibody to the thyroid-stimulating hormone receptor produces activation of the receptor with a resultant increase in the production of thyroid hormone) (Fig. 2.36).

Antibodies can cause lysis of the target cell by the mechanism of antibody-dependent cellular cytotoxicity (ADCC). Antibody bound to a cellular antigen exposes the Fc portion of the antibody. A subset of lymphocytes (possibly a subset of NK cells) have receptors for the Fc portion of IgG. When the lymphocyte binds to the

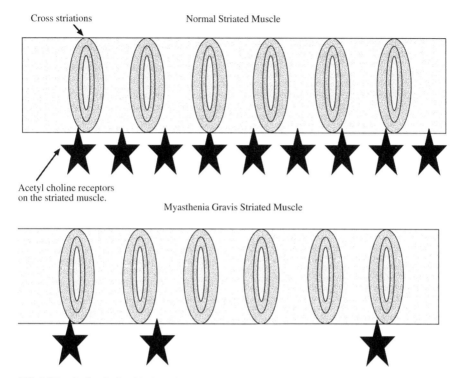

Cross striations

Normal Striated Muscle

Acetyl choline receptors
on the striated muscle.

Myasthenia Gravis Striated Muscle

FIG. 2.36 *Antibody that binds to the acetylcholine receptors causes a reduction in the number of receptors on the muscle surface. When acetylcholine is released from the motor nerve, it will have few receptors to bind to and, therefore, there is a decreased ability of the muscle to contract.*

cell bound antibody the lymphocyte exerts a cytotoxic enzyme mediated reaction on the tissue cell with the resultant killing of the cell. The lymphocyte is not sensitized to the target cell but becomes activated by binding to antibody. The phenomenon is called antibody-dependent cellular cytotoxicity (ADCC) (see Fig. 2.22).

Some immunological processes associated with type 2 reactions are:

Incompatible transfusion reactions
Autoimmune hemolytic anemia
Drug-induced hemolytic anemia
Autoimmune thrombocytopenic purpura
Goodpasture's disease
Autoimmune neutropenia

Hemolytic Disease of the Newborn. IgG antibodies are synthesized by a mother who is Rh negative to Rh antigens which the fetus inherits from an Rh positive father. If some of the fetal erythrocytes enter the maternal circulation the mother may make an antibody to the Rh antigen. This usually occurs after the first pregnancy as it is at the time of delivery that the fetal red cells enter the maternal circulation. Thus, the first Rh incompatible pregnancy is not at risk, but subsequent pregnancies are at risk. During the second pregnancies, the maternal IgG antibodies to Rh antigen are transported across the placenta into the fetal circulation. The resultant antibody-induced lysis of erythrocytes in the fetus leads to anemia and jaundice.

The disease is prevented by injecting the mother with an antibody to the Rh antigen at the time of delivery of each pregnancy. The antibody coats the fetal erythrocytes in the maternal circulation and causes their rapid removal (probably by neutrophils) before they can induce an immune response (neutrophils are not antigen presenting cells).

Autoimmune Hemolytic Anemia. An individual synthesizes IgG antibodies against their own red cells. Binding of the antibodies activates the complement system and the cells are either removed by phagocytosis or destroyed by lysis.

To achieve activation of complement, there have to be two IgG antibodies located adjacent to each other on the red cell membrane. This require as many as 800–1,000 molecules of IgG to be present on a red cell surface. Lesser amounts of IgG antibody will promote removal of the antibody-coated erythrocytes by the phagocytic cells of the spleen and liver, larger amounts will mediate lysis.

Autoimmune Thrombocytopenic Purpura and Autoimmune Agranulocytosis. Same mechanisms as for autoimmune hemolytic anemia, but the antibody has specificity for platelets or for polymorphonuclear leukocytes.

Drug-Induced Hemolytic Anemia. Some antibiotics (penicillin, cephalosporin) will nonspecifically adsorb to proteins on erythrocyte membranes, where they may function as a hapten (the protein serves as a carrier). If the hapten stimulates a B lymphocyte to produce antibody, a hemolytic anemia may occur if complement is activated or the cells will be ingested by the phagocytic cells and a nonhemolytic anemia will result.

Goodpasture's Disease. This disorder is characterized by antibodies directed against antigens located on the basement membrane of the glomeruli of the kidney or the alveoli of the lung. Bound antibody activates the complement system, leading to a glomerulonephritis of the kidney or alveolitis with hemorrhage into the alveoli of the lung.

Type 3 Reactions

Antigen–antibody (immune) complexes form when circulating antibody binds to the specific antigen that the antibody has specificity for. The phagocytic cells of the spleen, liver and lung normally remove immune complexes from the circulation. If there are more complexes formed than can be removed by mononuclear phagocytes, the complexes will become deposited in tissue. In tissue the complexes will activate the complement system. This will induce an inflammatory response and damage to the tissue that is caused by enzymes released from the inflammatory cells and anoxia (the lack of oxygen) caused by occlusion of small blood vessels.

Immune complex formation requires that their be an approximately equivalent amount of antigen and antibody present. The size of the complex that produces the most tissue damage is when there is slightly more antigen than antibody present. An excess of either antigen or antibody will prevent formation of immune complexes, as illustrated in Figure 2.37.

The amount of immune complex formed and the location of the complex determines the type of reaction. When the complexes are deposited in tissue near the site of an injected antigen, the reaction is called an "Arthus" reaction. Complexes formed in the bloodstream may deposit in blood vessel walls, the kidneys, synovium, and choroid plexus of the brain. Thus, systemic deposition of immune complexes is associated with a vasculitis, a nephritis, and an arthritis. This reaction is called "serum sickness."

Serum sickness can be either acute or chronic:

Acute serum sickness—occurs subsequent to the single injection of antigen. Clinical symptoms are short-lived and there is tissue healing after clearance of the complexes.

Chronic serum sickness—produced by repeated injection of antigen (or synthesis by an infectious agent) when there is circulating antibody present that binds to the antigen.

Immune complex-mediated pathology

1. Precipitating antibody binds to the antigen that elicited its production.
2. If the concentrations of the antigen and antibody lead to the formation of immune complexes in moderate antigen excess, the exposed Fc portion of the immunoglobulin molecule will activate the complement system. Complexes and activated complement deposit on basement membrane of the glomerulus and internal elastic lamina membrane of blood vessels.
3. Activation of the complement system will result in an inflammatory response.

    C3a, C4a, and C5a will cause increased vascular permeability

    C3a and C5a will attract PMN

    C3b will enhance phagocytosis
4. The release of enzymes from PMN, as they ingest the immune complexes, will damage tissue and cause necrosis (tissue death). Fibrinogen is activated with a resultant deposition of fibrin.
5. Either the lesion reverses after a single exposure to antigen or inflammation and tissue injury are maintained with the persistent formation of immune complexes.

Type 4 Reactions

Differs from the other three types of reactions in that no antibody is involved. It is a hypersensitivity reaction because it does not occur with the first exposure to an antigen. When the reaction does occur there is tissue destruction. This reaction is termed "delayed hypersensitivity" (DH) because it does not attain its maximum size in a lo-

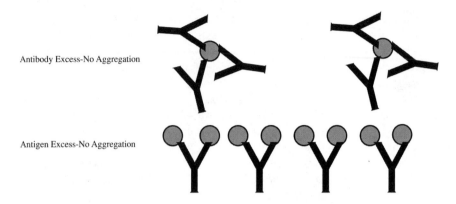

Antibody Excess-No Aggregation

Antigen Excess-No Aggregation

Equivalence-immune complex formed

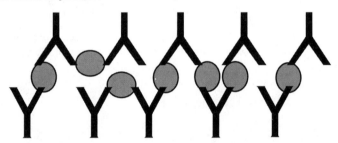

FIG. 2.37 *Each antibody molecule can bind to two sites on an antigen. Large amounts of antibody relative to the antigen will cover all of the antigenic sites without allowing lattice formation to occur. Similarly, excessive amounts of antigens will bind all of the antibody molecules, and lattice formulation will not occur. Immune complexes form when there are approximately equivalent amounts of antigen and antibody present.*

calized skin reaction site until approximately 48–72 hours after the antigen has been injected. The purpose of the DH reaction is to remove infectious agents that reside in intracellular locations where they are inaccessible to antibody (Fig. 2.38a–c).

There are in vitro correlates of DH. The in vitro assays evaluate the response of T lymphocytes to antigen.

Mechanism of localized delayed hypersensitivity reaction:

1. Conversion of a naive Th1 CD4 lymphocyte to an effector/memory lymphocyte occurs in lymph nodes or the spleen.

2. When the antigen to which the activated lymphocyte is reactive is introduced into the skin, the lymphocytes that have been sensitized to the antigen are activated, probably by antigenic peptides that have been processed and presented by dendritic cells in the skin.

3. IL-2 produced by the activated T cells may stimulate non-antigen reactive T cells to produce cytokines. Thus, the concentration of IL-2, IFN-γ, and TNF

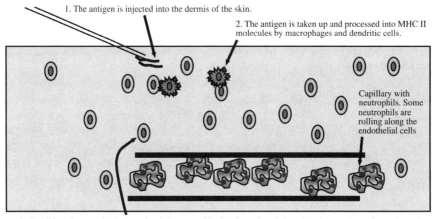

1. The antigen is injected into the dermis of the skin.

2. The antigen is taken up and processed into MHC II molecules by macrophages and dendritic cells.

Capillary with neutrophils. Some neutrophils are rolling along the endothelial cells

3. CD4 T lymphocytes that had previously been sensitized to the antigen in lymph nodes or spleen migrate through tissues, including the skin. If, by chance, a CD4 T lymphocyte that has been sensitized to the antigen samples the MHC II molecule containing the antigen, the CD4 T cell will remain at the point of cell interaction. As the CD4 cell is an effector cell, it does not require costimulatory molecules to become activated to release cytokines.

FIG. 2.38a   *Representation of a delayed hypersensitivity reaction occurring in the skin of an individual who has T lymphocytes that have been activated to an antigen.*

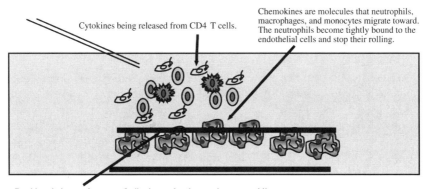

Cytokines being released from CD4 T cells.

Chemokines are molecules that neutrophils, macrophages, and monocytes migrate toward. The neutrophils become tightly bound to the endothelial cells and stop their rolling.

Cytokines induce an increase of adhesion molecules causing neutrophils to adhere to the endothelial cells at the site where c ytokines are being produced.

FIG. 2.38b   *Interacting through their TCR with the antigenic peptide that the T cells are sensitized to, the effector CD4 T lymphocytes begin to release cytokines. The cytokines increase the adhesion molecules on the endothelial cells in blood vessels near the site where the cytokines are being released. The adhesion molecules cause neutrophils to tightly adhere to the endothelial cells. Other cytokines attract the neutrophils and monocytes and macrophages to the site where the cytokines are being produced. Other cytokines induce mast cells to release histamine so that the blood vessels will become more permeable to fluid and the passage of cells.*

increases at the local site. MHC II expression on APC is increased by the presence of IFN-γ.

4. The activated lymphocytes begin to secrete cytokines. The cytokines diffuse to the endothelial cells lining the blood vessels at the site of the immune reaction. Adhesion molecules increase in concentration on the endothelial cells.

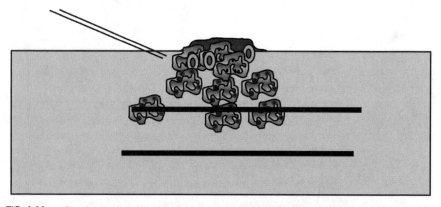

FIG. 2.38c *An elevated red area appears approximately 48 hours after the antigen was in-jected into the skin of an individual who had previously been sensitized to the antigen. The ele-vation (edema) is due to fluids leaking into the tissue from the blood vessels that had an increased permeability and to cells (neutrophils, lymphocytes, macrophages, eosinophils, and monocytes) being attracted to the site of antigen injection. The reaction usually begins to fade about 72 hours after the injection as the antigen is removed by the phagocytic cells and possibly by the appearance of substances (soluble or cellular) which inhibit the reaction to prevent ex-cessive tissue damage.*

Remember that different adhesion molecules will bind to different types of leukocytes.

5. Under the influence of the localized accumulation of cytokines, endothelial cells begin to: (a) produce soluble factors which mediate vascular dilation to increase the blood flow to the area, (b) generate adhesion molecules initially for neutrophils and then lymphocytes and monocytes [endothelial leukocyte adhesion molecule-1 (ELAM-1) and then intercellular adhesion molecule-1 (ICAM-1) and vascular cell adhesion molecule-1 (VCAM-1)], (c) produce IL-8 which stimulates leukocyte motility and helps get the leukocytes from the intravascular to the extravascular compartment (d) causing spaces to open up between the vascular endothelial cells to allow the leukocytes access to the extravascular spaces.

6. As monocytes enter the tissue some convert to large sized phagocytic macrophages. The monocytes/macrophages accumulating at the local site are activated by interferon-γ. The activated mononuclear phagocytes ingest foreign material that is present at the local site. In so doing, the monocytes/macrophages release lysosomal enzymes which cause tissue damage. In addition to the mononuclear phagocyte contribution to tissue destruction, these same cells produce factors which promote tissue healing by stimulating collagen production and new blood vessel formation (angiogenesis). If the antigen eliciting the DH reaction is rapidly removed, there may be little tissue destruction. Thus, fibrosis at the site of a DH response is an indication that the reaction has been present for a sufficient time to produce fibrous tissue.

Although the above description of the type 4 reaction has been described as a local reaction occurring in the skin, it is important to remember that this type of response to a foreign antigen can occur anywhere in the body. For example, if a foreign microorganism enters the lungs and is processed by antigen presenting cells and the antigen is presented in MHC II molecules, a DH response may occur in the lungs.

Cytotoxic T lymphocytes kill target cells by lysis (punching holes or "pores" in the target cell membrane). The pores are formed by a protein called perforin (pore forming protein), or other enzymes. Although the cytotoxic T cell mechanism of resistance to infectious agents is not a true delayed hypersensitivity response (lacks an inflammatory cell component) it is an important host defense mechanism and is therefore included as a cell mediated reaction.

WHEN THE IMMUNE SYSTEM DOESN'T WORK WELL

Autoimmunity

Autoimmunity occurs when the immune system reacts against one's own tissue (self tissue). There are various ways in which autoimmune reactions occur:

1. On occasion, lymphocytes responding to an infectious agent may coincidentally cross-react with self-tissue.
2. Sometimes, a virus, a drug, or a genetic mutation may alter the surface of a cell enough so that the cell appears to be foreign to the immune system.
3. An antigen which had been hidden from the immune system during embryogenesis so that tolerance did not occur to the antigen, may serve as an antigenic stimulus if the antigen is exposed to the immune system.

If the autoimmune reaction damages tissue, the event is considered an autoimmune disease.

Cancer

The "immune surveillance theory" suggests that the immune system is constantly detecting and destroying cells which have become malignant. If the immune system no longer works properly there is an increased likelihood of a malignancy developing as the malignant cells will not be destroyed by the immune system. Malignant cells may escape from immune surveillance by secreting immunosuppressive chemicals, not displaying MHC molecules on their surface, or lacking co-stimulation molecules.

Allergies

Allergies are hyper-reactive immune reactions to environmental antigens. The immune reaction associated with an allergy is very rapid and occurs in response to small amounts of antigens and can occur in a variety of areas of the body. The IgE class of immunoglobulins participates in allergic reactions by binding to the allergen while the IgE molecules is also anchored to a mast cell. The mast cells then release histamine and other inflammatory mediators.

Immunodeficiency Diseases

A deficiency of T lymphocyte function leads to susceptibility to viruses, some bacterial infections (particularly bacteria that multiply within cells), and cancer. B lymphocyte deficiencies increase susceptibility to infection with extracellular bacteria. Chapter 6 discusses each type of immunologically mediated disease and the relationship of stress to the disease.

LABORATORY TESTS USED TO EVALUATE THE IMMUNE SYSTEM

A variety of laboratory tests are used to determine the number of different types of lymphocytes present in blood and their function. Many of these tests have been mentioned in this chapter and will be repeatedly referred to in subsequent chapters and in all the scientific literature on immunology. The following section will present information about the tests to help your understanding of how the test is performed and what is learned from each. The list is not comprehensive but represents the tests most commonly used in psychoneuroimmunology research.

IN VITRO QUANTITATIVE TESTS

Immunoglobulin Quantitation

Method. The usual procedure to quantitate the amount of the major classes of immunoglobulin (IgG, IgA, IgM) is called "nephelometry." The procedure adds a known amount of antibody that binds to the heavy chain of the immunoglobulin class that is being measured. This forms an immune complex (with the antigen component of the complex being the antibody class that is being measured). The amount of precipitate that is formed relates to the concentration of the immunoglobulin class being measured. The amount of precipitate is compared to the amount produced by known concentrations of the antigen being measured.

Interpretation. The results are usually reported as milligrams of immunoglobulin in 100 ml of blood (mg/dl). Normal values are determined by quantitating the amount of each class of immunoglobulin in large numbers of normal individuals. The range of normal for adults for IgG, IgA, and IgM is broad. Children under the age of 16 have lower levels of immunoglobulin than adults. Therefore, when evaluating immunoglobulin levels in children, an age related normal must be used.

Information Learned. There are differences between the normal concentration determined statistically and the normal physiologic concentration (the amount of immunoglobulin needed to provide protection against infectious diseases). The physiological normal is lower than the normal determined from measuring immunoglobulin levels in large populations and determining the mean and standard deviation. Thus, a single number at a point in time provides little information regarding a biological significance for immunoglobulins, unless the amount detected is extremely low. Changes in immunoglobulin levels occur slowly and may be due to inadequate nutrition or loss. If stress or depression interfere with an individual obtaining adequate nutrition, low immunoglobulin levels could ensue. Quantitation of immunoglobulins does not provide information regarding what antigens the antibodies can react to and how much antibody is present to a given antigen. Immunoglobulins are proteins and low concentration of immunoglobulins occur in malnutrition

ELISA

Method. The enzyme-linked immunosorbent assay (ELISA) is used to quantitate either the amount of a specific antibody or the amount of specific antigen, that is present in a solution, such as blood. The method is described in Figure 2.39A and 2.39B.

Interpretation. Concentrations of antibody that are specific for a given antigen, or concentrations of an antigen, can be measured in blood by this assay.

Information Learned. This assay provides the opportunity to follow changes in antibody concentration to a specific antigen or, for example, the concentration of a viral antigen in plasma. It also provides the capabilities of comparing different populations of subjects. For example, following immunization to an antigen, the amount of antibody produced in a population of subjects experiencing high levels of stress in their lives can be compared with a population with low levels of stress.

Immunofluorescence Assay

Method. This assay is used to detect antibody in serum that reacts to antigens in tissue. This assay is frequently used to detect the presence of autoantibodies (self-reactive antibodies). The method is described in Figure 2.40.

Interpretation. The assay uses thin sections of different tissues placed onto microscope slides. Antibodies to several autoantigens are detected by this assay. Dilution of the serum to determine the highest dilution which provides positive fluorescence provides a rough idea of the concentration of the antibody in the patients serum.

Information Learned. The presence of antibody to self (auto) antigens and their approximate concentration (high or low amounts) is determined by this assay.

Lymphocyte Subset Quantitation (Flow Cytometry)

Method. This method provides quantitative information regarding the number of the different populations of lymphocytes that are present in blood (for example, CD4 cells, CD8 cells, B cells, NK cells). The method requires a single cell suspension of

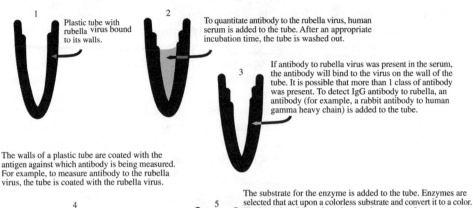

1 Plastic tube with rubella virus bound to its walls.

2 To quantitate antibody to the rubella virus, human serum is added to the tube. After an appropriate incubation time, the tube is washed out.

3 If antibody to rubella virus was present in the serum, the antibody will bind to the virus on the wall of the tube. It is possible that more than 1 class of antibody was present. To detect IgG antibody to rubella, an antibody (for example, a rabbit antibody to human gamma heavy chain) is added to the tube.

The walls of a plastic tube are coated with the antigen against which antibody is being measured. For example, to measure antibody to the rubella virus, the tube is coated with the rubella virus.

4 Enzyme

The anti-human IgG antibody added to the tube has an enzyme bound to it. When the antibody is added to the tube it will bind to the human IgG on the wall of the tube. The amount of the enzyme labeled antibody bound will depend on the amount of antibody bound to the virus.

5 The substrate for the enzyme is added to the tube. Enzymes are selected that act upon a colorless substrate and convert it to a color. The intensity of the color relates to the amount of enzyme present on the wall of the tube. By using standards with known amounts of antibody, and comparing the intensity of the color produced by the unknown serum specimen to the standards, the amount of antibody in the unknown specimen can be determined.

FIG. 2.39a   ELISA to quantitate specific antibody.

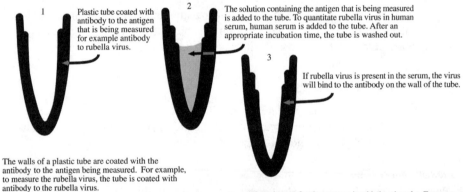

1 Plastic tube coated with antibody to the antigen that is being measured for example antibody to rubella virus.

2 The solution containing the antigen that is being measured is added to the tube. To quantitate rubella virus in human serum, human serum is added to the tube. After an appropriate incubation time, the tube is washed out.

3 If rubella virus is present in the serum, the virus will bind to the antibody on the wall of the tube.

The walls of a plastic tube are coated with the antibody to the antigen being measured. For example, to measure the rubella virus, the tube is coated with antibody to the rubella virus.

4 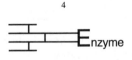 Enzyme

Antibody to the rubella virus is bound to the tube. When the antigen is added to the tube it will bind to the antibody on the wall of the tube. A second antibody to the virus, with an enzyme bound to it is then added. The amount of the enzyme labeled antibody bound will depend on the amount of virus bound to the tube.

5 The substrate for the enzyme is added to the tube. Enzymes are selected that act upon a colorless substrate and convert it to a color. The intensity of the color relates to the amount of enzyme present on the wall of the tube, which relates to the amount of antibody to the the virus, which relates to the amount of the virus bound to the wall of the tube. By using standards with known amounts of virus, and comparing the intensity of the color produced by the unknown serum specimen to the standards, the amount of virus in the unknown specimen can be determined.

FIG. 2.39b   ELISA to quantitate specific antigen.

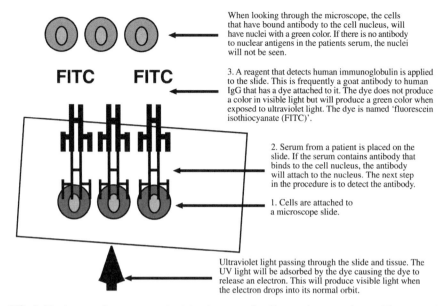

When looking through the microscope, the cells that have bound antibody to the cell nucleus, will have nuclei with a green color. If there is no antibody to nuclear antigens in the patients serum, the nuclei will not be seen.

FITC   FITC

3. A reagent that detects human immunoglobulin is applied to the slide. This is frequently a goat antibody to human IgG that has a dye attached to it. The dye does not produce a color in visible light but will produce a green color when exposed to ultraviolet light. The dye is named 'fluorescein isothiocyanate (FITC)'.

2. Serum from a patient is placed on the slide. If the serum contains antibody that binds to the cell nucleus, the antibody will attach to the nucleus. The next step in the procedure is to detect the antibody.

1. Cells are attached to a microscope slide.

Ultraviolet light passing through the slide and tissue. The UV light will be adsorbed by the dye causing the dye to release an electron. This will produce visible light when the electron drops into its normal orbit.

FIG. 2.40 *Immunofluorescence test to detect antibodies to tissue antigens. The example shown is the test for antinuclear antibodies.*

cells. Lymphocytes in blood or suspensions of the spleen or lymph nodes, are commonly studied. The method is described in Figure 2.41.

Interpretation. Each of the different subsets of lymphocytes can be quantitated by this procedure, provided that an antibody to a unique surface marker on the lymphocyte population is available. All T lymphocytes have the CD3 marker, all B lymphocytes have the CD19 marker, and NK lymphocytes have the CD56 marker. Additional surface markers are used to identify subgroups of the different populations. CD3 cells can be identified as helper (CD4$^+$) or cytotoxic (CD8$^+$). Surface markers to identify Th1 and Th2 are not yet available.

Information Learned. The quantitative information provides no information regarding whether a cell population is capable of carrying out a function. Numbers of different cells can be followed over time in a subject or group of subjects to determine whether an environmental situation (such as stress) alters the numbers of cells in that population. It is unusual to find an environmental situation (such as stress, divorce, death of a spouse) that will alter the numbers of a lymphocyte population so that the numbers are no longer in the normal range for that population. Thus, although statistically significant changes in lymphocyte population numbers may occur in response to an environmental situation, the numbers usually remain in the normal range of values (Fig. 2.41a–d).

Components of the flow cytometry procedure:
1. A single cell suspension of lymphocytes
2. An antibody to a CD marker on the lymphocytes
3. A dye coupled to the antibody that will absorb UV light and emit visible light. There are several dyes available that will emit different colors (usually green or red).
4. A flow cytometer that has the following capabilities:
   A) a laser that will emit the wave length of light that will excite the dye
   B) the mechanics to move the cells in a single line past the laser light
   C) a detection system that will characterize a cell passing the laser as to whether the cell is a lymphocyte or granulocyte and determine if the cell has been labeled with the dye bound to the antibody being used.

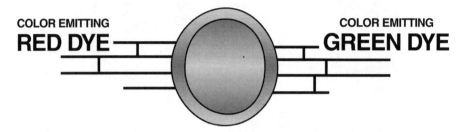

FIG. 2.41a   *Flow cytometry to quantitate different populations of lymphocytes. In this example, a lymphocyte has been incubated with two different antibodies. One antibody directed to the CD3 marker, which is present on all T lymphocytes, has been labeled with a red dye. The other antibody is directed to the CD4 marker, present on T-helper lymphocytes, has been labeled with a green dye.*

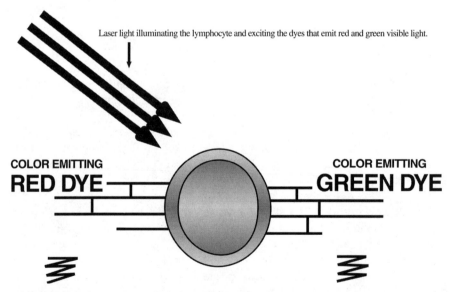

FIG. 2.41b   *Visible green and red light being emitted as the cell flows past photodetectors that characterize the cell as to its size and contents of granules. The information is received and analyzed by electronic means. The instrument can analyze 10,000 cells/second.*

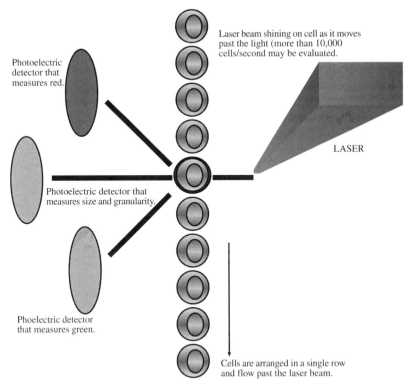

Laser beam shining on cell as it moves past the light (more than 10,000 cells/second may be evaluated.

Photoelectric detector that measures red.

LASER

Photoelectric detector that measures size and granularity.

Phoelectric detector that measures green.

Cells are arranged in a single row and flow past the laser beam.

FIG. 2.41c *As each cell is illuminated the laser beam is dispersed by the cell. The dispersion of the light relates to the size of the cell and its granularity. If the cell is labeled with a green dye (fluorescein isothiocyanate), a green color is generated which is detected by the appropriate photodetector. If the cell is labeled with a red dye (rhodamine), a red color is generated which is detected by the appropriate photodetector. All of these events are measured simultaneously.*

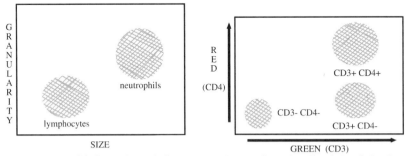

The electronics of the flow cyclometer look at each cell and characterize them according to their size and granularity. Each population of leukocytes has characteristics features. Neutrophils are larger than lymphocytes and have more granularity. Each of these cell populations are depicted on the graph above as they would appear in a flow cytometer.

The electronics are then able to look at the lymphocyte population and identify how many of the lymphocytes have the fluorescence label on them (either green or red). Some lymphocytes are CD3- and CD4-. These may be B lymphocytes or NK lymphocytes (there are specific antibodies that can identify these cell populations). Another ppopulation is CD3+ CD4-. This may be CD8 population of T cells. The final population is CD3+ and CD4+. This is the T helper population consisting of Th1 and Th2 cells. The number of cells in each population can also be determined.

FIG. 2.41d *Analysis of flow cytometry.*

IN VITRO FUNCTIONAL TESTS

Lymphocyte Response to Mitogens

Method. Lymphocytes are incubated with either nonspecific mitogens or specific mitogens and the amount of mitosis induced in the lymphocytes is measured. Non-specific mitogens are usually derived from plants and induce mitosis without the lymphocytes having to make an immune response to the plant substance. Specific mitogens are antigens that will only induce mitosis if the lymphocytes are derived from an individual who has previously made an immune response to the antigen (this may occur through immunization or natural infection). The method is described in Figure 2.42.

Interpretation. The ability of lymphocytes to respond to nonspecific mitogen is often difficult to relate to biological significance. Certainly, a child who is born with an immune deficiency disease and who has a response that is less than 10% of normal will be susceptible to the infectious disease against which the lymphocytes provide protection. However, environmental situations and acute laboratory stressors, although they may decrease lymphocyte mitogen responsiveness, do not alter the response to nonspecific mitogens out of the normal range. In addition, the normal range of values may not be the biological meaningful range.

Specific mitogenic stimulation is when lymphocytes are incubated with an antigen to which the subject has been immunized or to which there may have been a natural

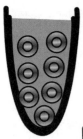

Blood is collected and total leukocytes (or) isolated lymphocytes are placed into tubes with tissue culture medium that supports growth of the cells. Normal human serum is often included as a source of nutrition. The mitogen is added to the growth medium. If the cells are responsive to the mitogen the cells will enlarge, and divide.

Non-specific mitogens are substances that induce lymphocytes to divide. Non-specific mitogens do not function as antigens as lymphocytes divide within hours of their first contact with the mitogen. Common non-specific mitogens are (1) Phytohemagglutinin (PHA), (2) Concanavalin-A (CON-A), and (3) Pokeweed mitogen (PWM).

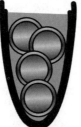

After approximately 48 hours of incubation the lymphocytes divide and assume the characteristics of a 'lymphoblast' which is a large cell with a large nucleus. Cell division is detected by adding radioactively labeled thymidine to the growth medium in the tube. Thymidine is incorporated into newly synthesized DNA. The more mitosis that is occurring, the more radioactive thymidine will be incorporated into the nuclei of the dividing cells.

Results of lymphocyte responsiveness to non-specific mitogens are usually reported as counts per minute (CPM) of radioactive thymidine in the cells incubated with the mitogen. As a control, the amount of radioactive thymidine uptake incorporated into cells incubated without mitogen are included for comparison.

FIG. 2.42   Determination of lymphocyte responsiveness to nonspecific mitogenic stimulation. Results of lymphocyte responsiveness to nonspecific mitogens are usually reported as counts per minute (CPM) of radioactive thymidine in the cells incubated with the mitogen. As a control, the amount of radioactive thymidine uptake incorporated into cells incubated without mitogen are included for comparison.

exposure. This assay can be used to determine whether an individuals lymphocytes have been sensitized to an antigen. A positive mitogenic response to an antigen in vitro, for example, *Candida* or tuberculin, would indicate that the individual has previously encountered the infectious agent.

Information Learned. Although the response to nonspecific mitogenic stimulation can be altered by stress, there is a lack of basic immunologic knowledge that allows the investigator to determine if the changes have meaning in regard to altering susceptibility to infection or on the course of an immune mediated disease. A positive response to a specific mitogen (eg, a fungal antigen) indicates that exposure has previously occurred to the agent.

Natural Killer Function

Method. NK cells are part of the innate host defense system. The method for determining their function is described in Figure 2.43.

Interpretation. The ability of NK cells to kill radioactively labeled target cells indicates that the cells are functional and that they should be able to contribute to resistance to viral infections and react against cells that become malignant. However, as with other immune functional assays, it is unclear as to how little or how much function is enough. Certainly, the lack of NK function is significant, but a reduction from normal is difficult to interpret in regard to biological meaning.

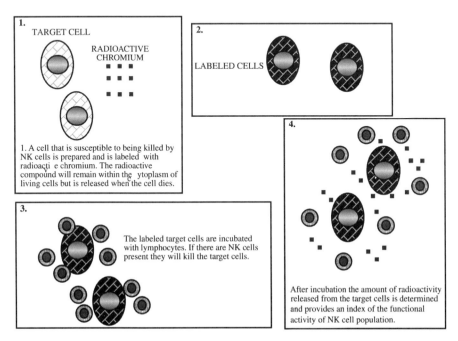

FIG. 2.43 *Determination of natural killer cell (NK) function.*

Information Learned. Alterations of NK function subsequent to a stressor are frequently reported and is a commonly used indicator of stressor effects on a component of the immune system.

Cytokine Production by Stimulated Lymphocytes

Method. The production of cytokines by lymphocytes is an important indication of their function. It currently is the method used to compare Th1 and Th2 cell function (eg, Th1 cells produce IFN-γ and Th2 cells produce IL-4). The procedure has two parts. The first is the generation of cytokines. The procedure is similar to lymphocyte response to mitogens with the culture medium being collected after stimulation of the lymphocytes. The second part of the procedure involves the quantitation of the cytokines in the supernatant. The procedure commonly used for this is ELISA using an antibody to a specific cytokine that is bound to the insoluble support. Different antibodies are used to quantitate different cytokines.

Interpretation. Cytokine production before and after exposure to an acute laboratory stressor has been shown to change. Again, as in other immune assays, there are limitations in regard to the biological interpretation of the data.

Information Learned. The effect of stress on altering cytokine production by a specific lymphocyte population can be determined.

IN VIVO TESTS

Antibody Response to a Specific Antigen

Method. The ability of an individual to produce antibody to a T-cell-dependent antigen provides a measure of the various components of the immune system and their functional interrelationship (antigen uptake, antigen processing, antigen presentation, T cell recognition of antigen, T-cell–B-cell interaction). Following immunization and after an appropriate time period serum is collected and assayed for antibody to the antigen. The ELISA procedure is frequently used for the antibody determination.

Interpretation and Information Learned. There is a wide range of responsiveness between individuals following immunization with a T-cell-dependent antigen. Comparison between groups of highly stressed in comparison to individuals experiencing low levels of stress have indicated that immunization of highly stressed individuals results in lower levels of antibody production.

Delayed Hypersensitivity Skin Test

Method. The method is described in Figure 2.38A–D.

Interpretation and Information Learned. A positive delayed hypersensitivity skin test indicates that the individual has T lymphocytes that have previously been sensitized to the antigen being studied. As the response depends on previous sensitization, there are two ways to use the test. If the question being asked is whether an individual has been sensitized to a specific antigen (eg, to determine whether an individual has been infected with *Mycobacterium tuberculosis*), testing with the particular antigen is done. A positive response indicates that the individual has T lymphocytes that have been sensitized to the antigen.

The second way to use the test is to determine whether the cell-mediated immune system of an individual is functional. This approach involves testing an individual for reactivity to at least five different antigens to which an individual is likely to have been exposed. The failure to respond to all the antigens is termed "anergy" and indicates a functional abnormality of the cellular immune system.

REFERENCES

Alm JS, Lilja G, Pershagen G, Scheynius A. Early BCG vaccination and development of atopy. Lancet. 350: 400–403, 1997.

Andervont HB. Influence of environment on mammary cancer in mice. Journal of the National Cancer Institute. 4: 579–581, 1944.

Ayensu WK, Pucilowski O, Mason GA, Overstreet DH, Rezvani AH, Janowsky DS. Effects of chronic mild stress on serum complement activity, saccharine preference, and corticosterone levels in Flinders lines of rats. Physiology and Behavior. 57: 165–169, 1995.

Benschop RJ, Rodriguezfeuerhahn M, Schedlowski M. Catecholamine-induced leukocytosis: Early observations, current research, and future directions. Brain, Behavior, and Immunity. 10: 77–91, 1996.

Carlson SL, Beiting DJ, Kiani CA, Abell KM, McGillis JP. Catecholamines decrease lymphocyte adhesion to cytokine-activated endothelial cells. Brain, Behavior, and Immunity. 10: 55–67, 1996.

Charlton B, Lafferty KJ. Th1/Th2 balance in autoimmunity. Current Opinion in Immunology. 7: 793–798, 1995.

Coe CL, Hall NR. Psychological disturbance alters thymic and adrenal hormone secretion in a parallel but independent manner. Psychoneuroendocrinology. 21: 237–247, 1996.

Cohen S, Tyrrell DA, Smith AP. Psychological stress and susceptibility to the common cold. New England Journal of Medicine. 325: 606–612, 1991.

Crucian B, Dunne P, Friedman H, Ragsdale R, Pross S, Widen R. Detection of altered T helper 1 and T helper 2 cytokine production by peripheral blood mononuclear cells in patients with multiple sclerosis utilizing intracellular cytokine detection by flow cytometry and surface marker analysis. Clinical and Diagnostic Laboratory Immunology. 3: 411–416, 1996.

Cunnick JE, Cohen S, Rabin BS, Carpenter AB, Manuck SB, Kaplan JR. Alterations in specific antibody production due to rank and social instability. Brain, Behavior, and Immunity. 5: 357–369, 1991.

Damjanov I, Linder, J (eds). Anderson's Pathology. 10th Ed. CV Mosby, St. Louis, 1990, p 1221.

Dardenne M, Boukaiba N, Gagnerault M, Homo-Delarche F, Chappuis P, Lemonnier D, Savino W. Restoration of the thymus in aging mice by in vivo zinc supplementation. Clinical Immunology and Immunopathology. 66: 127–135, 1993.

Daynes RA, Araneo BA. Contrasting effects of glucocorticoids on the capacity of T cells to produce the growth factors interleukin 2 and interleukin 4. European Journal of Immunology. 19: 2319–2325, 1989.

DeChambre RP, Gosse C. Individual versus group caging of mice with grafted tumors. Cancer Research. 33: 140–144, 1973.

Decker D, Schondorf M, Bidlingmaier F, Hirner A, Vonruecker AA. Surgical stress induces a shift in the type-1/type-2 T-helper cell balance, suggesting down regulation of cell-mediated and up-regulation of antibody-mediated immunity commensurate to the trauma. Surgery. 119: 316–325, 1996.

Dhabhar FS, Miller AH, McEwen BS, Spencer RL. Stress-induced changes in blood leukocyte distribution—Role of adrenal steroid hormones. Journal of Immunology. 157: 1638–1644, 1996.

Fricchione G, Bilfing r TV, Jandorf L, Smith EM, Stefano GB. Surgical anticipatory stress manifests itself in immunocyte desensitization: Evidence for autoimmunoregulatory involvement. International Journal of Cardiology. 53: S65–S73, 1996.

Goldberg ED, Dygai AM, Bogdashin IV, Sherstoboev EI, Shakov VP, Malaitsev VV. Role of humoral factors in the regulation of hemopoiesis is stress. Biulleten Eksperimentalnoi Biologii I Medisiny. 112: 15–18, 1991.

Grewal IS, Heilig M, Miller A, Sercarz EE. Environmental regulation of T-cell function in mice: Group housing of mice affects accessory cell function. Immunology. 90: 165–168, 1997.

Hadden J. Thymic endocrinology. International Journal of Immunopharmacology. 14:345–52, 1992.

Harmsen, AG, Turney TH. Inhibition of in vivo neutrophil accumulation by stress. Inflammation. 9: 9–20, 1985.

Herbert TB, Cohen S. Stress and immunity in humans: A meta-analytic review. Psychosomatic Medicine. 55: 364–379, 1993.

Herbert TB, Cohen S, Marsland AL, Bachen EA, Rabin BS, Muldoon MF, Manuck SB. Cardiovascular reactivity and the course of immune response to an acute psychological stressor. Psychosomatic Medicine. 56: 337–344, 1994.

Kallmann BA, Huther M, Tubes M, Feldkamp J, Bertrams J, Gries FA, Lampeter EF, Kolb H. Systemic bias of cytokine production toward cell-mediated immune regulation in IDDM and toward humoral immunity in Graves' disease. Diabetes. 46: 237–243, 1997.

Kiecolt-Glaser JK, Stephens RE, Lipetz PD, Speicher CE, Glaser R. Distress and DNA repair in human lymphocytes. Journal of Behavioral Medicine. 8: 311–320, 1985.

Kiecolt-Glaser JK, Glaser R, Strain EC, Stout JC, Tarr KL, Holliday JE, Speicher CE. Modulation of cellular immunity in medical students. Journal of Behavioral Medicine. 9: 5–21, 1986.

Kiecolt-Glaser JK, Fisher LD, Ogrocki P, Stout JC, Speicher CE, Glaser R. Marital quality, marital disruption, and immune function. Psychosomatic Medicine. 49: 13–34, 1987.

Kiecolt-Glaser JK, Dura JR, Speicher CE, Trask OJ, Glaser R. Spousal caregivers of dementia victims: Longitudinal changes in immunity and health. Psychosomatic Medicine. 53: 345–362, 1991.

Kiecolt-Glaser JK, Marucha PT, Malarkey WB, Mercado AM, Glaser R. Slowing of wound healing by psychological stress. Lancet. 346: 1194–1196, 1995.

Kita M, Iwaki H, Kitoh I, Imanishi J. The effect of stress on interferon production in mice. Comptes Rendus des Seances de la Societé de Biologie et de Ses Filiales. 183: 282–286, 1989.

Kobrynski LJ, Tanimune L, Kilpartick L, Campbell DE, Douglas SD. Production of T helper cell subsets and cytokines by lymphocytes from patients with chronic mucocutaneous candidiasis. Clinical and Diagnostic Laboratory Immunology. 3: 740–745, 1996.

Kroemer G, Hirsch F, Gonzalez-Garcia A, Martinez C. Differential involvement of Th1 and Th2 cytokines in autoimmune diseases. Autoimmunity. 24: 25–33, 1996.

Kruszewska B, Felten SY, Moynihan JA. Alterations in cytokine and antibody production following chemical sympathectomy in two strains of mice. Journal of Immunology. 155: 4613–4620, 1995.

Long CS, Hartogensis WE, Simpson PC. Beta-adrenergic stimulation of cardiac non-myocytes augments the growth-promoting activity of non-myocyte conditioned medium. Journal of Cellular and Molecular Cardiology. 25: 915–925, 1993.

McKinnon W, Weisse CS, Reynolds CP, Bowles CA, Baum A. Chronic stress, leukocyte subpopulations, and humoral response to latent viruses. Health Psychology. 8: 389–402, 1989.

Manuck SB, Cohen S, Rabin BS, Muldoon MF, Bachen EA. Individual differences in cellular immune response to stress. Psychological Science. 2: 1–5, 1991.

Maestroni GJ. The immunoneuroendocrine role of melatonin. Journal of Pineal Research. 14: 1–10, 1993.

Maisel AS, Knowlton KU, Fowler P, Rearden A, Ziegler MG, Motulsky HJ. Adrenergic control of circulating lymphocyte subpopulations. Journal of Clinical Investigation. 85: 462–467, 1990.

Meyer RJ, Haggerty RJ. Streptococcal infections in families: Factors altering individual susceptibility. Pediatrics. 29: 539–549, 1962.

Michalopoulos GK, DeFrances MC. Liver regeneration. Science. 276: 60–66, 1997.

Mocchegiani E, Bulian D, Santarelli L, Tibaldi A, Muzzioli M, Pierpaoli W, Fabris N. The immuno-reconstituting effect of melatonin or pineal grafting and its relation to zinc pool in aging mice. Journal of Neuroimmunology. 53: 189–201, 1994a.

Mocchegiani E, Bulian D, Santarelli L, Tibaldi A, Pierpaoli W, Fabris N. The zinc–melatonin interrelationship. A working hypothesis. Annals of the New York Academy of Sciences. 719: 298–307, 1994b.

Mocchegiani E, Fabris N, Age-related thymus involution: Zinc reverses in vitro the thymulin secretion defect. International Journal of Immunopharmacology. 17: 745–749, 1995a.

Mocchegiani E, Santarelli L, Muzzioli M, Fabris N. Reversibility of the thymic involution and of age-related peripheral immune dysfunctions by zinc supplementation in old mice. International Journal of Immunopharmacology. 17: 703–718, 1995b.

Moyna. NM, Acker GR, Fulton JR, Weber K, Goss FL, Robertson RJ, Tollerud DJ, Rabin BS. Lymphocyte function and cytokine production during incremental exercise in active and sedentary males and females. International Journal of Sports Medicine. 17: 585–591, 1996.

Naliboff BD, Benton D, Solomon GF, Morley J, Fahey JL, Bloom E, Makinodan T, Gilmore S. Immunological changes in young and old adults during brief laboratory stress. Psychosomatic Medicine. 53: 121–132, 1991.

Nicholson LB, Kuchroo VK. Manipulation of the Th1/Th2 balance in autoimmune disease. Current Opinion in Immunology. 8: 837–842, 1996.

Nystrom L, Dahlquist G, Ostman J, Wall S, Arnqvist H, Blohme G, Lithner F, Littorin B, Schersten B, Wibell L. Risk of developing insulin-dependent diabetes mellitus (IDDM) before 35 years of age: Indications of climatological determinants for age at onset. International Journal of Epidemiology. 21: 352–358, 1992.

Olsson T. Cytokine-producing cells in experimental autoimmune encephalomyelitis and multiple sclerosis. Neurology. 45(suppl 6): S11–S15, 1995.

Palmblad J, Cantell K, Strander H, Froberg J, Karlsson C, Levi L, Granstrom M, Unger P. Stressor exposure and immunological response in man: Interferon producing capacity and phagocytosdis. Journal of Psychosomatic Research. 20: 193–199, 1976.

Persengiev S, Patchev V, Velev B. Melatonin effects on thymus steroid receptors in the course of primary antibody responses: Significance of circulating glucocorticoid levels. International Journal of Biochemistry. 23: 1487–1489, 1991.

Peterson PK, Chao CC, Molitor T, Murtaugh M, Strgar F, Sharp BM. Stress and pathpgenesis of infectious disease. Reviews of Infectious Diseases. 13: 710–720, 1991.

Pierpaoli W. Pineal grafting and melatonin induce immunocompetence in nude (athymic) mice. International Journal of Neuroscience. 68: 123–131, 1993.

Pierpaoli W, Regelson W. Pineal control of aging: Effect of melatonin and pineal grafting on aging mice. Proceedings of the National Academy of Sciences USA. 91: 787–791, 1994.

Plaut SM, Ader R, Friedman SB, Ritterson AI. Social factors and resistance to malaria in the mouse: Effects of groups versus individual housing on resistance to plasmodium berghei infection. Psychosomatic Medicine. 31: 536–552,1969.

Poon AM, Liu ZM, Pang CS, Brown GM, Pang SF. Evidence for a direct action of melatonin on the immune system. Biological Signals. 3: 107–117, 1994.

Provinciali M, Di Stefano G, Bulian D, Tibaldi A, Fabris N. Effect of melatonin and pineal grafting on thymocyte apoptosis in aging mice. Mechanisms of Aging Development. 90: 1–19, 1996.

Rabin BS, Lyte M, Epstein LH, Caggiula AR. Alteration of immune competency by number of mice housed per cage. Annals of the New York Academy of Science. 496: 492–500, 1987.

Rodriguez AB, Barriga C, De la Fuents M. Phagocytic function of blood neutrophils in sedentary young people after physical exercise. International Journal of Sports Medicine. 12: 276–280, 1991.

Saha AR, Hadden EM, Hadden JW. Zinc induces thymulin secretion from human thymic epithelial cells in vitro and augments splenocyte and thymocyte responses in vivo. International Journal of Immunopharmacology. 17: 729–733, 1995.

Salvin SB, Rabin BS, Neta R. Evaluation of immunologic assays to determine the effects of differential housing on immune reactivity. Brain, Behavior, and Immunity. 4: 180–188, 1990.

Sanders VM, Street NE, Fuchs BA. Differential expression of the beta-adrenoreceptor by subsets of T helper lymphocytes. FASEB Journal. 8: A114, 1994.

Schedlowski M, Falk A, Rohne A, Wagner TO, Jacobs R, Tewew U, Schmidt RE. Catecholamines induce alterations of distribution and activity of natural killer (NK) cells. Journal of Clinical Immunology. 13: 344–351, 1993.

Shirakawa T, Enomoto T, Shimazu S, Hopkin JM. The inverse association between tuberculin responses and atopic disorder. Science 275: 77–79, 1997.

Shurin MR, Kusnecov AW, Hamill E, Kaplan S, Rabin BS. Stress-induced alteration of polymorphonuclear leukocyte function in rats. Brain, Behavior, and Immunity. 8: 163–169, 1994.

Soave OA. Reactivation of rabies virus in a guinea pig due to the stress of crowding. American Journal of Veterinary Research. 25: 268–269, 1964.

Sonnenfeld G, Gould CL, Williams J, Mandel AD. Inhibited interferon production after space flight. Acta Microbiologica Hungarica. 35: 411–416, 1988.

Sonnenfeld G, Cunnick JE, Armfield AV, Wood PG, Rabin BS. Stress-induced alterations in interferon production and class II histocompatibility antigen expression. Brain, Behavior, and Immunity. 6: 170–178, 1992.

Spratt ML, Denney DR. Immune variables, depression, and plasma cortisol over time in suddenly bereaved parents. Journal of Neuropsychiatry and Clinical Neurosciences. 3: 299–306, 1991.

Tonnesen E, Brinklov MM, Christensen NJ Olesen AS, Madsen T. Natural killer cell activity and lymphocyte function during and after coronary bypass grafting in relation to the endocrine stress response. Anesthesiology. 68: 526–533, 1987.

Vandenbark AA, Chou YK, Whitham R, Mass M, Buenafe A, Liefeld D, Kavanagh D, Cooper S, Hashim GA, Offner H, Bourdette DN. Treatment of multiple sclerosis with T-cell receptor peptides: Results of a double-blind pilot trial. Nature Medicine. 2: 1109–1115, 1996.

Yokota K, Shineha R, Nisihira T, Mori S. Perioperative alterations in polymorphonuclear function of gastrointestinal surgery. Tohoku Journal of Experimental Medicine. 169: 103–112, 1993.

Zwilling BS, Dinkins M, Christner R, Faris M, Griffin A, Hilburger M, McPeek M, Pearl D. Restraint stress induced suppression of major histocompatibility class II expression by murine peritoneal macrophages. Journal of Neuroimmunology. 29: 125–130, 1990.

Zwilling BS, Brown D, Pearl D. Induction of major histocompatibility complex class II glycoproteins by interferon-gamma: Attenuation of the effects of restraint stress. Journal of Neuroimmunology. 37: 115–122, 1992.

3

The Nervous System—
Immune System Connection

Responses to situations presented by an individual's environment that are perceived as stress are associated with activation of neurons in the brain. Through neuronal and chemical pathways, subsequent modification of the function of the immune system may occur. This chapter presents evidence that establishes the presence of a nervous system–immune system connection and discusses events that occur within the brain that are linked to this connection. In addition, the mechanism of communication from the immune system to the brain is presented. Part of homeostasis involves the immune system using cytokine messengers to inform the brain that the immune system is active. The brain may respond by releasing hormones that prevent excessive activation of the immune system.

THE AUTONOMIC NERVOUS SYSTEM

This section presents a brief review of the autonomic nervous system. The autonomic nervous system regulates many of the functions of the body. The reactions of the autonomic nervous system occur without conscious decisions or awareness.

The autonomic nervous system may be considered to have its origin in peripheral tissues that signal the brain, by afferent (going from the periphery of the body to the brain) pathways. The brain responds by sending regulatory signals that modulate tissue function. There are two components to the autonomic nervous system: the sympathetic and the parasympathetic nervous system. In broad terms, the sympathetic nervous system prepares the body to cope with emergencies, while the parasympathetic nervous system helps the body conserve energy.

Axons (fibers carrying impulses away from the neuronal cell body) from autonomic system neurons in the brain terminate on neurons in the lateral gray portion of the spinal cord and on motor nuclei of cranial nerves. The neurons receiving the input from the autonomic neurons in the brain are termed *preganglionic* neurons. Axons from the preganglionic neurons leave the spinal cord and synapse (the site at the termination of an axon where a chemical is released that modulates the function of the cell where the axon terminates) on another neuron, which is termed the *postganglionic* neuron. Postganglionic neurons cluster together in accumulations called *ganglia* (these are masses of nerve cells that form clump-like structures outside the central nervous system [CNS]). The autonomic nervous system ganglia are located adjacent to the spinal cord (paravertebral), adjacent to the origin of large blood vessels in the abdomen, and within the walls of tissues and organs. Both afferent (from tissue to brain) and efferent (from brain to tissue) pathways comprise the autonomic nervous system.

The sympathetic and parasympathetic autonomic nervous systems have different anatomical characteristics, use different chemical transmitters, and have different physiological effects. Efferent preganglionic sympathetic nerve fibers originate in the lateral gray portion of the spinal cord between the first thoracic to the second lumbar segment. The parasympathetic preganglionic neurons are found in the third, seventh, ninth, and tenth cranial nerves and in the gray matter of the second through fourth sacral segments of the spinal cord.

The postganglionic fibers of the parasympathetic system are short, while those of the sympathetic system are long. Therefore, the parasympathetic ganglia (where the preganglionic axon terminate on the postganglionic neuron) are located within the tissue that they innervate, or close to the tissue. The sympathetic ganglia are located close to the spinal cord or near the branching of large blood vessels from the aorta in the peritoneal (abdominal) cavity. All preganglionic neurons release acetylcholine, which activates the postganglionic neurons. The postganglionic neurons of the parasympathetic system release acetylcholine, while most sympathetic postganglionic neurons release norepinephrine (acetylcholine is released by the sympathetic nervous system at sweat glands) (Figs. 3.1 and 3.2).

Examples of differences between the effect of the sympathetic and parasympathetic systems are presented in Table 3.1.

The sympathetic nervous system and the emotions are interrelated. When emotions indicate that the body needs to be prepared for a *fight-or-flight* response, the sympathetic nervous system increases the heart rate, dilates the pupils of the eyes, directs an increased flow of blood to the skeletal muscles, brain, and heart, by constricting blood vessels in the skin and intestines, causes hair to stand on end, constricts sphincters, and induces sweating. In addition, the activity of the immune system decreases with a resultant increased susceptibility to infection.

Why does the sympathetic nervous system decrease immune function at the same time it is preparing for a *fight-or-flight* response? Logically, you would ex-

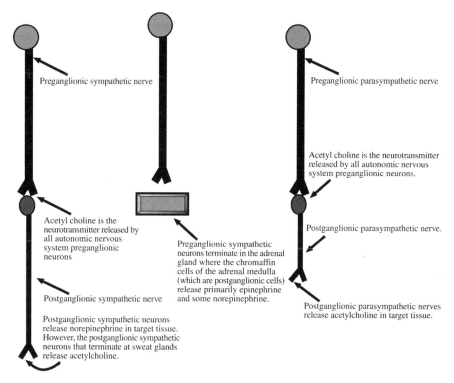

FIG. 3.1 *Diagram of the cell structure and the hormones released by the sympathetic and parasympathetic nervous systems.*

pect more resistance to infectious diseases, to promote a better state of health. Keeping the immune system working well would contribute to better health. It could be argued that *flight* requires energy, and activation of the immune system drains metabolic energy from the body. Minimizing the function of the immune system could provide more energy to flee. Some of the behavioral changes that occur during an immune response to an infectious agent are tiredness, loss of appetite, and fever—all undesirable if *flight* is needed. Possibly, a diminished immune response would avoid these effects allowing the person to feel better as they

TABLE 3.1   Sympathetic and Parasympathetic Effects

Tissue	Sympathetic Effect	Parasympathetic Effect
Pupil of eye	Dilates	Constricts
Heart rate	Increases	Decreases
GastroIntestinal peristalsis	Decreases	Increases

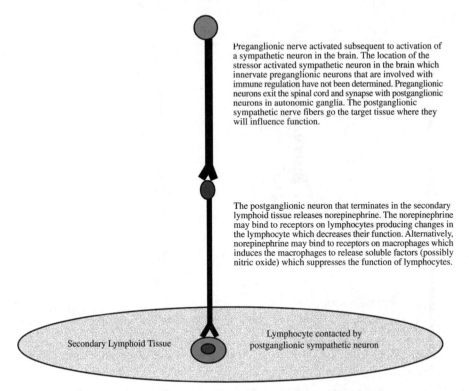

Preganglionic nerve activated subsequent to activation of a sympathetic neuron in the brain. The location of the stressor activated sympathetic neuron in the brain which innervate preganglionic neurons that are involved with immune regulation have not been determined. Preganglionic neurons exit the spinal cord and synapse with postganglionic neurons in autonomic ganglia. The postganglionic sympathetic nerve fibers go the target tissue where they will influence function.

The postganglionic neuron that terminates in the secondary lymphoid tissue releases norepinephrine. The norepinephrine may bind to receptors on lymphocytes producing changes in the lymphocyte which decreases their function. Alternatively, norepinephrine may bind to receptors on macrophages which induces the macrophages to release soluble factors (possibly nitric oxide) which suppresses the function of lymphocytes.

Secondary Lymphoid Tissue

Lymphocyte contacted by postganglionic sympathetic neuron

FIG. 3.2   *Sympathetic neurons terminate in secondary lymphoid tissues adjacent to lymphocytes and macrophages. When the neurons are activated there is modulation of function of the immune cells.*

flee. However, an increased risk of infection would not be advantageous. Thus, there is no definitive explanation regarding the biological advantage provided by stressor-induced immune alteration.

STRESS AND THE IMMUNE SYSTEM

Stress-induced alteration of the immune system occurs in the secondary lymphoid tissues (spleen, lymph nodes, and mucosal-associated lymphoid tissues), where effector T cells are produced from naive T cells, and T-cell help is provided to B lymphocytes. A stress-related influence on the activation and function of effector lymphocytes in parenchymal tissues is likely due to stress-induced changes in the hormonal milieu in which the immune system resides. Glucocorticoids and catecholamines are among the principal hormones that contribute to these functional alterations.

There are different processes involved in activation of naive lymphocytes within secondary lymphoid tissue in comparison to activation of effector lymphocytes in parenchymal tissues (see Chapter 2). Whether there are different hormones or different concentrations of hormones that alter the initial activation of the immune response has not been determined. For example, if a neuropeptide decreased the concentration of costimulatory molecules on antigen-presenting cells (APC), there would not be an effect on the CD4 T-cell-mediated delayed hypersensitivity response, where costimulation is not required. However, there would be an effect upon the primary activation of CD4 T cells in secondary lymphoid tissues. Therefore, generalizations regarding the effect on immune function of a stress-related hormone on a cell surface molecule or a biochemical pathway must be avoided. The specific immune reactions in different lymphoid compartments or in parenchymal tissues need to be individually evaluated.

The anatomical structure of secondary lymphoid tissues may also influence stress hormone effects on lymphoid cells. The spleen is a filter through which the blood passes. The red pulp and marginal zones and sinuses may be bathed in higher concentrations of plasma hormones than are the cells of the white pulp, which is a dense accumulation of lymphocytes. The lymph node has a blood supply, but it must diffuse through the endothelial cells. Whether concentrations of hormones derived from plasma are similar in the spleen and lymph nodes, and whether different anatomical parts of the spleen and lymph nodes receive the same concentrations of plasma hormones, is unknown.

There are numerous components of the immune system that may be modified by stress hormones. Often, primary and secondary immune responses, as well as effector immune responses, are occurring simultaneously, but to different antigens. Research that studies the effect of stress on immune system modification is usually limited by having to select a single immune compartment (spleen, lymph node, or blood in experimental animals, but confined to blood in humans) and a limited number of responses (primary or secondary, T cell, B cell, natural killer [NK] cell, APCs) for study. Finding changes of immune function in the spleen during a primary immune response, or of a component of the innate defense system, must be interpreted with caution, as lymphocytes in the lymph nodes or blood may or may not be undergoing the same changes.

Another concern relates to how baseline immune function is established. Is it in a dark room with the subject resting and listening to pleasant music? Or is baseline immune function the function that is measured when a subject is going about their daily activities and is experiencing the stress that they normally encounter? If an experimental stress is imposed on a subject, is more information learned by imposing it on a resting subject or a subject engaged in their daily activities? Possibly each approach is correct, depending on the question being asked.

How is baseline hypothalamic–pituitary–adrenal (HPA) and sympathetic nervous system (SNS) activity defined? As will be described, both HPA-derived and SNS-derived hormones influence immune system function. As baseline function of the HPA axis and SNS cannot be easily defined or established in experimental studies of stress and the immune system, baseline immune function becomes a semantic situation, possibly relating to whatever HPA and SNS conditions exist at the time of baseline measurements.

Different immune compartments, different characteristics of the immune response, and the imposition of a stressor on immune systems that may already be influenced by stress, all contribute to the complexities of the brain–immune system interaction. For example, an acute stressor-induced change in NK cell numbers and function differs when comparing male subjects who have or do not have high levels of stress in their daily lives, although NK levels are the same in both groups before exposure to the acute stressor (Pike et al, 1997). Individuals experiencing chronic stress in their lives have less of an acute stressor elevation of NK function than occurs in those with low levels of daily stress

It has been shown that subjects who are under stress are more susceptible to upper respiratory viral infection (Cohen et al, 1991) and have a decreased ability to produce antibody to an antigen that they are immunized with (Glaser et al, 1992). There are also suggestions from epidemiological studies that individuals who are under stress are at an increased risk of the development of an autoimmune disease or the exacerbation of an autoimmune disease (see Chapter 6). Thus, it is both logical and important to define the areas of the brain that are associated with regulation of immune function in order to develop hypotheses related to a means of modulating CNS function to prevent stress from producing alterations of immune function that will predispose to an increased susceptibility to disease. Understanding the interactions within the brain and how the brain facilitates or inhibits stressor-induced suppression of immune function will help in understanding the mechanisms of stressor-induced immune alteration and suggest ways in which stressor-induced immune alteration can be prevented.

WHAT AREAS OF THE BRAIN ARE ACTIVATED BY STRESS?

Experimental procedures may be used to alter the functional activity of selected brain areas. Some brain areas that are activated during stress induce a change in the hormonal or sympathetic nervous system, or both, that influence the function of the immune system. Other areas that may be activated by stress do not alter immune system function.

The c-Fos proto-oncogene produces a protein that appears in the nucleus of activated cells. Synthesis of this protein can be used as a marker of activation of neurons that are responsive to an environmental stimulus, such as stress. Antibody to the c-Fos protein has been used in immunohistochemical assays to identify stress-activated neurons in the brain (Fig 3.3).

Interpretation of the biological significance, with regard to immune function, of an area of the brain that is found to be c-Fos positive subsequent to stress must be done with caution:

C-fos positive neurons may have no involvement in immune function regulation.

A neuron that is activated by stress and that becomes c-Fos positive may be transmitting signals to preganglionic neurons and through postganglionic neurons to the lymphoid tissues, where catecholamine is released.

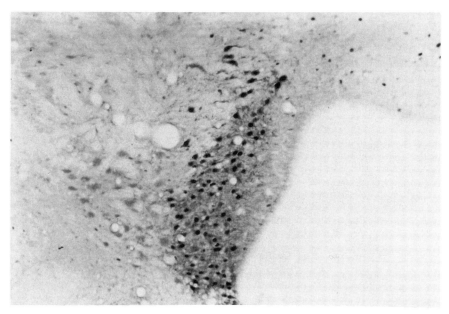

FIG. 3.3   *Example of c-fos-positive brain cells induced by stress in a rat, showing the area of the locus coeruleus. The dark-staining area in the cell nucleus is a positive reaction.*

The c-Fos-positive neuron may transmit signals to another area of the brain that will activate postganglionic neurons that release catecholamines in lymphoid tissue. Or, a c-Fos-positive area of the brain may inhibit the activity of another area of an area of the brain, which, in turn, may regulate catecholamine release in secondary lymphoid tissue.

It is also possible that areas of the brain that are activated by stress do not synthesize c-Fos, even though they are functionally activated as determined by measurements of their electrical activity. Thus, finding c-Fos in various areas of the brain will only indicate the minimum number of brain areas that are activated and has limitations with regard to defining the function of the brain area in regard to its influence on altering the immune system.

The presence of c-Fos in the neurons of the rat brain has been used to identify activated neurons after foot-shock stress, or re-exposure to a conditioned aversive stimulus (Pezzone et al, 1992, 1993). Study of a conditioned response provides a means of determining whether c-Fos activation occurs in animals that experience fear but are not exposed to a stimulus that causes physical discomfort. Conditioned fear can be created by placing a rat in a shock box, sounding a tone, and delivering a brief electric foot-shock of 1.6 mA for 5 seconds. Approximately 10–16 shocks are delivered over a 1-hour period. Several weeks later, returning the rat to the box and sounding the tone but not delivering foot-shock, results in stressor-induced immune alteration of the same magnitude as does foot-shock.

Neurons in areas of the forebrain that are activated in the rat brain after footshock or exposure to a conditioned stimulus include the following:

Medial parvocellular division of the hypothalamus (in neurons containing corticotropin, releasing hormone [CRH])

Periphery of the posterior magnocellular division of the hypothalamus (these neurons likely contain oxytocin)

Dorsomedial nucleus of the hypothalamus

Lateral hypothalamus

Dorsal border of the supraoptic nucleus (these neurons likely contain oxytocin)

Medial nucleus of the amygdala

Lateral edges of the central nucleus of the amygdala

Ventral subdivision of the lateral septal area

Dorsomedial nucleus and basal ganglia of the thalamus

Neurons in areas of the brain stem (portion of the brain connecting to the spinal cord) that are activated in the rat brain following footshock or exposure to a conditioned stimulus include the following:

Catecholamine-containing neurons of the ventral lateral medulla

Nucleus of the solitary tract

Noradrenergic neurons of the A5 area

Noradrenergic neurons of the A7 area

Locus coeruleus

Periaqueductal gray

Raphe nuclei

Many of the areas of the brain stem that become c-Fos-positive are involved with activation and regulation of the autonomic nervous system (the ventral lateral medulla, nucleus of the solitary tract, A5, A7, and the locus coeruleus).

Although the precise function of each of the c-Fos-positive neurons cannot be determined from a immunohistological approach, some information regarding the function of the various areas is known. Whether the known functions are related to stressor-induced immune alteration is unknown. Regardless, the following information is provided to give a functional orientation to the c-Fos-positive areas.

CRH-containing neurons in the medial parvocellular division of the hypothalamus—this area of the hypothalamus contains small neurons (parvocellular neurons). Parvocellular neurons contain several hormones that increase or decrease the release of other hormones from the anterior lobe of the pituitary gland. The c-Fos-activated CRH-containing neurons are likely to be associated with stress inducing an increase in the plasma concentration of cortico-sterone.

Periphery of the posterior magnocellular division of the hypothalamus (these neurons likely contain oxytocin)—these magnocellular neurons project to the posterior lobe of the pituitary. Oxytocin is important in lactation and uterine contraction during labor. Stressor-induced activation of oxytocin-containing neurons during stress may be involved in stimulation of autonomic brain nuclei in the brain stem or may participate in behavioral modifications during stress. There is no evidence for a direct effect of oxytocin on lymphocyte function, although oxytocin may contribute to interleukin-1 (IL-1)-induced adrenocorticotropic hormone (ACTH) release from the pituitary (Watanobe et al, 1995).

Dorsomedial nucleus of the hypothalamus—axons from these neurons of the hypothalamus mainly terminate within the various nuclei of the hypothalamus. Activation of this area stimulates motility in the intestine and may regulate emotional fear responses to stressors and cardiovascular responses to emotional stimuli.

Lateral hypothalamus—interaction between the neurons of the lateral hypothalamus and immune function has been indicated. The lateral hypothalamus may participate in the regulation of delayed hypersensitivity skin test reactivity, NK cell numbers in the blood, and NK cell function (Wrona et al,1994; Juzwa et al, 1995; Wenner et al, 1996). Both hunger and thirst are regulated by neurons of the lateral hypothalamus. How the hormones responsible for hunger and thirst interact with the function of the immune system remains to be evaluated.

Dorsal border of the supraoptic nucleus (these neurons likely contain oxytocin)—there is no evidence that this area is involved in immune regulation.

Medial nucleus of the amygdala—activation of this brain area may be induced by pain and may contribute to activation of ACTH release. It may therefore participate in stressor-induced increases of glucocorticoids.

Lateral edges of the central nucleus of the amygdala—the function of this area is unclear, but it may be related to the experience of fear. Whether there are nerve pathways from this area that participate in inducing the release of glucocorticoids or neuropeptides has not been established.

Ventral subdivision of the lateral septal area—activation is associated with the development of anxiety.

Dorsomedial nucleus and basal ganglia of the thalamus—the thalamus consists of several groups of cells that connect to areas of the cortex involved with muscle movement (motor areas), the perception of sensations, and cognition (perceiving, thinking, and memory). The dorsomedial nucleus connects to the frontal lobe of the brain, the hypothalamus, and other areas of the thalamus. It is involved in relating emotional feelings to sensory information. The basal ganglia of the thalamus are involved in the control of movement.

Catecholamine-containing neurons of the ventral lateral medulla—their function has not been defined.

Nucleus of the solitary tract—this brain area is associated with regulation of heart rate.

Noradrenergic neurons of the A5 and A7 areas—projections from these areas to the spinal cord may contribute to the activation of preganglionic neurons which innervate secondary lymphoid tissues.

Locus coeruleus (LC)—an accumulation of norepinephrine-containing neurons that sends projections to many areas of the brain including the amygdala, thalamus, and hypothalamus. The LC is involved in producing a decreased sensation of pain. Its activation has been shown to suppress lymphocyte function in the spleen and peripheral blood of rats.

Periagueductal gray (PAG)—part of the brain surrounding the cerebral aqueduct in the midbrain. Injection of morphine into discrete parts of the PAG will alter the function of lymphocytes and NK cells. The pathways that induce these changes are not defined.

Raphe nuclei—neurons are involved in producing analgesia.

ALTERATION OF DIFFERENT AREAS OF THE BRAIN CAN ALTER THE IMMUNE SYSTEM

An important question regarding the areas of the brain that are activated by stress, as well as the effect of this activation on the immune system, is whether a stress-activated area of the brain can modify immune function. The CNS regulation of immune function can be considered under two conditions: (1) immune function when a stress is not encountered, and (2) immune function when a stress is encountered. The following discussion reviews studies that have provided insight into some brain areas that influence the immune system. The studies inhibited or activated selected areas of the brain and determined how components of the immune system were affected.

However, before presenting the data, it should be noted that there are several reasons why the data obtained from the studies may be difficult to interpret. For example, when a surgical lesion of the CNS is created (damage produced by electrical current, cutting with a knife, or damage by trauma such as the twirling of a small probe), the specific cells or neuronal pathways that are disrupted are difficult to identify. A knife lesion will cut nerve fibers from all areas that are passing through the lesioned area, and the precise pathways disrupted may not be apparent. Thus, although the result of a lesion may result in a functional alteration of the immune response, the specific CNS pathways that result in the immune change may not be easy to identify, especially if several pathways are cut.

Another way to study CNS regulation is to use chemicals to suppress the activity of selected areas of the brain. However, this approach is not without problems. Some chemicals, such as lidocaine, will suppress neuronal activity but will also suppress the ability of axons that are passing through the area of lidocaine infusion to transmit impulses. This makes interpretation of the effects of injection of lidocaine into an area of the brain difficult.

Chemicals such as ibotenic acid and kainic acid are analogs of glutamic acid, the precursor of γ-aminobutyric acid (GABA). When bound by receptors on neurons, they cause destruction of the neuron. Muscimol, a GABA agonist, binds directly to GABA receptors and will suppress neuronal activity without killing neurons or altering the activity of axons passing through the injected area. However, precise placement of the chemical and injection of amounts that do not diffuse into areas other than those that are being studied present technical difficulties requiring carefully conducted procedures.

A final way to study the influence of the CNS on immune function is to activate areas of the brain selectively by injection of chemical activators. These studies require careful placement of the chemicals and must control for diffusion beyond the area being evaluated.

Given the concerns that make interpretation of the data far from precise, data from some published studies follow. The studies provide support for different areas of the CNS able to alter immune function. However, it is important to remember that the only immune parameters shown to be altered were those that were measured in each study. Comprehensive evaluations of the immune system were not made in any of the reported studies.

FACTOID

Study of innate, primary, secondary, or effector immune response: Innate (does not have to be activated; is always present from birth).

Species (and strain) studied: Male Fischer 344 rats.

Brain region modified: Periaqueductal gray matter. (The periaqueductal gray matter consists of neurons and the proximal process of the neurons as well as glial cells which surround the aqueduct in the midbrain. Activation of this area of the brain is associated with pain relief (analgesia).

How modified: Injection of morphine. Morphine will produce analgesia. It binds to opioid receptors in the brain. Its effect on neuropeptide production that could influence immune function have not been defined.

Tissue studied: Spleen.

Immune parameters changed: Baseline NK cell function decreased.

Comments: It was not determined whether morphine injection increased or decreased the concentration of stress responsive hormones in the blood or altered the release of neuropeptides from the sympathetic nerves of the spleen. Injection of morphine into the hypothalamus, arcuate nucleus, medial amygdala, medial thalamus, or dorsal hippocampus had no effect on the function of NK cells. Thus, an area of the brain was identified that, when injected with morphine, caused a decrease of the baseline activity of NK cells. However, the hormonal mechanism responsible for the altered function was not identified.

Source: Weber and Pert (1989).

FACTOID

Study of innate, primary, secondary, or effector immune response: Non-specific lymphocyte mitogenic stimulation was measured after activation of the locus coeruleus. This will be classified as intrinsic function of lymphocytes that cannot be further classified as being part of the primary, secondary, or effector immune response.

Species (and strain) studied: Male Wistar rats.

Brain region modified: Locus coeruleus (the locus coeruleus contains a large number of neurons that synthesize norepinephrine. Projections from these neurons go throughout the brain. LC neurons are active during awake time and decrease their activity during slow-wave sleep. LC neurons are involved in the control of vigilance and attention).

How modified: Injection of CRH into the LC, which produces activation of the LC.

Tissue studied: Spleen and blood.

Immune parameters changed and comments: Lymphocyte responsiveness to stimulation with nonspecific mitogens was decreased in the spleen and blood. Plasma concentration of ACTH, corticosterone, and IL-6 increased. The hormonal and immune changes are the same as those that result from electric foot-shock stressor or conditioned stress.

CRH activation of the LC probably activates the HPA axis and sympathetic nervous system. However, connections from LC to preganglionic neurons that innervate lymphoid tissues have not been identified.

Source: Rassnick et al (1994).

FACTOID

Study of innate, primary, secondary, or effector immune response: Primary antibody response.

Species (and strain) studied: Male and female Sprague-Dawley rats.

Brain region modified: Lateral septal area or hippocampus (The septal area is a pleasure-generating area and stimulation of it produces a sense of well-being and destruction of it produces a sense of displeasure. Projections go from the septum to the brain stem, hippocampus and hypothalamus).

How modified: Kainic acid, domoic acid, or electrolytic ablation to remove functional activity.

Tissue studied: Antibody response to immunization with albumin.

Immune parameters changed and comments: In a 1987 study, which included only female rats, the IgG, IgA, and IgM antibody response was lower in the lateral septal kainic acid lesioned animals in comparison to the electrolytic lesioned and control animals. The electrolytic lesioned and control animals had comparable antibody responses. This finding suggests that the neurons whose activity was eliminated by kainic acid resulted in an increase of hormones or neuropeptides that inhibited activation of the immune system. Possibly, the function of these neurons is to inhibit release of immune-suppressing hormones.

A kainic acid lesion in the hippocampus resulted in a significant increase of IgG and IgM, but not IgA, antibody responses to ovalbumin. This would suggest that the lesion prevented Th2 lymphocytes from releasing cytokines, which produced class switching of immunoglobulin from IgM and IgG, to IgA. The increased amount of IgG and IgM antibodies may indicate more antigen uptake and processing, more T:B lymphocyte interaction, or more proliferation of antibody-producing B lymphocytes.

The failure to reduce antibody responses in the electrolytic-lesioned animals, which would destroy neurons and axons passing through the area, suggests the possibility that the alterations produced by destruction of neurons and axons may have canceled each other out with a resultant normal antibody response.

A 1991 study used both male and female rats. The prior data of a reduced antibody response in kaininc acid lesioned females was reproduced. However, the lesion failed to alter the immune response in male rats. Thus, an influence of sex hormones interacting with the hormonal response to stress is suggested. Lesions produced by the neurotoxin domoic acid failed to alter the immune response in either male or female rats.

Kainic acid and domoic acid bind to different receptors and therefore, are likely to produce lesions of different types of neurons (Keinanen et al, 1990). The data from this study suggest that the neurons within those areas of the brain that are involved with the regulation of immune function are going to be difficult to identify due to admixture with neurons that may not influence immune function.

The failure of kainic acid lesions to alter antibody responsiveness in male rats highlights the known differences in immune function in male and females. A dramatic example of this difference is seen in the age of onset of the spontaneous autoimmune disease systemic lupus erythematosus (SLE) in the NZB/NZW strain of mice. The female mice develop SLE at approximately 2–3 months of age and male mice develop disease at approximately 6 months of age. Ovariectomy of the female mice converts them to the time course of disease of males. Similarly, in humans, there are significant differences in the percentage of males and females who develop autoimmune diseases such as multiple sclerosis (10:1 female-to-male ratio), rheumatoid arthritis (3:1 female-to-male ratio), Grave's disease (4:1 female-to-male ratio), or SLE (10:1 female-to-male ratio). It is apparent that sex hormones can contribute to the modification of immune system function (Ansar et al, 1985). Consideration may have to be directed to a possible differential effect of stress on altering immune function in males and females.

The mechanism of lateral septal lesion alteration of the antibody response can be related to an influence at several stages of the immune response. Included are an altered function or expression of costimulatory molecules by antigen-presenting cells (APC), alteration of the reactivity of naive T cells with the APC, altered antigen uptake and presentation by B lymphocytes, and altered reactivity of activated T with antigen presenting B lymphocytes (including an alteration of cytokine release by the T lymphocytes involved in class switching of the antibody produced by the B lymphocyte). Studies that report a stressor-induced alteration of specific antibody production to an antigen fail to identify which of the many components of the immune system are modified. However, these studies contribute to the realization that the immune system does not function in a manner independent of the influence of the CNS.

Source: Nance et al (1987); Wetmore and Nance (1991).

FACTOID

Study of innate, primary, secondary, or effector immune response: Innate.
Species (and strain) studied: Male Wistar rats.
Brain region modified: Lateral and medial hypothalamus. The hypothalamus sends projections that participate in the regulation of the autonomic nervous system and endocrine organs. Neuronal input to the hypothalamus is from other areas of the brain and tissues of the body. The lateral and medial areas of the hypothalamus each consist of several nuclei.
How modified: Electrolytic lesion.
Tissue studied: Function of NK cells in the blood.
Immune parameters changed and comments: Electrolytic lesions placed in the lateral, but not the medial hypothalamus of rats altered NK function. NK cytotoxicity changed from depression (2nd postoperative day) through enhancement (5th postoperative day) to depression (21st postoperative day).

The lateral hypothalamus primarily produces CRH and sends neurons to the brain stem to innervate the locus coeruleus. Thus, modification of the HPA axis or activation of the sympathetic nervous system by the lesion influenced NK function. The fluctuation from depressed, to enhanced, to depressed function may have been due to different hormonal changes being induced at different times or different populations of NK cells being released from the bone marrow or spleen at different times after placing the lesion.

The number of NK cells was not controlled for, and fluctuations of NK numbers may have influenced the functional data.

No significant change in NK cytotoxicity was found after destruction of the medial hypothalamus. The medial hypothalamus mainly produces CRH and secretes it into the hypophysial portal system, where it induces ACTH production. As this lesion did not affect NK function in the blood, and lesion of the lateral hypothalamus did, it is possible that the major effect of the lateral lesions ability to alter NK function was due to an effect on activation of the sympathetic nervous system.

Source: Wrona et al (1994).

FACTOID

Study of innate, primary, secondary, or effector immune response: Secondary cell-mediated immune reactions.

Species (and strain) studied: C3H/He and C5BL/6 mice.

Brain region modified: Preoptic nucleus (located in the anterior hypothalamic areas and involved in the integration of homeostatic functions such as temperature regulation and the sleep–wake cycle) and arcuate nuclei (located in the periventricular area of the ventral part of the third ventricle and sends projections to the blood vessels in the median eminence of the hypothalamus. May be involved in the enhancement of analgesia) of the hypothalamus.

How modified: Monosodium glutamate (MSG) injection subcutaneously, which destroys neurons in the preoptic and arcuate nuclei.

Tissue studied: Delayed-type hypersensitivity skin responses after sensitization by immunization with antigens of *Mycobacterium tuberculosis.*

Immune parameters changed and comments: The MSG-treated mice had a significantly decreased ability of the T cells to produce delayed hypersensitivity reactions. The functional defect was suggested to be related to the inability of the T cells from the lesioned animals to release cytokines that mediate the delayed hypersensitivity response. However, as delayed hypersensitivity reactions involve many different activation steps and interactions, the precise mechanisms cannot be precisely defined.

Source: Kato et al (1986).

FACTOID

Study of innate, primary, secondary, or effector immune response: Nonspecific lymphocyte mitogenic stimulation was measured after lesioning of the paraventricular nucleus of the hypothalamus. This will be classified as intrinsic function of lymphocytes that cannot be further classified as part of the primary, secondary, or effector immune response.

Species (and strain) studied: Male Lewis rats.

Brain region modified: Paraventricular nucleus (PVN) of the hypothalamus. Area of the brain where oxytocin is synthesized. The area of the hypothalamus where the PVN is located also contains the preoptic nucleus, anterior nucleus, suprachiasmatic nucleus, dorsomedial nucleus, ventromedial nucleus, arcuate nucleus, and posterior nucleus. It is difficult to localize a knife lesion to a specific area.

How modified: Rotation of a knife.

Tissue studied: Spleen and peripheral blood lymphocyte response to nonspecific mitogenic stimulation after footshock stress.

Immune parameters changed and comments: Footshock-induced suppression of peripheral blood lymphocyte responsiveness to nonspecific mitogenic stimulation was attenuated as compared with sham-operated controls. Footshock-induced suppression of spleen lymphocyte responsiveness to nonspecific mitogenic stimulation was increased in comparison with sham-operated controls.

Producing a lesion by knife cuts removes neuronal cells and axons passing through the area. Therefore, multiple pathways were likely to have been altered by this procedure. It is possible that the effect of the damage led to an increase of stressor-induced catecholamine, or other neuropeptide release in the spleen. Lesioning of the PVN has been reported to result in an enhancement of stressor-induced epinephrine release from the adrenal (Darlington et al, 1988). If the lesion also enhanced norepinephrine release in the spleen, the spleen lymphocytes would have been expected to show a more marked decline of mitogenic function than that of intact rats. In addition, a lesion of the PVN, resulting in a decrease of stressor-induced corticosterone production, may increase catecholamine release through removal of a negative feedback mechanism (Kvetnansky et al, 1993).

The attenuation of the suppression of the peripheral blood mitogenic response was probably due to an attenuation of the corticosterone elevation by the stressor in the lesioned animals. Alterations of CRH, arginine vasopressin (AVP), and oxytocin concentrations, as well as activation of the sympathetic nervous system, were likely after the lesion was placed. Therefore, specific mechanisms responsible for the altered immune function are difficult to identify.

Source: Pezzone et al (1994).

FACTOID

Study of innate, primary, secondary, or effector immune response: Nonspecific lymphocyte mitogenic stimulation was measured after lesioning of the anterior hypothalamus, ventromedial hypothalamus mamillary bodies, or fornix. This will be classified as intrinsic function of lymphocytes that cannot be further classified as being part of the primary, secondary, or effector immune response.

Species (and strain) studied: Male Fischer 344 rats.

Brain region modified: Anterior hypothalamus (the paraventricular, preoptic, and suprachiasmatic nuclei are located in this area), ventromedial hypothalamus (the middle part of the hypothalamus, which sends projections to many areas, including the amygdaloid body and periaqueductal gray), mamillary bodies (located in the posterior hypothalamus and have a function related to memory), and fornix (the boundary between the medial and lateral hypothalamus)

How modified: Electrolytic lesion.

Tissue studied: Spleen.

Immune parameters changed and comments: A lesion placed in the anterior hypothalamus decreased the ability of Concanavalin A (Con A) to induce spleen lymphocyte mitosis. Mitosis was increased by lesions in the amygdaloid complex, and mamillary bodies. No alterations were induced by lesions in the ventromedial hypothalamus or fornix. Thus, depending on the site of the lesion, different functional alterations were produced. The functional changes were present 4 days after the lesion and gone by 7 days.

Function could be decreased due to fewer lymphocytes in the spleen, a shift of subpopulations with fewer Con A responsiveness cells, or hormonal changes in the plasma reducing the responsivity of lymphocytes to Con A. The data do not permit determination of the mechanism.

Source: Brooks et al (1982).

The above studies add much and little to our understanding of the interaction between the brain and the immune system. Reducing the activity of selected brain areas by lesioning or chemical toxicity for neurons can modify pathways that regulate hormones and neuropeptide release in lymphoid tissues. However, specific mechanisms and pathways cannot be determined. An increase of antibody production after alteration of neuronal activity in the brain may be due to an effect on one of many parts of the immune system. Finding a change does not explain why the change occurred. However, in a very positive sense, the studies cited above establish an interaction between the brain and both baseline and stressor altered immune function.

A further question relates to whether the above studies have a biological counterpart. Do stress, fear, anxiety, or happiness, produce changes in neuronal activity that are analogous to any of the changes produced by the above models? It is unlikely that stress will only activate a single location of neurons in the brain. Indeed, c-Fos studies have shown that numerous brain areas are activated by stress, although not all are involved in stressor-induced immune alteration. Specific site lesioning or activation studies fail to evaluate modulating effects produced when multiple brain areas are activated and that may modify functional alterations produced by site-specific alterations.

It is possible to hypothesize functional implications for some of the areas of the brain which are induced by stress to express c-Fos.

Activation of CRH-containing neurons in the hypothalamus are responsible for corticosterone elevation through the HPA axis. Corticosterone may modify the function of lymphocytes and mononuclear phagocytic cells by binding to glucocorticoid receptors which alter the production of cytokines and lymphocyte trafficking. How stress activates the CRH neurons is unclear.

Activation of the hypothalamus may activate the autonomic nervous system through neuronal connections from the hypothalamus to the locus coeruleus and spinal cord. This may activate catecholamine release in lymphoid tissues with a subsequent alteration of immune cell function and trafficking.

The dorsomedial nucleus of the hypothalamus innervates sympathetic preganglionic nuclei in the brain stem and spinal cord. These may activate postganglionic neurons, which terminate in primary and secondary lymphoid tissue with subsequent release of catecholamines.

Activation of neurons in the amygdala and lateral septal area result from fear and emotionality introduced by pain or fear. Footshock causes pain and reexposure to the conditioned footshock stressor is likely to cause fear. Therefore, activation of these brain areas would be expected.

The activated thalamic nuclei probably are associated with increased motor activity, which occurs during a painful stimulus.

ALTERATION OF THE BRAIN BY STRESS

There is evidence that the elevation of cortisol to the high normal range can have an effect on the hippocampus (if this study is confirmed the normal range of cortisol may have to be redefined for different biological effects of cortisol). The size of the hippocampus is smaller in individuals who experience higher levels of stress and recent memory tasks that depend on a functional hippocampus are performed less well in those individuals experiencing high stress levels (Lupien et al, 1998). The hippocampus is involved in functions related to recent memory.

Urinary cortisol levels have been correlated with memory performance (Seeman et al, 1997). The amount of urinary cortisol excretion in men was not associated with memory performance. However, in women, higher urinary cortisol excretion was associated with poorer memory, and increased cortisol excretion over time was associated with a decline of memory. Memory improvement over time was associated with a decrease of urinary cortisol excretion. This raises the interesting question regarding whether cortisol kills neurons or is the alteration of memory a pharmacological effect where higher levels of cortisol interfere with neuron function, in a reversible manner.

A recent report indicates that in nonhuman primates there is continuous production of new neurons in the hippocampus, and the production of new neurons is inhibited by stress (Gould et al, 1998). Until there are studies that evaluate the biological significance of interference with neuronal cell generation it will be impossible to know whether there is an influence of generation of new neurons on stressor induced immune alteration. However, if a disruption of the neuroanatomy of the brain occurs, it is possible that immune function would become altered.

THE LOCUS COERULEUS AND STRESSOR-INDUCED IMMUNE ALTERATION

Regardless of the hypothesized contributions of each c-Fos-positive area to altering immune function, altering the functional properties of selected c-Fos-positive areas can be used to determine the potential contribution of each activated area to stress-induced immune alteration, bearing in mind the previously expressed cautions. Following are examples of studies that focus on the locus coeruleus.

Selected c-Fos positive areas can be chemically activated or treated to prevent their activation. We have initiated such an approach. This is based on our observation that pretreatment of rats with benzodiazepine prior to exposing them to a conditioned stress procedure, prevents the alteration of lymphocyte mitogenic responsiveness that occurs in the spleens of rats pretreated with saline. In addition, stressed benzodiazepine treated rats do not activate c-Fos in the LC or A5 areas of the brain stem. Benzodiazepine is an anxiolytic agent that provides symptomatic relief from anxiety and tension.

Activation of the LC by infusing corticotropin-releasing factor (CRF) into the LC produces the same immune and hormonal alterations as does footshock or a conditioned aversive stressor (Rassnick et al, 1994). These data suggest that the LC may be an important anatomical site that must be activated for stress to alter the immune system. If the LC is important in stressor-induced immune alteration, the pathways that produce activation of the locus coeruleus and projections from the locus coeruleus will be important to identify, as pharmacological alteration of their function may interfere with stressor-induced immune alteration. It is important to emphasize that (1) extensive research must still be done before these pathways can be conclusively implicated as the major pathways contributing to stressor-induced immune alteration, and (2) there may be more than a single pathway associated with stress-induced alteration of the immune system.

LC activity is influenced by a variety of neurotransmitters, with the most influential being an excitatory input from the paragigantocellularis nucleus (PGi) and an inhibitory input from the prepositus hypoglossi (PrH) nucleus in the brain stem, both of which are located in the rostral portion of the medulla. The PGi is readily activated by footshock stress, producing a marked activation of the LC (Ennis et al, 1992). The fact that (1) the PGi is c-Fos positive after the footshock regimen that produces stressor-induced immune alteration, (2) is retrogradely labeled when PRV is injected into the spleen (see following section), (3) sends both glutamatergic and CRH-containing projections to the LC, each of which activates the LC, and, (4) has been suggested to play a prominent role in autonomic function, support the idea that PGi afferents to the LC may be important to the phenomenon of stressor-induced immune alteration (Ennis et al, 1992; Chiang and Aston-Jones G, 1993; VanBockstaele et al, 1993).

INNERVATION FROM THE SPLEEN TO THE BRAIN

Certain techniques can be used to identify the neuronal areas of the brain linked to specific peripheral sites. Pseudorabies virus (PRV) a swine α-herpes virus, is an example of a procedure that can be used to map neuronal circuitry. After injection of PRV into a tissue, it passes through neurons in a retrograde direction to the brain. The virus is then identified in neuronal cell bodies by an immunohistochemical procedure (Card et al, 1993). Our preliminary studies found that PRV placed into the spleen produces retrograde labeling of neurons in the A5 region of the brain stem, the PGi, and parts of the PVN.

PRV injected into different sympathetic ganglia (an accumulation of nerve cell bodies outside the central nervous system) or the adrenal produces labeling in the PVN, A5, PGi, caudal raphe region, rostral ventral medulla, and ventromedial medulla (Loewy, 1991). Thus, certain areas of the brain are connected to multiple tissue sites that are innervated by the sympathetic nervous system. However, there are also unique sets of neurons in the brain that become labeled when different peripheral sites are injected with PRV (Loewy, 1991). Thus, there may be discrete sites within the brain that are only linked to innervation of single peripheral tissues (Strack et al, 1989).

It is important to determine whether there are specific brain sites for autonomic innervation of the spleen. This will suggest areas of the brain whose regulation may be able to modulate stressor-induced immune alteration with minimal effects on other autonomic functions.

CHARACTERISTICS OF THE INNERVATION PRESENT IN LYMPHOID TISSUE

Neurons associated with altering immune function are activated in the brain. The result of this activation in lymphoid tissues is the release of hormones that alter immune function. The primary (bone marrow and thymus gland) and the secondary lymphoid tissues (spleen and lymph nodes) receive innervation from the sympathetic nervous system. Lymphocytes and macrophages have receptors for norepinephrine (NE) (studies have not been performed on dendritic cells). Other neuropeptides such as neuropeptide Y, substance P (SP), or vasoactive intestinal peptide (VIP) may also modify immune function if the appropriate cells have receptors for these neuropeptides.

Pattern of Innervation of the Bone Marrow

Sympathetic nerve fibers containing norepinephrine (NE) and substance P (SP) enter the marrow along with the arteriolar vasculature. The nerve terminals are found in the sinuses of the marrow and among the pluripotent stem cells that form the red cells, granulocytes, and lymphocytes. The specific role of the innervation in stimulating growth factor synthesis and release, maturation of pluripotent stem cells, maturation of the various lines of leukocytes, and release of mature leukocytes from the marrow has not been defined.

However, studies have been reported that suggest that stress hormones can modify the maturation of bone marrow stem cells and the production of growth factors for bone marrow cells (Tseilikman et al, 1995; Khlusov et al, 1993; Dygai et al, 1992). These studies suggest that the production of leukocytes from the bone marrow and of cytokine growth factors by bone marrow cells is altered by stress. Stressor-induced migration of mature T lymphocytes into the marrow that are able to influence hematopoiesis has also been reported (Gol'dberg et al, 1990).

Pattern of Innervation of the Thymus

Studies of the innervation of the thymus have primarily been performed in rats where there is both a sympathetic and parasympathetic innervation. The area of the cortex below the capsule of the thymus and the corticomedullary junction contain the largest input of sympathetic nerve fibers with parasympathetic fibers predominating in the medulla (Kendall and Al-Shawaf, 1991). There are also neuropeptide-containing nerves with SP, neuropeptide Y, VIP, and calcitonin gene-related protein identified (Muller and Weihe, 1991) adjacent to areas of the thymus where mast cells are located. Even though synapses between the nerve endings and lymphocytes have not been observed in the thymus (Vizi et al, 1995) diffusion of neuropeptides from the sympathetic nerve terminals is likely to modify lymphocyte function in the thymus. The human thymus also contains sympathetic innervation, although the distribution may differ from the rat, which has a larger sympathetic innervation present in the medulla (deLeeuw et al, 1992).

The precise function of the innervation of the thymus is unclear. Whether it has a biologically significant influence on maturation or release of lymphocytes from the thymus, or has a significant regulatory effect on the production of thymic hormones from the epithelial cells, remains to be determined. Depletion of sympathetic innervation by the injection of 6-hydroxydopamine results in a significant decrease of lymphocyte numbers in the thymic cortex but not the thymic medulla. Catecholamine agonists may accelerate the maturation of thymic lymphocytes (Singh, 1979). Release of lymphocytes from the thymus has been shown to be inhibited by cutting of the parasympathetic innervation and to be increased by stimulation of the parasympathetic innervation (Antonica et al, 1994). Protection of thymic cells from the cytolytic activity of glucocorticoids has been suggested for vasoactive intestinal peptide (Ernstrom et al, 1995).

As the thymus decreases in mass and thymic hormone production decreases during the aging process, it will be of interest to determine whether this process is altered by the concentration of neuropeptides in the thymus. Does stress influence the age associated involution of the thymus? If there is a relationship, it is possible that one mechanism of stress-associated immunologic disease is through an acceleration of thymic involution? Do individuals with low levels of stress in their lives maintain thymic hormone production and normal maturation of T lymphocytes longer than individuals with high levels of stress in their lives? Does stress accelerate the aging process by accelerating an age-related decline of immune function?

Studies have used hormonal replacement in aged rats to restore thymic architecture and function (Lesnikov et al, 1992). The effect of these hormonal manipulations on thymic innervation would be of interest. If there is a loss of the normal pattern of innervation during aging, and a restoration of innervation by hormonal replacement, the effect of hormonal replacement on the innervation of lymphoid tissue and a possible maintenance of function should be determined. Of course, identification of the appropriate hormones and whether they are best used singly or in combination would have to be determined—not an easy task.

The specific neuropeptide receptors expressed at various stages of thymic lymphocyte maturation are unknown. Release of neuropeptide at the site of a cell that lacks receptors for the neuropeptide would have no influence on the function of the cell. It is also possible that thymus lymphocytes develop receptors for different neuropeptides at different stages of their maturation. This would be similar to the appearance, and loss, of different CD markers at different stages of their maturation. Although general aspects of thymic lymphocyte maturation are known, the precise events which occur during thymic lymphocyte maturation have not been clarified (Scollay and Godfrey, 1995). Therefore, defining the events occurring at the cortico-medullary junction (which is rich in sympathetic innervation) that may be influenced by the various neuropeptides present in the nerve terminals cannot be done with any degree of reliability.

Pattern of Innervation of the Spleen

Studies of splenic innervation have primarily been performed in rats. The postganglionic sympathetic innervation of the spleen comes from the superior mesenteric coeliac ganglion. The nerve fibers form the splenic nerve that travel along the splenic artery entering the spleen at the hilus. More than 95% of the splenic nerve fibers contain norepinephrine (NE). Some also contain neuropeptide Y (NPY). Upon entering the spleen, some of the nerve fibers spread out to the capsule of the spleen, while most continue along the vasculature to the periarteriolar lymphocyte sheath, consisting primarily of T lymphocytes and dendritic cells that have carried antigen into the white pulp. Synaptic contact between nerve fibers and CD4+ and CD8+ lymphocytes have been identified.

Some nerve fibers extend through the white pulp to the marginal sinus and marginal zone. The marginal sinus contains dendritic cells, macrophages, and T and B lymphocytes. Surrounding the marginal sinus is the "marginal zone," which covers the periarteriolar lymphocyte sheath (PALS). Additional nerve fibers are found in proximity to the outer portions of the B cell containing follicles with few nerve fibers within the B-cell-rich follicles.

From anatomical studies it appears that the innervation and neuropeptides released from sympathetic nerves would have their major effect on dendritic cells and T lymphocytes. As the innervation within the follicles is sparse, it would be anticipated that neuropeptide effects on B cells in the follicles would depend on diffusion rather than release at the lymphocyte membrane. Alteration of the function of APC and T lymphocytes would have an effect on antibody production.

Whether diffusion of catecholamines from blood into the lymphoid compartments of the spleen contribute to the functional alteration of spleen lymphocytes is unlikely. In rodents in which high concentrations of plasma catecholamines have been achieved without activation of the sympathetic innervation to the spleen, spleen lymphocyte mitogenic responsiveness is normal. Thus, plasma catecholamines probably do not diffuse into secondary lymphoid tissues and the alteration of immune function in secondary lymphoid tissue is due to the local release of catecholamines.

It is interesting to compare the relative numbers of β-adrenergic receptors on different populations of lymphocytes with the anatomy of splenic innervation. Different populations of lymphocytes have different numbers of adrenergic receptor (Khan et al, 1986; Maisel et al, 1989). The NK cell population has the largest number of adrenergic receptors, and B lymphocytes have the next highest number. CD8 lymphocytes have fewer adrenergic receptors than B lymphocytes, but a greater number of receptors than the CD4 lymphocyte population, which has the fewest number of receptors (NK>B>CD8>CD4).

FACTOID

A naturally occurring biological situation in which the effect of chronic cate-cholamine elevation on immune function can be assessed occurs in individuals with congestive heart failure. A study of 38 subjects who had approximately twice the normal plasma norepinephrine levels found no quantitative differences of blood lymphocyte subset numbers or nonspecific mitogenic responses in comparison to controls (Hwang et al, 1993). However, significant differences were present when the mitogenic response of lymphocytes to an antigen, tetanus toxoid, was measured with the subjects having significantly less reactivity than the controls. Antigenic-specific stimulation requires the presentation of the antigen by phagocytic cells (in this case monocytes which are present in the blood) in MHC II molecules, to previously sensitized CD4 lymphocytes. Thus, although nonspecific mitogenic function was normal, a norepinephrine dependent alteration of antigen presentation or antigen-specific T-cell responsiveness may be present in these subjects.

Disregarding NK cells, the largest number of β-adrenergic receptors are found on B lymphocytes, where the least amount of innervation is found. In the T-cell areas there is more extensive innervation and the lymphocytes contain lower numbers of β-adrenergic receptors. Thus, it is possible that the concentration of locally released norepinephrine influences the number of β-adrenergic receptors on lymphocytes. High concentrations of catecholamines decrease receptor expression.

Electron microscopic studies have investigated the anatomical relationship between the nerve terminals and lymphocytes and macrophages (Felten and Olschowka, 1987). There appear to be direct contacts between the nerve terminals, determined to be catecholaminergic by the presence of tyrosine hydroxylase, and the outer membrane of lymphocytes with a gap distance between the nerve and lymphocyte of approximately 6 nanometers (nm). At the point of contact the membranes of both the nerve terminal and lymphocyte were slightly thickened. There were also some apparent points of contact between the nerve terminals and macrophages. The small size of the gap between the nerve terminal and cell membrane suggests that released norepinephrine (NE) from the nerve would have the opportunity to rapidly bind to the lymphoid cell adrenergic receptors. It is unlikely that plasma catecholamine concentrations reflect the concentration that may occur at the synapse.

In addition to nerve terminals ending at lymphocyte and macrophage membranes, other terminals do not appear to be adjacent to cells. Release of NE from these terminals may increase the NE concentration in the extracellular tissue spaces of the spleen and potentially bathe the immune cells in a concentration of NE that is increased over basal levels (remembering that basal levels may differ depending upon the current life stressors than an individual is experiencing). For example, in rats exposed to immobilization stress, there is an increase of free NE in the spleen (Hori et al, 1995). Approximately 20 minutes after initiation of the immobilization, NE concentrations increase seven- to eightfold before decreasing.

Many of the same nerve fibers that contain NE also contain NPY. Other nerve fibers contain the neuropeptides vasoactive intestinal peptide (VIP), substance P (SP), and somatostatin. Although parasympathetic innervation in the spleen has been looked for, there is no convincing evidence that the parasympathetic nervous system innervates the spleen.

Pattern of Innervation of the Lymph Node

The innervation of lymph nodes have been studied with similar findings regardless of location of the node (Ackerman et al, 1987). Norepinephrine-containing nerve fibers enter the node at the hilus and extend to the paracortical region (where T lymphocytes interact with antigen-presenting dendritic cells) with some fibers terminating in the capsule of the node, the subcapsular sinus where lymphocytes, dendritic cells, and macrophages enter the node from the afferent lymphatic system, and the medullary cords (where plasma cells are located). There is little, if any, innervation of the B-cell-containing follicles. Thus, as in the spleen, the primary area in which immune function is likely to be affected by NE release is where T lymphocytes interact with antigen presenting cells.

Pattern of Innervation of the Mucosal Associated Lymphoid Tissue

There is innervation of the mucosa-associated lymphoid tissues with NE, NPY, SP, and calcitonin gene-related peptide containing nerve fibers (Nohr and Weihe, 1991). As with the innervation of other lymphoid tissue, the functional significance of the innervation remains to be determined and will be dependent on the presence of hormone receptors on lymphoid cells.

EFFECT ON IMMUNE FUNCTION OF INTERRUPTION OF THE INNERVATION TO LYMPHOID TISSUE

Effect on Immune Function by Catecholamine Depletion in Peripheral Tissue by Surgical Means

An interesting model that takes advantage of the separate innervation of lymph nodes located on two sides of the body was done in mice. Surgical interruption of the sympathetic innervation to the submaxillary lymph node on one side of the neck was performed, and a sham procedure was done on the other side (Alito et al, 1987; Esquifino and Cardinali, 1994). The content of norepinephrine in the sympathetic denervated lymph node decreased approximately 90% by 20 days postsurgery.

Several immune responses were measured in the nodes, including the number of B lymphocytes producing antibody in response to the injection of sheep erythrocytes, a delayed hypersensitivity response to a chemical hapten (1-chloro-2,4-dinotrobenzene (DNCB)), growth of tumor cells injected into the ear of the mice, and the response of lymphocytes in the node to Con A, a nonspecific mitogen.

Mice were immunized to sheep erythrocytes 10–20 days after surgery. There was an approximate twofold greater number of B lymphocytes releasing antibodies to sheep erythrocytes in the node from the side that had disruption of the sympathetic innervation in comparison with the sham-operated side. The explanation for the increased number of antibody-producing B lymphocytes has not been determined. Possibilities would include increased numbers or function of APCs, increased numbers of helper CD4 lymphocytes, increased numbers of B lymphocytes in the follicles, or increased mitosis of antibody producing B lymphocytes subsequent to their activation.

At 11 days after surgery, the mice were sensitized to DNCB and reexposed to the DNCB 9 days later. Delayed hypersensitivity reactivity was evaluated by the amount of swelling which took place in the ear of the denervated and sham-denervated sides. The ear of the denervated side had significantly more swelling than the sham side.

The growth of injected tumor cells was significantly less in the ear of the denervated side. These observations can be explained by mechanisms similar to the increase in antibody production, which involve increased numbers or function of APCs and increased numbers and function of the Th1 population of CD4 lymphocytes.

The response of the lymphocytes from the submaxillary lymph nodes to nonspecific mitogenic stimulation did not differ. However, the function of the cells that Con A induces to divide is unknown. They may provide help to B cells for antibody production, or participate in delayed-type hypersensitivity reactions, or they may not function as helper cells.

Thus, in this experimental system, decreased sympathetic innervation was associated with (1) an increase of antibody-producing B lymphocytes, (2) increased delayed hypersensitivity reactions, and (3) increased resistance to tumor growth. The data suggest that the sympathetic nervous system suppresses the function of the immune system. Other supportive studies have found enhancement of the immune response to antigen injection and enhanced nonspecific responses to mitogens and NK function after surgical interruption of the sympathetic innervation to lymphoid tissue (Besedovsky et al, 1979; Alito et al, 1985; Wan et al, 1993; Hori et al, 1995).

Catecholamine content of the spleen decreases at the time of the maximum increase of antibody-producing B lymphocytes in the spleens of rats immunized with sheep erythrocytes, suggesting an inverse relationship between catecholamine content and immune reactivity (Besedovsky et al, 1979). Thus, it is likely that the concentration of catecholamines in the secondary lymphoid tissues contribute to the characteristics (both qualitative and quantitative) of immune function. By extrapolation, it may be assumed that psychological factors that modulate catecholamine release in lymphoid tissues will also modulate immune function.

Activation of the splenic nerve, which occurs during stress (Shimizu et al, 1994), has been shown to increase the amount of free norepinephrine present in the spleen. Cutting of the splenic nerve with resultant denervation of the spleen prevents stress from modifying splenic immune function (Wan et al, 1993), confirming the importance of the peptides released from the splenic nerve as immune modulators.

It is likely that autonomic activity of the brain is involved in regulation of the amount of catecholamine and other peptides released into lymphatic tissues. Indeed, this is one of the foundations of psychoneuroimmunology. However, the above studies do not provide information regarding the actual part of the immune activation pathway that is modulated by catecholamines. Regardless of the mechanism, these studies indicate that modulation of catecholamine concentrations in lymphoid tissues, modifies immune function.

Effect on Immune Function by Catecholamine Depletion in Peripheral Tissue by Chemical Means

The influence of a hormone on regulating the function of cells of the immune system can be assessed by procedures that (1) reduce the concentration of the hormone in an experimental subject or (2) by inhibiting the binding of the hormone to its receptor. However, as in surgical studies that cut the innervation to secondary lymphatic tissue, the precise mechanism responsible for immune changes may be difficult to identify on a cellular level. For example, a decrease of the ability of T lymphocytes to respond to nonspecific mitogenic stimulation may be due to alterations of calcium flux, cyclic nucleotide formation, or protein phosphorylation. On a more biological basis, a decreased ability to produce antibody to antigenic challenge may be due to alterations at the antigen-processing stage, antigen presentation, or T-cell interaction with B cells. Regardless, this experimental approach provides a means that allows insight into the hormones that can influence the function of immune cells.

Injection of the chemical 6-hydroxydopamine (6-OHDA) decreases the amount of NE present in tissue by damaging the peripheral nerves that release NE. Repeated injection of newborn rats with 6-OHDA, followed by adrenalectomy (to remove epinephrine, which may be produced in higher concentrations when NE concentrations are low) and then immunization of the treated animals when adults, results in an enhanced antibody response to sheep erythrocytes (Besedovsky et al, 1979). In neonatal animals, this approach has been reproducible (Williams et al, 1981). This further suggests that NE impairs immune activation and an enhanced immune response occurs with catecholamine depletion.

Based on the above studies using 6-OHDA in neonatal animals, lowering of the concentration of catecholamines by 6-OHDA would be expected to be associated with an enhanced immune response. However, an inhibition, rather than an enhancement, of the antibody response after treatment of adult rats with 6-OHDA has been reported (Hall et al, 1982; Livnat et al, 1985; Felten et al, 1987). This may suggest that in the adult animal catecholamines are needed to maintain proper antigen uptake-processing and presentation by APCs, or that interaction of APCs with T lymphocytes and sensitized T lymphocytes with B lymphocytes require catecholamines for a functional immune response to occur. Obviously, the proper explanation can not be provided, as the necessary experiments have not been done.

Another explanation for the inhibition of the immune response seen in adult animals with 6-OHDA catecholamine depletion is that there may be sparing of nerve terminals that release neuropeptides other than NE. If only NE release is depleted, other neuropeptides, such as substance P, NPY, or VIP may continue to be released with a resultant alteration of immune function, possibly an inhibition. Thus, a possible complexity to the influence of hormones on the immune system is suggested to be related to the influence of multiple hormones simultaneously binding to receptors on single lymphocytes.

Another possible explanation for the differences in immune responsiveness to sheep erythrocytes between newborn or adult animals treated with 6-OHDA may be that the adult animals were having a secondary response and the alteration of the secondary antibody response differs in its susceptibility to catecholamines in comparison to the primary antibody response. As previously described in Chapter 2, there are different requirements for primary and secondary immune activation. A natural exposure of animals to antigens in the environment that are also present on sheep erythrocytes may have sensitized adult animals.

Sheep erythrocytes contain an antigen, the Forssman antigen, that is also present on a variety of plant substances. Indeed, many humans have antibodies to the Forssman antigen subsequent to ingestion of foods containing the antigen. Adult animals may have been exposed to the Forssman antigen which would result in T and B lymphocytes that were sensitized to the antigen. Whether this could account for the differences between the type of alteration induced by chemical sympathectomy in adult and young animals has not been explored. However, in support of this possibility, catecholamine depletion of experimental animals at the time of primary immunization does not alter a secondary immune response to sheep erythrocytes (Kasahara et al, 1977). This suggests that the secondary immune response is not as susceptible to stressor-induced alteration as is the primary response. In addition, the above study did not find an effect of catecholamine depletion on altering the immune response to a T-cell-independent antigen, further implicating the antigen processing cells or their interaction with T lymphocytes as being susceptible to catecholamine-dependent immune alteration.

An additional reason for different responses to catecholamine depletion in the adult and young animals is that there are differences in the immune system at these ages. B lymphocytes from newborn animals have a reduced ability to stimulate antigen-specific T-cell lines to secrete IL-2 (Bonomo et al, 1993). Although the ability to bind antigen and internalize it and present the antigen in MHC II molecules is the same in neonatal and adult B cells (Morris et al, 1992), the B lymphocytes of newborns have low levels of CD40, and the T lymphocytes of newborns have low levels of CD40L expression (Durandy et al, 1995). Thus, catecholamine depletion study comparison between newborn and adult animals may not be comparing apples and oranges because of differences in the development of the immune system and the possibility that secondary responses may be activated in the adult but not in the neonatal animal.

The function of T cells, measured by delayed-type hypersensitivity skin testing, has been determined in catecholamine depleted mice. Experimental animals were depleted of catecholamines by 6-OHDA after which a chemical hapten was placed onto their skin. The process is the same as occurs when skin reactivity occurs to poison ivy. Reactivity to the chemical was determined by placing the chemical on the ear of the experimental animal and measuring the amount of swelling that occurred. The swelling is produced by T lymphocytes that have become sensitized to the chemical.

The T lymphocytes migrate into the ear and release cytokines that increase vascular permeability (resulting in fluid flow into tissue). 6-OHDA-treated mice had a significant reduction in the amount of ear swelling (Madden et al, 1989). T lymphocytes from these animals were studied in vitro and were found to have a decreased ability to produce cytotoxic T lymphocytes and a reduced ability to produce IL-2. The data suggest that catecholamines were needed to maintain the proper function and interactions between the antigen-processing stages, the antigen presenting stages, and the activation and effector functions of the CD4 lymphocytes. These data, of course, differ from the findings previously described in surgically denervated animals.

When animals that had been sensitized to the chemical hapten were treated with 6-OHDA after sensitization, but before being challenged with the antigen, suppression of the ear swelling response was also found. This suggests that the effector phase of the CD4 lymphocytes (see delayed hypersensitivity skin testing, in Chapter 2) is impaired with catecholamine depletion. However, previously cited studies using surgical interruption of the sympathetic innervation to lymph nodes have found an enhanced delayed hypersensitivity response to chemical sensitization as well as an enhanced antibody response (Alito et al, 1987; Esquifino et al, 1994). Whether the different methods of catecholamine depletion affect different phases of the immune system or 6-OHDA effects immune cell function through pathways that are in addition to its effect on the sympathetic nervous system, are unresolved. However, the data indicate that catecholamines participate in the regulation of immune function. Much remains to be learned about the mechanisms of the interaction. Carefully designed experimental systems that control for primary versus secondary immune responses, baseline stress levels, age of the experimental animals, and maturation of the immune system are some of the parameters that need to be considered.

Effect of Catecholamine Infusion on Immune Function

Infusion of catecholamine into humans or experimental animals and measuring the quantitative and functional changes in lymphocytes can provide information regarding the effect of catecholamine elevations on immune function (Crary et al, 1983; De Blasi et al, 1986; van Tits et al, 1990). Epinephrine infusion into humans increases the concentration of CD8 lymphocytes and NK lymphocytes in the blood. A decreased responsiveness of lymphocytes to mitotic stimulation with nonspecific mitogens also occurs. This may be related to an alteration the relative distribution of different lymphocyte subsets or to direct effects of epinephrine on second messenger pathways that decrease the ability of lymphocytes to be induced into mitosis. These early studies were unable to consider alterations of the Th1 and Th2 populations as mediators of the altered response to mitogens because this cell population had not yet been identified.

In humans who experience an acute laboratory stressor, the same changes caused by the injection of epinephrine are found in the peripheral blood (Manuck et al, 1991; Bachen et al, 1992; Naliboff et al, 1991).

To confirm that catecholamines are responsible for the alterations of the peripheral blood lymphocyte populations following a stressor, subjects have been pretreated with an adrenergic receptor antagonist before being exposed to the psychological stressor (Bachen et al, 1995). Lymphocyte subsets, natural killer cell function, and the responsiveness of T lymphocytes to stimulation with nonspecific mitogens were compared in specimens obtained both before and after the mental stressor in subjects who received an injection of saline or the adrenergic antagonist. Both quantitative and qualitative alterations of the immune system occurred in those subjects who were exposed to the stressor and injected with saline. However, in those subjects who received the adrenergic antagonist the psychological stressor failed to produce alterations of immune function.

In another study, a group of healthy individuals, with a mean age of 27 years, were given an adrenergic antagonist (propranolol) for 7 consecutive days (Maisel et al, 1991). The propranolol treatment led to an increase in the percentage T lymphocytes, an increased response to stimulation with nonspecific mitogen, and an increased production of IL-2. These studies strongly suggest that, in humans, the immunological response of peripheral blood lymphocytes to psychological stress is mediated by activation of the sympathetic nervous system.

An experimental rodent model that maintains a high level of catecholamines and presents a chance to study an equivalent of infusion of catecholamines is the spontaneously hypertensive rat (SHR). These animals have increased concentrations of catecholamines in tissue and a reduced responsivity of spleen B and T lymphocytes to stimulation with nonspecific mitogens. Removal of cells which had the characteristics of mononuclear phagocytic cells (monocytes and macrophages) restored the lymphocyte reactivity to normal. In addition, when the mononuclear phagocytic cells were mixed with normal lymphocytes, the ability of the normal lymphocytes to respond to nonspecific mitogenic stimulation was suppressed (Pascual et al, 1992). Thus, in these animals baseline immune function is modified in comparison to normotensive animals from which they were derived, indicating that baseline immune function may be related to endogenous levels of catecholamines, and that the mononuclear phagocytic cell may mediate the interaction between catecholamines and lymphocytes.

ACUTE VERSUS CHRONIC STRESS—SIMILAR OR DIFFERENT IMMUNE CHANGES?

An appropriate question relates to whether the acute stressor-induced immune changes are the same as those found in association with chronic stress. Chronic stress may lead to a prolonged exposure of lymphoid cells to catecholamines, with the possibility that the alterations that occur are different from those induced by an acute stress. Indeed, that is apparently what happens.

A meta-analysis of studies of the influence of stress on immune function in humans provides interesting data regarding an effect of the duration of a stressor on immune parameters (Herbert and Cohen, 1993). When the effect on quantitative numbers of lymphocyte populations was determined, both acute experimental laboratory stress and long-term stress experienced as part of one's life had similar effects on the number of circulating CD4 and B lymphocytes, with decreased numbers found. Lymphocyte responsiveness to stimulation with nonspecific mitogens was decreased by either acute laboratory or naturalistic long duration, stress. CD8 lymphocytes showed a different pattern of change in association with acute or long-term stress. CD8 lymphocyte numbers increase in the blood after an acute laboratory stressor but are decreased in subjects who have a high level of naturalistic stress in their lives.

Different responses to acute and chronic stress occur within the CNS. Examples are:

1. Exposure of cats to a loud noise activates the locus coeruleus (LC), but the electrical activity decreases with repeated exposures to the noise (Abercrombie and Jacobs, 1987). This suggests that repeated exposure to the same stressor modifies the ability of the LC to become activated.

2. Activation of the LC either by stress or by injection with CRH has been shown to alter the reactivity of the LC to subsequent exposure to the activating stimulus or another stimulus. If a rat is given a single session of footshock stress, the response of the LC to localized CRH injection is altered as the LC has a reduction of its normal electrical activation to CRH injection. However, if the rat is given five stress sessions, the sensitivity of the LC to low concentrations of CRH is increased but the magnitude of activation is decreased (Curtis et al, 1995).

3. Injection of CRH into the LC alters its reactivity to subsequent injections of CRH (Conti and Foote,1995). A single CRH injection attenuated the response of the LC to a second injection of CRH for 72 hours. Rats given 8 daily injections of CRH into the LC had a decreased LC reactivity to subsequent CRH injection 7 days later. The data indicate that reactivity of the LC to an acute stressor will be altered if the LC experiences prolonged CRH exposure induced by chronic stress. Whether, and specifically how, this alteration of LC activity relates to immune differences in response to acute and chronic stress remains to be determined.

4. The activation of c-Fos within neurons is different in response to acute or chronic stress. Both acute restraint and shaking activated c-Fos in the locus coeruleus, midbrain raphe nuclei, paraventricular nuclei, and central gray matter. Repeated restraint stress for 14 days produced habituation to restraint stress but not to shaking, in all areas other than the LC. Habituation to both stressors was seen in the locus (Watanabe et al, 1994).

5. Another study also found decreased c-Fos activation with repeated restraint stress in the paraventricular nucleus and medial amygdala but not in other areas such as the locus coeruleus, lateral septum and lateral preoptic area. These studies suggest that the reactivity of some brain areas that are repeatedly activated by stress may eventually habituate when assayed by c-Fos activation. Whether the neurons are still functionally active in regard to their ability to influence the immune system cannot be extrapolated from the c-Fos data. However, the investigators did measure plasma corticosterone concentrations after 1 or 10 daily stress sessions and found an attenuation of corticosterone elevations with repeated stress. Thus, it is possible that repeated stress does modify the CNS response to the same stressor.

Another mechanism that could be associated with different immune alterations associated with acute versus chronic stress is a change of function at the level of the cells of the immune system. Binding of catecholamines to the β-adrenergic receptor may lead to a change in the number of receptors, their affinity for catecholamine, or their functionality, as evaluated by a reduction in the amount of second messengers they stimulate. A variety of studies indicate that physiological process which increase catecholamine production, or treatment of subjects with β-adrenergic ligands, lead to decreased sensitivity of the β-adrenergic receptor (Brodde et al, 1992; Smiley and Vulliemoz, 1992; Brodde et al, 1990; Marty et al, 1990). There has also been a report that the IL-1 receptor-mediated activation of CD4 lymphocytes can undergo desensitization with a resultant decrease of receptor mediated function (McKean et al, 1994).

Acute footshock stress can reduce the percentage of peripheral blood T lymphocytes and delayed-type hypersensitivity skin reactions in rats. However, if the rats experience 7 consecutive days of restraint and are then exposed to footshock, there is no alteration of immune function (Basso et al, 1994). This may suggest that repeated stress prevented activation of areas of the brain that are activated by acute stress or the immune system has been modified by the repeated stress so that it no longer responds to the hormonal changes induced by the acute stress.

Differences in the number of occupied glucocorticoid receptors in the cytoplasm of spleen cells in rats undergoing different intensities of chronic stress have been reported (Spencer et al, 1996). The data suggest that the rats undergoing greater levels of chronic stress had fewer glucocorticoid receptors that were unoccupied in the cytoplasm of spleen cells. Thus, an acute stressor would have less of a physiological effect in regard to the glucocorticoid system in the animals experiencing the greater level of chronic stress as more of their glucocorticoid receptors are already occupied.

These data raise the interesting question regarding what baseline immune function the alterations of hormonal concentrations induced by stress are acting on. If an individual is experiencing chronically high levels of stress, are the baseline functions of lymphocytes the same in that individual as in an individual who has low levels of stress-related hormones in their plasma? If the number of adrenergic receptors differs on the lymphocytes of an individual who is experiencing high levels of chronic stress in comparison with an individual with low stress levels, will each individual's immune function be altered to the same extent by an acute stressor? If the concentration of adhesion molecules differs on both the surface of lymphocytes and on endothelial cells of high versus low stress subjects, what are the implications for an acute stress altering the relative percentages of the various lymphocyte populations in blood and in tissues of each category of subject? Thus, both quantitative and functional differences may be found when comparing the effect of stress on the immune system in individuals who have high or low levels of stress in their daily lives.

Alteration of the function of several different immune parameters after acute stress has been studied in subjects who were experiencing high or low levels of stressors in their lives. Individuals who experience more hassles in their lives have a greater decrease of peripheral blood T and NK lymphocytes in comparison to individuals who experience fewer hassles in their lives (Brosschot et al, 1994). It has also been reported that an acute stressor may alter some parameters of the immune system in subjects experiencing high levels of life stress, but the cardiovascular system of the same individuals responds to the same extent as the cardiovascular system of individuals experiencing low life stressors (Benschop et al, 1994). Thus, if chronic stress elevates hormones and the concentration and function of hormonal receptors are subsequently altered, it is possible that different tissues undergo different alterations.

A functional assay of NK cells of subjects exposed to an acute laboratory stressor differed between individuals experiencing high or low levels of stress in their lives. NK cell function decreased significantly more in subjects with high levels of life stress than in those without (Pike et al, 1997). Thus, the definition of immune baseline will have to depend on an individual's own particular life events.

It is important to determine whether chronic exposure to the same stress has a different effect on brain and immune function than does sequential exposure to different chronic stressors. Repeated exposure to the same stress may decrease the amount of NE released in the brain. However, if there is repeated exposure to the same stress, followed by exposure to a novel new stressor, there may be increased release of NE that is significantly greater than the amount of NE released when a nonstressed animal is exposed to the novel stressor (Nissenbaum et al, 1991; Gresch et al, 1984; Konarska et al, 1989). Thus, chronic stress must be evaluated with regard to the uniqueness of the chronic stressor. Being stressed by one's spouse for a week, financial concerns the next week, a medical problem the next week, and job performance the following week may produce different effects in the brain and on the immune system than does 4 weeks of worrying about one's spouse.

HYPOTHESIS

Certain analogies can be used to help understand possible differences between acute and chronic stress on the nervous system. The analogy that I will use characterizes the primary antibody response as an acute stressor. When antigen is reinjected into a subject who is undergoing a primary immune response, a comparison with the imposition of an acute stress on an existing chronic stress can be made.

Activation of the primary antibody response requires antigen processing by dendritic cells, presentation of the antigenic peptides to naive CD4 cells, binding of costimulatory molecules, and cytokine production. Antibody production occurs when the appropriate activated CD4 cell interacts with antigen presented by MHC molecules of the B cell. Initially IgM, and then other classes of antibody, are produced. Chronic activation of the B cells occurs when antigen is retained on the follicular dendritic cells (FDC). Thus, if the introduction of antigen is equated with an acute stressor, chronicity of the antibody (or, in this analogy, the stressor) is maintained by the persistence of antigen on the FDC.

The antibody response to reintroduction of the antigen (the secondary response) has different requirements and parameters of activation than does the primary response. The activated T cells and activated B cells are already present. Thus, once the antigen is processed and presented by the B cells, there is a rapid increase of IgG antibody and the amount produced is greater than that produced by a primary response.

The antibody response has been changed by the first response to the antigen. However, if an unrelated antigen is injected, there will be a primary response to the new antigen. A secondary response will only occur if the same antigen is injected.

Similar to the immune system, an acute stress response imposed on an individual who is already experiencing a chronic stress may have different parameters of induced change and activation than does an acute stress response imposed on an individual who is not experiencing chronic stressors. Whether there are differences when an acute stress is imposed on an individual experiencing the same stress in a chronic state (such as would be caused by an increased intensity of the stress) in comparison with an individual who is experiencing chronic stress being exposed to a different acute stressor has not been unequivocally resolved.

CYTOKINE COMMUNICATION TO THE BRAIN—SICKNESS BEHAVIOR

The maintenance of homeostasis of the immune system requires prevention of the uncontrolled activation of the immune system. Neuropeptides and hormones released by the CNS contribute to the homeostasis of the immune system. Without knowledge that the immune system has been activated, the CNS would not know when to modulate the activity of immune cells. The mechanism of communication from the immune system to the brain likely involves cytokines released from cells of the immune system. The cytokines enter the CNS and signal the brain regarding the state of activation of the immune system. Evidence of communication from the immune system to the brain has been established by several approaches:

1. There is an increase in plasma catecholamines at the peak of the antibody response following injection of a T-dependent antigen into an experimental animal (Besedovsky and Sorkin, 1977a,b). It is likely that plasma levels of catecholamines and lymphoid tissue concentrations of catecholamines increase when the immune system signals the brain that the immune system is activated.

2. CNS electrical activity during an immune response has been measured for some areas of the brain (Saphier et al, 1987). Recording electrodes that measured electrical activity were placed into the preoptic area of the anterior hypothalamus and into the dorsal medial paraventricular nucleus of male rats. Animals were immunized with an intraperitoneal injection of sheep erythrocytes. Electrical activity was measured for several days after the injection. Saline-injected controls were also studied. Alterations in electrical activity were detected as shown in Table 3.2.

   The peak of the immune response after the intraperitoneal injection of sheep erythrocytes occurs at 4–6 days after injection. It is possible that cytokines released into the systemic circulation by APCs and CD4 T lymphocytes gained entry to the CNS and altered the activation of the areas whose electrical activity was being monitored. Whether the modulation of electrical activity was related to release of ACTH and catecholamines, is speculative.

3. IL-1 is capable of activating the HPA axis (Besedovsky et al, 1986, 1991; Bereknbosch et al, 1987). The essential points of these studies are that:

Systemic injection of purified IL-1 into rodents resulted in an increase of plasma ACTH and corticosterone.

Injection of IL-1 into mice that lacked T cells also produce an increase of corticosterone, indicating that the IL-1 did not induce T lymphocytes to release soluble factors that were responsible for the elevation of ACTH and corticosterone.

Injection of mice with IL-2 or IFN-γ did not elevate corticosterone.

The effect of IL-1 is not directly on adrenal cells, as neutralization of CRH prevented the IL-1-induced increase in corticosterone.

The effect of IL-1 is primarily on cells which produce CRH as IL-1 did not increase plasma concentrations of prolactin, melanocyte-stimulating hormone, or growth hormone.

Injection of rats with IL-1, IL-6, or tumor necrosis factor-α (TNF-α) each produced increases of plasma ACTH and corticosterone. However, IL-6 and TNF-α were much less potent, as 20-fold higher doses in comparison to IL-1 did not elevate ACTH or corticosterone as much as did IL-1

Cytokines communicating information to the CNS are IL-1, IL-6, and TNF-α, which induce a temperature increase and CRH and arginine vasopressin (AVP) release from the hypothalamus (Harbuz and Lightman, 1992; Reichlin, 1993). IL-1, IL-6, and TNF-α activate the hypothalamus by binding to cytokine receptors (Chrousos, 1995) but may also have a direct effect on the ACTH-synthesizing cells of the pituitary (Kapcala et al, 1995).

Uncontrolled release of cytokines by an activated immune system can have deleterious effects on health. For example, excessive amounts of the cytokine TNF-α produces systemic vasodilation with plasma extravasation into tissues and hypotensive shock. Small blood clots may form which consume the coagulation factors resulting in a tendency to bleed. The kidneys, liver, lungs, and heart may have inadequate perfusion and fail to function. Thus, a mechanism to decrease cytokine production is essential.

TABLE 3.2   Brain Activity Associated with Immune System Activation

Day after Immunization	Anterior Hypothalamus	PVN
2	Baseline	Decrease
3	Decrease	Decrease
4	Increase	Baseline
5	Increase	Baseline
6	Baseline	Increase
7	Baseline	Increase
8	Decrease	Decrease

One mediator of suppression of excessive cytokine production is probably a glu-cocorticoid effect on mononuclear cell cytokine messenger RNA (mRNA) transcription (Munck et al, 1984). Indeed, differences in production of cytokines and cytokine receptors are found when comparing patients with hypercortisolism and hypocortisolism (Sauer et al, 1994). Hypercortisolism suppresses cytokine production.

The intravenous injection of either IL-1 or TNF-α elevated plasma ACTH (Sharp et al, 1989). However, the CNS location of receptors for IL-1 and TNF-α may differ as IL-1 infusion into the median eminence of the pituitary elevates plasma ACTH levels while infusion of TNF-α into the same site does not elevate ACTH. This finding suggests that the principal binding site for TNF-α is either outside the CNS or that there is a mechanism to transport the TNF-α into an appropriate site within the CNS.

Fever is a response of the body to infection, often functioning as an indicator of infection. Fever is caused by cytokines produced by mononuclear phagocytic cells (IL-1, IL-6, and TNF-α), altering the thermoregulatory properties of the preoptic anterior hypothalamus (Kluger et al, 1995; Luheshi et al, 1996). The specific sequence of cytokines interaction with the hypothalamus and the relative importance of each cytokine on fever elevation is under investigation. The cytokines may function by initiating release of prostaglandin, as fever elevation is prevented by inhibitors of prostaglandin synthesis. Cytokine release of corticotropin-releasing factor (CRF) may also contribute to fever elevation.

Another cytokine-mediated effect on behavior is the feeling of sleepiness. Numerous publications which have characterized both IL-1 and IL-6 as participants in sleep induction. TNF-α may also participate (Darko et al, 1995; Kruger and Majde, 1995; Takahashi et al, 1996). There is also an indication that individuals who experience excessive daytime sleepiness have elevated levels of either TNF-α or IL-6 in their circulation (Vgontzas et al, 1997).

Other sickness-associated behavioral changes that occur at the time of infectious illness, when it is likely that cytokine production in increased, include a loss of appetite, decreased social interaction, and decreased reproductive drive. These behavioral changes are distinct from the joint and muscle discomfort (likely to be caused by immune complex deposition in the vasculature of the joints and muscles with the subsequent activation of the complement system and the attraction of neutrophils to ingest the immune complexes) that are also mediated by an immune reaction. All the sickness-associated behaviors are probably caused by cytokine influences within the CNS (Bluthe et al, 1995; Bluthe et al, 1997; Montkowski et al, 1997; Propes and Johnson, 1997; Segreti et al, 1997).

A final question in regard to the communication between the immune system and the brain relates to how the cytokines gain access to the CNS. One possible pathway is for cytokines to diffuse out of blood vessels across the vascular endothelial cells and into the choroid plexus and the brain. However, blood vessels in the CNS are tightly adherent to each other, are entirely surrounded by a basement membrane, and have foot processes from choroidal epithelial cells or astrocytes adherent to the outside of the basement membrane. This forms a highly impermeable barrier. Although the blood–brain and blood–CSF barrier is poorly developed at the circumventricular organs at the base of the fourth ventricle near the opening to the central canal (where the pineal gland, posterior lobe of the pituitary, area postrema, and the organum vasculosum of the lamina terminalis are located), it is unlikely that adequate amounts of cytokine diffuse into the CNS to exert a physiological function. However, transport mechanisms to actively move IL-1, IL-6, and TNF-α from the vasculature to the CSF have been reported (Banks et al, 1995).

Another possible means of transmission of information regarding the presence of cytokines in the systemic circulation is by transmission through the nervous system to the brain. It has been found that intraperitoneal injection of IL-1 or TNF-α will produce behavioral changes in rodents. However, if the afferent branches of the subdiaphragmatic portion of the vagus nerve are surgically severed before cytokine injection, there are no behavioral effects (Goehler et al, 1995; Bluthe et al, 1996a,b). Although the mechanism of transmission has not been fully defined, it may involve the binding of cytokine to specific receptors on paraganglia located adjacent to the hepatic branch of the afferent vagus nerve.

BRAIN LATERALITY AND IMMUNE FUNCTION

The preceding discussion has presented information indicating that the brain is activated by stress, that experimental manipulation of stress activated areas of the brain alter immune function and that the immune system communicates with the brain. Another interesting way to look at the influence of the brain on immune reactivity is to consider immune function in relationship to right or left hemispheric dominance.

A variety of neurohormonal and anatomic differences exist between right and left handed individuals as the two hemispheres of the brain are not totally symmetrical. The hemisphere that is dominant for motor control determines hand preference. Approximately 90% of humans have left hemisphere dominance, making them right handed.

A perfectly round ball rolls in a straight line. A ball that has unequal weight on each side will wobble when it rolls. The human brain is not equal on both sides. If it were, we would probably all be ambidextrous. Because the brain is unequal on each side, we become either right handed or left handed. The imposition of handedness by the asymmetry of the brain appears to extend to the influence of immune function. This is a further indication that the anatomy and physiology of the brain contributes to the environment in which the immune system works and participates in the regulation of the immune system.

Lesions placed in the right or left brain cortex of mice had opposite effects on lymphocyte responsiveness to nonspecific mitogenic stimulation and production of IgG antibodies. Left-sided lesions suppressed lymphocyte responsiveness and antibody production, while right-sided lesions either had no effect or enhanced responsiveness (Renoux et al, 1983; Neveu et al, 1986). Left frontoparietal lesions in mice reduce NK activity (Bardos et al, 1981). In humans who have brain tumors, a tumor affecting the left side of the brain is associated with an impairment of in vitro lymphocyte responsiveness to mitogenic stimulation. However, right-sided cerebral tumors do not affect lymphocyte responsiveness (Blomgren et al, 1986). Intracranial tumors may interfere with the function of certain centers in the brain that are involved in the regulation of lymphocyte responses.

Animals can be characterized as having a predominant right or left side of the brain by showing a paw preference when food is displayed to them. An influence of sex hormones on brain asymmetry related immune parameters has also emerged (Betancur et al, 1991). Female, but not male, C3H/He mice displaying left paw preference had a higher nonspecific lymphocyte mitogenic activity than did right paw preference mice. However, male mice with left paw preference had lower NK activity than right paw preference mice or ambidextrous mice. Baseline levels of plasma corticosterone are higher in left paw preference mice as were corticosterone levels after restraint stress (Neveu and Moya, 1997). Whether the hormonal response directly affects the immune response and whether there are differences in sympathetic nervous system activity in animals with right or left cerebral dominance have not been determined.

Dopmaine levels have been found to differ in the nucleus accumbens of the two hemispheres of the brain in mice that express right or left paw preference (Cabib et al, 1995). However, no difference were found in regard to function of the HPA axis between right and left paw-preferenced animals (Betancur et al, 1992).

There is also variability between different strains of rodents (Neveu, 1993). Obviously, animal models of stressor-induced immune alteration have to be identified as to the sex and strain and paw preference. However, as discussed in Chapters 2 and 8, additional factors, such as the mother's experience of stressors during gestation, housing conditions (quite vs noisy; rough handling vs careful handling by animal caretakers; temperature control), shipping conditions if animals purchased from a supplier, can all have an influence on basal brain and immune function and therefore modulate the effect of stress on altering immune function.

An influence of cerebral asymmetry as manifested by right or left hand preference on immune function has been suggested in humans (Witelson, 1980; Geschwind and Behan, 1982, 1984; Pennington et al, 1987). However, not all studies have supported an association between handedness and immune function in humans (Meyers and Janowitz, 1985; McManus et al, 1990). There has also been the suggestion that some, but not all, autoimmune diseases are more common in left-handed individuals (McManus et al, 1993).

In humans, different immune function has been reported in association with brain asymmetry, which was defined by α power (8–13 Hz) on electroencephalographic (EEG) recording (Kang et al, 1991). The subjects were 20 healthy females college students, each having right-hand preference. The subjects with the highest right frontal activation had significantly lower NK cell function than that of subjects with the highest left frontal activation. No differences were detected in the response of lymphocytes to nonspecific mitogenic stimulation. The immune parameters were measured under baseline conditions, without the subjects being exposed to a stressor. Plasma cortisol and anxiety and depression-related symptomatology were the same for both groups.

Determination of the effect of stressor-induced changes on immune function in groups with differences in cerebral dominance was also determined (Liang et al,

1997). The subjects were right-handed males age 14–16. All subjects were exposed to a brief psychological stress task. An interaction between recent stress producing life events and right or left frontal brain asymmetry, determined by EEG, on immune function was determined. When exposed to the laboratory stress task, subjects with greater left frontal activation had an increase in lymphocyte mitogenic function and a decrease in NK function. Life events did not influence how a subject with right frontal activation responded to a laboratory stressor. These data suggest that the physiological characteristics of the brain, in addition to the stressors in an individual's environment, participate in determining whether an acute stressor will alter immune function.

We have studied several aspects of immune function in right- and left-handed normal individuals and in individuals with schizophrenia. Significantly more left-handed males, but not females, were found to have autoantibodies present in their serum. The amount of IL-2 released from lymphocytes, stimulated with nonspecific mitogen in vitro, was significantly lower in left-handed individuals. The mean serum concentration of IL-6 in left-handed individuals was significantly lower in left- than in right-handed individuals. However, we did not find an association between IL-2 production and the presence of autoantibodies (Chengappa et al, 1992a,b, 1994).

The cell communication and hormonal mechanisms responsible for the immune alterations associated with brain lesions and asymmetry are unknown. Whether endocrine hormone production is modified or whether the activity of the sympathetic nervous system innervating the bone marrow, thymus, and secondary lymphoid tissues is responsible for the immune effects has not been determined.

It is unlikely that every brain is anatomically the same. An analogy would be a baseball team. The anatomy of the catcher clearly differs from the anatomy of the short stop. Both players look different and function differently. With regard to the individuality of different parts of the brain, it may be expected that the size and shape of the locus coeruleus in different brains may influence their function and their impact on the immune system.

REFERENCES

Abercrombie ED, Jacobs BL. Single unit response of adrenergic neurons in locus coeruleus of freely moving cats. II. Adaptation to chronically presented stressful stimuli. Journal of Neuroscience. 7: 2844–2848, 1987.

Ackerman KD, Felten SY, Bellinger DL, Livnat S, Felten DL. Noradrenergic sympathetic innervation of spleen and lymph nodes in relation to specific cellular compartments. Progress in Immunology. 6: 588–600, 1987.

Alito AE, Carlomagno MA, Cardinali DP, Braun M. Effect of regional sympathetic denervation on local immune reactions. Federation Proceedings. 44: 564, 1985.

Alito AE, Romeo HB, Baler R, Chuluyan HE, Braun M, Cardinali DP. Autonomic nervous system regulation by local surgical sympathetic and parasympathetic denervation. Acta Physiology and Pharmacology, Latinoamerica. 37: 305–319, 1987.

Ansar AS, Penhale WJ, Talal N. Sex hormones, immune responses, and autoimmune diseases: Mechanism of sex hormone actions. American Journal of Pathology. 121: 531–551, 1985.

Antonica A, Magni F, Mearini L, Paolocci N. Vagal control of lymphocyte release from rat thymus. Journal of the Autonomic Nervous System. 48: 187–197, 1994.

Bachen EA, Manuck SB, Marsland AL, Cohen S, Malkoff SB, Muldoon MF, Rabin BS. Lymphocyte subsets and cellular immune responses to a brief experimental stressor. Psychosomatic Medicine. 54: 673–679, 1992.

Bachen EA, Manuck SB, Cohen S, Muldoon MF, Raibel R, Herbert TB, Rabin BS. Adrenergic blockade ameliorates cellular immune responses to mental stress in humans. Psychosomatic Medicine. 57: 366–372, 1995.

Banks WA, Kastin AJ, Broadwell RD. Passage of cytokines across the blood–brain barrier. Recent Progress in Neuroimmunomodulation. 2: 241–248, 1995.

Bardos P, Degenne D, Lebranchu Y, Biziere K, Renoux G. Neocortical lateralization of NK activity in mice. Journal of Scandanavian Immunology. 13: 609–611, 1981.

Basso AM, Depiantedepaoli M, Cancela L, Molina VA. Chronic restraint attenuates the immunosuppressive response induced by novel aversive stimuli. Physiology and Behavior. 55: 1151–1155, 1994.

Benschop RJ, Brosschot JF, Godaert GLR, DeSmet M, Geenen R, Olff M, Heijnen CJ, Ballieux RE. Chronic stress affects immunologic but not cardiovascular responsiveness to acute psychological stress in humans. American Journal of Physiology. 266: R75–80, 1994.

Bereknbosch F, Oers J, Del Rey A, Tilders F, Besedovsky H. Corticotropin-releasing factor in the rat activated by interleukin-1. Science. 238: 524–526, 1987.

Besedovsky HO, Sorkin E. Hormonal control of immune processes. Endocrinology. 2: 504–513, 1977a.

Besedovsky HO, Sorkin E. Network of immune–neuroendocrine interactions. Clinical and Experimental Immunology. 27: 1–12, 1977b.

Besedovsky H, Del Rey A, Sorkin E, Da Prada M, Keller HH. Immunoregulation mediated by the sympathetic nervous system. Cellular Immunology. 48: 346–355, 1979.

Besedovsky H, Del Rey A, Sorkin E, Dinarello CA. Immunoregulatory feedback between interleukin-1 and glucocorticoid hormones. Science. 233: 652–654, 1986.

Besedovsky HO, Del Rey A, Klusman I, Furukawa H, ArditiGM, Kabiersch A. Cytokines as modulators of the hypothalamus–pituitary–adrenal axis. Journal of Steroid Biochemistry and Molecular Biology. 40: 613–618, 1991.

Betancur C, Neveu PJ, Le Moal M. Strain and sex differences in the degree of paw preference in mice. Behavioural Brain Research. 45: 97–101, 1991.

Betancur C, Sandi C, Vitiello S, Borrell J, Guaza C, Neveu PJ. Activity of the hypothalamic–pituitary–adrenal axis in mice selected for left- or right-handedness. Brain Research. 589: 302–306, 1992.

Blomgren HM, Blom V, Ullen H. Relation between the site of primary intracranial tumors and mitogenic responses of blood lymphocytes. Cancer Immunology and Immunotherapy. 21: 31–38 1986.

Bluthe RM, Beaudu C, Kelley KW, Dantzer R. Differential effects of IL-1ra on sickness behavior and weight loss induced by IL-1 in rats. Brain Research. 677: 171–176, 1995.

Bluthe RM, Michaud B, Kelley KW, Dantzer R. Vagotomy attenuates behavioural effects of interleukin-1 injected peripherally but not centrally. Neuroreport. 7: 1485–1488, 1996.

Bluthe RM, Michaud B, Kelley KW, Dantzer R. Vagotomy blocks behavioural effects of interleukin-1 injected via the intraperitoneal route but not via other systemic routes. Neuroreport. 7: 2823–2827, 1996.

Bluthe RM, Dantzer R, Kelley KW. Central mediation of the effects of interleukin-1 on social exploration and body weight in mice. Psychoneuroendocrinology. 22: 1–11. 1997.

Bonomo A, Kehn PJ, Shevach EM. Premature escape of double-positive thymocytes to the periphery of young mice. Possible role in autoimmunity. Journal of Immunology. 152: 1509–1514, 1993.

Brodde OE, Daul A, Michel-Reher M, Boomsma F, Man in't Veld AJ, Schlieper P, Michel MC. Agonist-induced desensitization of beta-adrenoceptor function in humans. Subtype selective reduction in beta 1- beta-2-adrenoceptor mediated physiological effects by xamoterol or procaterol. Circulation. 81: 914–921, 1990.

Brodde OE, Michel-Reher M, Oefler D, Sarikouch S, Michel MC. Terbutaline-induced down-regulation of beta-2-adrenoceptors without Gi-protein alterations in human lymphocytes. Journal of Cardiovascular Pharmacology. 20: 785–789, 1992.

Brooks WH, Cross RJ, Roszman TL, Markesbery WR. Neuroimmunomodulation: Neural anatomical basis for impairmerment and facilitation. Annals of Neurology. 12: 56–61, 1982.

Brosschot JF, Benschop RJ, Godaert GLR, Olff M, DeSmet M, Heijnen CJ, Ballieux RE. Influence of life stress on immunological reactivity to mild psychological stress. Psychosomatic Medicine. 56: 216–224, 1994.

Cabib S, D'Amato FR, Neveu PJ, Deleplanque B, LeMoal M, Puglisi-Allegra S. Paw preferene and brain dopamine assymetries. Neuroscience. 64: 427–432, 1995.

Card JP, Rinaman L, Lynn RB, Meade RP, Miselis RR, Enquist LW. Pseudorabies virus infection of the rat central nervous system: Ultrastructural characterization of viral replication, transport, and pathogenesis. Journal of Neurosciences. 13: 2515–2539, 1993.

Chengappa KNR, Ganguli R, Ulrich R, Rabin BS, Cochran J, Brar JS, Yang ZW, Deleo M. The prevalence of autoantibodies among right and left handed schizophrenic patients and control subjects. Biological Psychiatry. 32: 803–811, 1992a.

Chengappa KNR, Ganguli R, Yang ZW, Schurin G, Cochran J, Brar JS, Rabin B. Non-right sidedness: An association with lower IL-2 production. Life Sciences. 51: 1843–1849, 1992b.

Chengappa KNR, Ganguli R, Yang ZW, Schurin G, Brar JS,Rosenbleet JA, Rabin BS. Differences in serum interleukin-6 (IL-6) between healthy dextral and non-dextral subjects. Neuroscience Research. 20: 185–188, 1994.

Chiang C, Aston-Jones G. Response of locus coeruleus neurons to footshock stimulation is mediated by neurons in the rostral ventral medulla. Neuroscience. 53: 705–715, 1993.

Chrousos GP. The hypothalamic–pituitary–adrenal axis and immune-mediated inflammation. New England Journal of Medicine. 332: 1351–1362, 1995.

Cohen S, Tyrrell DAJ, Smith AP. Psychological stress and susceptibility to the common cold. New England Journal of Medicine. 325: 606–612, 1991.

Conti LH, Foote SL. Effects of pretreatment with corticotropin-releasing factor on the electrophysiological responsivity of the locus coeruleus to subsequent corticotropin-releasing factor challenge. Neuroscience. 69: 209–219, 1995.

Crary B, Hauser SL, Borysenko M, Kutz I, Hoban C, Ault KA, Weiner HL, Benson H. Epinephrine induced changes in the distribution of lymphocyte subsets in peripheral blood of humans. Journal of Immunology. 131: 1178–1181, 1983.

Curtis AL, Pavcovich LA, Grigoriadis DE, Valentino RJ. Previous stress alters corticotropin-releasing factor neurotransmission in the locus coeruleus. Neuroscience. 65: 541–550, 1995.

Darko DF, Mitler MM, Henriksen SJ. Lentiviral infection, immune response peptides, and sleep. Advances in Neuroimmunology. 5: 57–77, 1995.

Darlington DN, Shinsako J, Dallman MF. Paraventricular lesions: Hormonal and cardiovascular responses to hemorrhage. Brain Research. 439: 289–301, 1988.

De Blasi, Maisel AS, Feldman RD, Ziegler MG, Fratelli M, DiLallo M, Dmith DA. In vivo regulation of beta-adrenergic receptors on human mononuclear leukocytes: Assessment of receptor number, location, and function after posture change, exercise, and isoproterenol infusion. Journal of Clinical Endocrinology and Metabolism. 63: 847–853, 1986.

deLeeuw FE, Jansen GH, Batanero E, van Wichen DF, Schuurman HJ. The neural and neuroendocrine component of the human thymus. I. Nerve-like structures. Brain, Behavior, and Immunity. 6: 234–248, 1992.

Durandy A, De Saint Basile G, Lisowska-Grospierre B, Gauchat JF, Forveille M, Kroczek RA, Bonnefoy FA. Undetectable CD40 ligand expression on T cells and low B cell responses to CD40 binding agonists in human newborns. Journal of Immunology. 154: 1560–1568, 1995.

Dygai AM, Gol'dberg ED, Shakhov VP, Ivasenko IN, Khlusov IA. Compensation-adaptation reactions of hemopoiesis-inducing microenvironment of bone marrow in stress. Gematologiia I Transfuziologiia. 37: 3–5, 1992.

Ennis M, Aston-Jones G, Shiekhattar R. Activation of locus coeruleus neurons by nucleus paragigantocellularis or noxious sensory stimulation is mediated by intracoerulear excitatiry amino acid neurotransmission. Brain Research. 598: 185–195, 1992.

Ernstrom U, Gafvelin G, Mutt V. Rescue of thymocytes from cell death by vasoactive intestinal peptide. Regulatory Peptides. 57: 99–104, 1995.

Esquifino AI, Cardinali DP. Local regulation of the immune response by the autonomic nervous system. Neuroimmunomodulation. 1: 265–273, 1994.

Felten DL, Felten SY, Bellinger DL, Carlson SL, Ackerman KD, Madden KS, Olschowki JA, Livnat S. Noradrenergic sympathetic neural interactions with the immune system: Structure and function. Immunological Reviews. 100: 225–260, 1987.

Felten SY, Olschowka J. Noradrenergic sympathetic innervation of the spleen. II. Tyrosine hydroxylase (TH) positive nerve terminals form synaptic contacts on lymphocytes in the splenic white pulp. Journal of Neuroscience Research. 18: 37–44, 1987.

Geschwind N, Behan P. Left handedness: Association with immune disease, migraine and developmental learning disorders. Proceedings of the National Academy of Science USA. 79: 5097–5100, 1982.

Geschwind N, Behan PO. Laterality, hormones and immunity. In Cerebral Dominance: The Biological Foundations. Geschwind N, Galaburda AM (eds). Harvard University Press, Cambridge, pp 211–224, 1984.

Glaser R, Kiecolt-Glaser J, Bonneau R, Malarkey W, Kennedy S, Hughes J. Stress-induced modulation of the immune response to recombinant hepatitis B vaccine. Psychosomatic Medicine. 54: 22–29, 1992.

Goehler LE, Busch CR, Tartaglia N, Relton J, Sisk D, Maier SF, Watkins LR. Blockade of cytokine induced conditioned taste aversion by subdiaphragmatic vagotomy: Further evidence for vagal mediation of immune-brain communication. Neuroscience Letters. 185: 163–166, 1995.

Gol'dberg ED, Dygai AM, Shakhov VP, Bogdashin IV, Mikhlenko AV. Lymphocytic mechanisms of myelopoiesis regulation under stress. Biomedical Science. 1: 366–372, 1990.

Gould E, Tanapat P, McEwen BS, Flugge G, Fuchs E. Proliferation of granule cell precursors in the dentate gyrus of adult monkeys is diminishes by stress. Proceedings of the National Academy of Sciences USA. 95: 3168–3171, 1998.

Gresch PJ, Sved AF, Zigmond MJ, Finlay JM. Stress-induced sensitazation of dopmaine and norepinephrine efflux in medial prefrontal cortex of the rat. Journal of Neurochemistry. 63: 575–583, 1984.

Hall NR, McClure JE, Hu S, Tare NS, Seals CM, Goldstein AL. Effects of 6-hydroxydopamine upon primary and secondary thymus dependent immune responses. Immunopharmacology. 5: 39–48, 1982.

Harbuz MS, Lightman SL. Stress and the hypothalamo–pituitary–adrenal axis: Acute, chronic and immunological activation. Journal of Endocrinology. 134: 327–339, 1992.

Herbert TB, Cohen S. Stress and immunity in humans: A meta-analytic review. Psychosomatic Medicine. 55: 364–379, 1993.

Hori T, Katafuchi T, Take S, Shimizu N, Niijima A. The autonomic nervous system as a communication channel between the brain and the immune system. Neuroimmunomodulation. 2: 203–215, 1995.

Hwang S, Harris TJ, Wilson NW, Maisel AS. Immune function in patients with chronic stable congestive heart failure. American Heart Journal. 125: 1651–1658, 1993.

Juzwa W, Gnacinska G, Rawicz-Zegrzda I, Kaczmarek J. Modulation of cellular immunity by a lesion of the lateral hypothalamic area (LHA) in rats. Experimental and Toxicologic Pathology. 47: 403–408, 1995.

Kang DH, Davidson RJ, Coe CL, Wheeler RE, Tomarken AJ, Ershler WB. Frontal brain asymmetry and immune function. Behavioral Neuroscience. 105: 860–869, 1991.

Kapcala LP, Chautard T, Eskay RL. The protective role of the hypothalamic–pituitary–adrenal axis against lethality produced by immune, infectious, and inflammatory stress. Annals of the New York Academy of Sciences. 771: 419–437, 1995.

Kasahara K, Tanaka S, Ito T, Hamashima Y. Suppression of the primary response by chemical sympathectomy. Research Communications in Chemical and Pathological Pharmacology. 16: 687–694 1977.

Kato K, Hamada N, Mizukoshi N, Yamamoto KI, Kimura T, Ishihara C, Fujioka Y, Kato K, Fujieda K, Matsuura N. Depression of delayed-type hyperesnsitivity in mice with hypothalamic lesion induced by monosodium glutamate: Involvement of neuroendocrine system in immunomodulation. Immunology. 58: 389–395, 1986.

Keinanen K, Wisdon W, Sommer B, Werner P, Herb A, Verdoorn TA, Sakmann B, Seeburg PH. A family of AMPA selective glutamate receptors. Science. 249: 556–560, 1990.

Kendall MD, Al-Shawaf AA. Innervation of the rat thymus gland. Brain, Behavior, and Immunity. 5: 9–28, 1991.

Khan MM, Sansoni P, Silverman ED, Engleman EG, Melmon KL. Beta-adrenergic receptors on human suppressor, helper, and cytolytic lymphocytes. Biochemical Pharmacology. 35: 1137–1142, 1986.

Khlusov IA, Dygai AM, Gol'dberg ED. The adrenergic regulation of interleukin production by bone marrow cells during immobilization stress. Biulleten Eksperimentalnoi Biologii I Meditsiny. 116: 570–572, 1993.

Kluger MJ, Kozak W, Leon LR, Soszynski D, Conn CA. Cytokines and fever. Recent Progress in Neuroimmunomodulation. 2: 216–223, 1995.

Konarska M, Stewart RE, McCarty R. Sensitization of sympathetic-adrenal responses to a novel stressor in chronically stressed laboratory rats. Physiology and Behavior. 46: 129–135, 1989.

Kruger JM, Majde JA. Cytokines and sleep. International Archives of Allergy and Applied Immunology. 106: 97–100, 1995.

Kvetnansky R, Fukuhara K, Pacak K, Cizza G, Goldstein DS, Kopin IJ. Endogenous glucocorticoids restrain catecholamine synthesis and release at rest and during immobilization stress in rats. Endocrinology. 133: 1411–1419, 1993.

Lesnikov VA, Korneva EA, Dall'ara A, Pierpaoli W. The involvement of pineal gland and melatonin in immunity and aging. II. Thyrotropin-releasing hormone and melatonin forestall involution and promote reconstitution of the thymus in anterior hypothalamic area (AHA)-lesioned mice. International Journal of Neuroscience. 62: 141–153, 1992.

Liang SW, Jemerin JM, Tschann JM, Wara DW, Boyce WT. Life events, frontal electroencephalogram laterality, and immune status after acute psychological stressors in adolescents. Psychosomatic Medicine. 59: 178–186, 1997.

Livnat S, Felten SY, Carlson SL, Bellinger DL, Felten DL. Involvement of peripheral and central catecholamine systems in neural–immune interactions. Journal of Neuroimmunology. 10: 5–30, 1985.

Loewy AD. Forebrain nuclei involved in autonomic control. Progress in Brain Research. 87: 253–268, 1991.

Luheshi G, Rothwell N. Cytokines and fever. International Archives of Allergy and Applied Immunology. 109: 301–307, 1996.

Lupien SJ, de Leon M, de Santi S, Convit A, Tarshish C, Nair NPV, Thakur M, McEwen BS, Hauger RL, Meaney MJ. Cortisol levels during human aging predict hippocampal atrophy and memory deficits. Nature Neuroscience. 1: 69–73, 1998.

Madden KS, Felten SY, Felten DL, Sundarsan PR, Livnat S. Sympathetic neural modulation of the immune system. I. Depression of T cell immunity in vivo and in vitro following chemical sympathectomy. Brain, Behavior, and Immunity. 3: 72–89, 1989.

Maisel AS, Fowler P, Rearden A, Motulsky HJ, Michel MC. A new method for isolation of human lymphocyte subsets reveals differential regulation of beta-adrenergic receptors by terbutaline treatment. Clinical Pharmacology and Therapeutics. 46: 429–439, 1989.

Maisel AS, Murray D, Lotz M, Rearden A, Irwin M, Michel MC. Propranolol treatment affects parameters of human immunity. Immunopharmacology. 22: 157–164, 1991.

Manuck SB, Cohen S, Rabin BS, Muldoon MF, Bachen EA. Individual differences in cellular immune responses to stress. Psychological Science. 2: 1–5, 1991.

Marty J, Nimier M, Rocchiccoli C, Mantz J, Luscombe F, Henzel D, Loiseau A, Desmonts JM. Beta-adrenergic receptor function is acutely altered in surgical patients. Anesthesia and Analgesia. 71: 1–8, 1990.

McKean DJ, Huntoon C, Bell M. Ligand induced desensitization of interleukin 1 receptor-initiated intracellular signaling events in T helper lymphocytes. Journal of Experimental Medicine. 180: 1321–1328, 1994.

McManus IC, Naylor J, Brooker BL. Left-handedness and myasthenia gravis. Neuropsychologia. 28: 947–955, 1990.

McManus IC, Bryden MP, Bulman-Fleming MB. Handedness and autoimmune disease. Lancet. 341: 891–892, 1993.

Meyers S, Janowitz HD. Left-handedness in inflammatory bowel disease. Clinical Gastroenterology. 7: 33–35, 1985.

Montkowski A, Landgraf R, Yassouridis A, Holsboer F, Schobitz B. Central administration of

IL-1 reduces anxiety and induced sickness behavior in rats. Pharmacology, Biochemistry, and Behavior. 58: 329–336, 1997.

Morris JF, Hoyer JT, Pierce SK. Antigen presentation for T cell interleukin-2 secretion is a late acquisition of neonatal B cells. European Journal of Immunology. 22: 2923–2928, 1992.

Muller S, Weihe E. Interrelation of peptidergic innervation with mast cells and ED-1 positive cells in rat thymus. Brain, Behavior, and Immunity. 5: 55–72, 1991.

Munck A, Guyre PM, Holbrook NJ. Physiological functions of glucocorticoids in stress and their relation to pharmacological actions. Endocrine Reviews. 5: 25–44, 1984.

Naliboff BD, Benton D, Solomon GF, Morley JE, Fahey JL, Bloom ET, Makinodan T, Gilmore SL. Immunological changes in young and old adults during brief laboratory stress. Psychosomatic Medicine. 53: 121–132, 1991.

Nance DM, Rayson D, Carr RI. The effect of lesions in the lateral septal and hippocampal areas on the humoral immune response of adult female rats. Brain, Behavior, and Immunity. 1: 292–305, 1987.

Neveu P, Taghzouti K, Dantzer R, Simon H, Le Moal M. Modulation of mitogen induced lymphoproliferation by cerebral neocortex. Life Sciences. 38: 1907–1913, 1986.

Neveu PJ. Brain lateralization and immunomodulation. International Journal of Neuroscience. 70: 135–143, 1993.

Neveu PJ, Moya S. In the mouse, the corticoid response depends on lateralization. Brain Research. 749: 344–346, 1997.

Nissenbaum LK, Zigmond MJ, Sved AF, Abercrombie ED. Prior exposure to chronic stress results in enhanced synthesis and release of hippocampal norepinephrine in response to a novel stressor. Journal of Neuroscience. 11: 1478–1484, 1991.

Nohr D, Weihe E. The neuroimmune link in the bronchus-associated lymphoid tissue (BALT) of cat and rat: Peptides and neural markers. Brain, Behavior, and Immunity. 5: 84–101, 1991.

Pascual VH, Oparil S, Eldridge JH, Jin H, Bost KL, Pascual DW. Spontaneously hypertensive rat: Lymphoid depression is age dependent and mediated via a mononuclear cell population. American Journal of Physiology. 262: R1–7, 1992.

Pennington BF, Smith SD, Kimberling WJ, Green PA, Haith MM. Left-handedness and immune disorders in familial dyslexics. Archives of Neurology. 44: 434–439, 1987.

Pezzone MA, Lee WS, Hoffman GE, Rabin BS. Induction of c-Fos immunoreactivity in the rat forebrain by conditioned and unconditioned aversive stimuli. Brain Research. 597: 41–50, 1992.

Pezzone MA, Lee WS, Hoffman GE, Pezzone KM, Rabin BS. Activation of brainstem catecholaminergic neurons by conditioned and unconditioned aversive stimuli as revealed by c-Fos immunoreactivity. Brain Research. 608: 310–318, 1993.

Pezzone MA, Dohanics J, Rabin BS. Effects of footshock stress upon spleen and peripheral blood lymphocyte mitogenic responses in rats with lesions of the paraventricular nuclei. Journal of Neuroimmunology. 53: 39–46, 1994.

Pike JL, Smith TL, Hauger RL, Nicassio PM, Patterson TL, McClintick BS, Costlow C, Irwin MR. Chronic life stress alters sympathetic, neuroendocrine, and immune responsivity to an acute psychological stressor in humans. Psychosomatic Medicine. 59: 447–457, 1997.

Propes MJ, Johnson RW. Role of corticosterone in the behavioral effects of central interleukin-1 beta. Physiology and Behavior. 61: 7–13, 1997.

Rassnick S, Sved AF, Rabin BS. Locus coeruleus stimulation by corticotropin-releasing hormone suppresses in vitro cellular immune responses. Journal of Neuroscience. 14: 6033–6040, 1994.

Reichlin S. Neuroendocrine–immune interactions. New England Journal of Medicine. 329: 1246–1253, 1993.

Renoux G, Biziere K, Renoux M, Guillaumin JM, Degenne D. A balanced brain asymmetry modulates T cell mediated events. Journal of Neuroimmunology. 5: 227–238, 1983.

Saphier D, Abramsky O, Mor G, Ovadia H. Multiunit electrical activity in conscious rats during an immune response. Brain, Behavior, and Immunity. 1: 40–51, 1987.

Sauer J, Stalla GK, Muller OA, Arzt E. Inhibition of interleukin-2 mediated lymphocyte activation in patients with Cushing's syndrome: A comparison with hypocortisolemic patients. Neuroendocrinology. 59: 144–151, 1994.

Scollay R, Godfrey DI. Thymic emigration: Conveyor belts or lucky dips? Immunology Today. 16: 268–273, 1995.

Seeman TE, McEwen BS, Singer BH, Albert MS, Rowe JW. Increase in urinary cortisol excretion and memory declines: MacArthur studies of successful aging. Journal of Clinical Endocrinology and Metabolism. 82: 2458–2465, 1997.

Segreti J, Gheusi G, Dantzer R, Kelley KW, Johnson RW. Defect in interleukin-1beta secretion prevents sickness behavior in C3H/HeJ mice. Physiology and Behavior. 61: 873–878, 1997.

Sharp BM, Matta SG, Peterson PK, Newton R, Chao C, Mcallen K. Tumor necrosis factor-alpha is a potent secretagogue: Comparison to interleukin-1-beta. Endocrinology. 124: 3131–3133, 1989.

Shimizu N, Hori T, Nakane H. An interleukin 1b-induced noradrenaline release in the spleen is mediated by brain corticotropin releasing factor: An in vivo microdialysis study in conscious rats. Brain, Behavior, and Immunity. 7: 14–23, 1994.

Singh U. Effect of catecholamines on lymphopoiesis in fetal mouse thymic explants. Journal of Anatomy. 129: 279–292, 1979.

Smiley RM, Vulliemoz Y. Cardiac surgery causes desensitization of the beta-adrenergic receptor system of human lymphocytes. Anesthesia and Analgesia. 74: 212–218, 1992.

Spencer RL, Miller AH, Moday H, McEwen BS, Blanchard RJ, Blanchard DC, Sakai RR. Chronic social stress produces reductions in available splenic type II corticoidreceptor binding and plasma corticosteroid binding globulin levels. Psychoneuroendocrinology. 21: 95–109, 1996.

Strack AM, Sawyer AB, Hughes JH, Platt KB, Loewy AD. A general pattern of CNS innervation of the sympathetic outflow demonstrated by transneuronal pseudorabies viral infections. Brain Research. 491: 156–162, 1989.

Takahashi S, Kapas L, Fang JD, Seyer JM, Wang Y, Krueger JM. An interleukin-1 receptor fragment inhibits spontaneous sleep and muramyl dipeptide-induced sleep in rabbits. American Journal of Physiology. 271: R101–R108, 1996.

Tseilikman VE, Volchegorskii IA, Kolesnikova OL, Gienko IA, Viazovskii IA, Lifshits RI. The formation of blood system tolerance in rats to the repeated action of a stressor stimulus. Fiziologicheskii Zhurnal Imeni I M Sechenova. 81: 88–94, 1995.

VanBockstaele EJ, Akaoka H, Aston-Jones G. Brainstem afferents to the rostral nucleus paragigantocellularis: Integration of exteroceptive and interoceptive sensory inputs in the ventral tegmentum. Brain Research. 603: 1–18, 1993.

van Tits LJH, Michel MC, Wilde H, Happel M, Eigler FW, Soleman A, Brodde OE. Catecholamines increase lymphocyte beta-2-adrenergic receptors via a beta-2-adrenergic, spleen dependent process. American Journal of Physiology. E. 258: 191–201, 1990.

Vgontzas AN, Papanicolaou DA, Bixler EO, Kales A, Tyson K, Chrousos GP. Elevation of plasma cytokines in disorders of excessive daytime sleepiness: role of sleep disturbance and obesity. Journal of Clinical Endocrinology & Metabolism. 82: 1313–1316, 1997.

Vizi ES, Orso E, Osipenko ON, Hasko G, Elenkov IJ. Neurochemical, electrophysiological and immunocytochemical evidence for a noradrenergic link between the sympathetic nervous system and thymocytes. Neuroscience. 68: 1263–1276, 1995.

Wan W, Vriend CY, Wetmore L, Gartner JG, Greenberg AH, Nance DM. The effects of stress on splenic immune function are mediated by the splenic nerve. Brain Research Bulletin. 30: 101–105, 1993.

Watanoabe H, Sasaki S, Takebe K. Involvement of oxytocin and cholecystokinin-8 in interleukin-1 beta-induced adrenocorticotropin secretion in the rat. Neuroimmunomodulation. 2: 88–91, 1995.

Watanabe Y, Stone E, McEwen BS. Induction and habituation of c-fos and zif/268 by acute and repeated stressors. Neuroreport. 5: 1321–1324, 1994.

Weber RJ, Pert A. The periaqueductal gray matter mediates opiate-induced immunosuppression. Science. 245: 188–190, 1989.

Wenner M, Kawamura N, Miyazawa H, Ago Y, Ishikawa T, Yamamoto H. Acute electrical stimulation of lateral hypothalamus increases natural killer cell activity in rats. Journal of Neuroimmunology. 67: 67–70, 1996.

Wetmore L, Nance DM. Differential and sex-specific effects of kainic acid and domoic acid lesions in the lateral septal area of rats on immune function and body weight regulation. Experimental Neurology. 113: 226–236, 1991.

Williams JM, Peterson RG, Shea PA, Schmedtje JF, Bauer DC, Felten DL. Sympathetic innervation of murine thymus and spleen: Evidence for a functional link between the nervous and immune systems. Brain Research Bulletin. 6: 83–94, 1981.

Witelson SF. Neuroanatomical asymmetry in left-handers: A review and implications for functional asymmetry. In Neuropsychology of Left-Handedness. Herron J (ed). Academic Press, New York, pp 79–113, 1980.

Wrona D, Jurkowski MK, Trojniar W, Staszewska M, Tokarski J. Electrolytic lesions of the lateral hypothalamus influence peripheral blood NK cytotoxicity in rats. Journal of Neuroimmunology. 55: 45–54, 1994.

4

The Study of Stress and Immunity

This chapter will present studies that use both laboratory stressors delivered as part of an experimental protocol and stress encountered within the daily activities of an individual's life, in an effort to identify components of the immune system that are susceptible to alteration by stress.

There are a number of concerns that you should be aware of regarding the interpretation of the studies that will be reported. The concerns relate to parameters that influence an individual subjects responsiveness to a stressor. Consideration needs to be directed to:

1. Prior stressors experienced by subjects in animal studies, including noise in the animal room, temperature extremes when housed, shipping conditions if the animals were shipped from a breeder, and disturbed sleep patterns

2. Innate characteristics of the subject, including strain, species, age, and sex of an experimental animal and age and sex of a human subject

3. Coping skills of a human subject

4. Physical fitness of the subject

5. Characteristics of the stressor, including the intensity and duration of the stressor

6. Whether the stress is of an acute nature or a chronic nature

7. How acute and chronic stressors are defined in subjects with different intensities and durations of daily stressors in their lives and in individuals who have different coping skills

As described in Chapter 2, the immune system consists of multiple components that interact to produce responses that eliminate infectious disease-causing organisms. Stress changes many of the quantitative and qualitative aspects of the immune system. In evaluating the effect of stress on immune function, it is important to remember that a stressor-induced change in a component of the immune system must be interpreted only within the context of the study. For example, a stressor-induced change in the numbers of CD4 or CD8 cells can be determined by flow cytometry (see Chapter 2). Going beyond this presentation of the data will lead to speculation that cannot be supported. For example, does an increase of CD8 cells alter susceptibility to infectious disease? No one knows! Biological interpretations should not be determined from alterations of numbers of lymphocyte subpopulations.

Another question relates to whether the stressor-induced changes produce (1) statistical, or (2) functional abnormalities of immune function. Statistical abnormalities are easy to detect. However, statistics use normal populations to establish the upper and lower limits of normality. Such factors as race, age, sex, diet, and health influence immune measures in a "normal" population. "Normal" statistical ranges that can be applied to specific populations are very difficult to obtain for immune parameters. Even obtaining blood specimens from "normal" individuals to determine normal statistical ranges is difficult.

As the director of a large clinical immunology laboratory that provides testing to a major university medical center, this is a problem that I have to deal with on a constant basis. Thus, imprecision can be introduced when collecting data from experimental subjects and comparing the data with a "normal" population, unless the normal population is accurately matched to the subjects. This is a luxury that is usually not available.

Stressor-induced change of an immune parameter within a subject can be measured. This allows alterations of immune function to be measured without referral to a normal value. Interestingly—and importantly—stressor-induced immune changes in humans do not alter any immune functions, so that the immune function no longer lies within "the normal range." However, even if stress were able to produce changes outside the "normal" statistical range, the function might still be adequate for resistance to infectious or other immune-mediated disease.

Functional implications for stressor-induced immune alterations are difficult to characterize. For example, as discussed in Chapter 1, the normal concentration of IgG in an adult is approximately 1,000 mg/dl. Two standard deviations (2 SD) below the mean is approximately 600 mg/dl. If a subject has an IgG concentration of 300 mg/dl, which is markedly below the lower limits of the normal range, it may be assumed that clinical problems associated with the abnormally low IgG level will occur. However, there is a marked difference between the statistical abnormality and the physiological concentration of IgG, which is needed to protect an individual from becoming infected with bacteria. A concentration of 200 mg/dl of IgG is adequate to protect against infectious diseases.

Lymphocyte function tests also have significant difficulties in regard to their interpretation. I don't know what the difference between counts per minute (cpm) of 100,000 and 300,000 (see Chapter 2 for a description of lymphocyte mitogenic stimulation test) in a lymphocyte mitogenic response to phytohemagglutinin (PHA) means. I know that if there are 10,000 cpm, there is a functional defect of T cells. However, counts greater than 50,000, even though below the normal statistical range, are difficult to interpret with regard to whether there is an associated altered susceptibility to disease.

It is not known whether multiple abnormalities of immune function act additively or synergistically to alter susceptibility to immune mediated disease. If a stressor alters more than one immune function, even though each immune function by itself may not alter disease susceptibility, there may be increased disease susceptibility, possibly even if each immune parameter were not moved out of the normal range.

There are no studies in the stress literature that have performed comprehensive evaluations of the changes in all the immune parameters produced by stress. Even if these studies had been performed, their interpretation would be difficult with regard to determining whether there would be an influence on the changes of susceptibility to disease.

There is also a sampling problem in humans. The only immune compartment easily obtained and studied is the blood. This excludes the entire mucosal immune system, lymphocytes within parenchymal tissues, lymph nodes, and the spleen. The only blood cells that are sampled are those that are not adherent to the endothelial cells. This sampling situation would not be significant if all immune compartments were to experience the same stressor-induced immune changes. However, this is not likely to be the case (Cunnick et al, 1988). Studies in rats have suggested that different hormonal systems may be involved in altering of lymphocyte function in different lymphoid compartments and that different populations of lymphocytes may be altered by different hormones.

The only immune parameters that can be measured that are reflective of a summation of the activity of all the immune compartments for either humoral or cellular immunity is the amount of serum antibody to an antigen and delayed hypersensitivity skin test reactivity.

Immunization with an antigen and quantitating the serum antibody to the antigen would provide an indication of the function of several components of the immune system. Indeed, the amount of antibody produced in response to immunization is decreased when subjects experiencing higher versus lower levels of stress are studied (Glaser et al, 1992; Kiecolt-Glaser et al, 1996). However, the reason for the decreased total amount of antibody has not yet been determined. Possibilities include one, several, or all of the following: antigen uptake, antigen degradation, antigen presentation, CD4–dendritic cell interaction, CD4–B-cell interaction, cytokine production, or costimulatory molecule interaction.

Another possible effect on antibody production, other than the total amount of IgG produced, is an alteration of the subtypes of IgG produced. Cytokines produced by CD4 Th1 lymphocytes stimulate B lymphocytes to produce IgG1, IgG2, and IgG3, while cytokines produced by CD4 Th2 lymphocytes stimulate production of IgG4. Because IgG4 does not activate the complement system, a decrease of the complement activating subtypes and an increase of IgG4 would decrease resistance to bacterial infection.

There are several approaches to determining the effect of stress on delayed hypersensitivity responsiveness. Chemical substances can be applied to the skin to induce activation of cellular immunity. Reapplication of the chemical will elicit a delayed hypersensitivity reaction if the delayed skin-test reaction is intact. The use of a chemical allows the time of sensitization to be controlled, hence the effect of stress on either sensitization or the effector phase of the delayed hypersensitivity reaction to be evaluated. A second approach is to challenge an individual with several antigens present in the environment and to which sensitization should have occurred as a result of environmental exposure. Testing with recall antigens requires evaluation of the response to several antigens (usually five to six) to be certain of including at least one antigen that the subject is sensitized to.

As already suggested, not every experimental subject—whether human or animal—will respond to stress with the same immunological alterations. Before presenting studies of stressor-induced immune alteration, some of the factors that may contribute to individual differences will be discussed.

HLA AND THE IMMUNE RESPONSE

Chapter 2 discussed the major histocompatibility complex (MHC) molecules and their role in antigen presentation. Unless an antigenic peptide can fit into the groove of an HLA molecule, the peptide cannot be presented to T lymphocytes for initiation of the immune response. However, there may be another influence of HLA on the immune system with individuals who are HLA-B8 and/or DR3 positive having different immune function than individuals who do not possess these HLA molecules. In the United States, approximately 16% of the population is HLA-B8, 21% HLA-DR3, and 10% HLA-B8/DR3.

Differences between HLA-B8 and/or DR3-positive individuals and those who do not possess these antigens include:

1. A decreased total lymphocyte number and increased spontaneous apoptosis is found in normal individuals who are positive for both HLA markers (Caruso et al, 1997). The percentage of each lymphocyte subpopulation was the same in all groups regardless of HLA indicating that the decreased number of lymphocytes was due to a decrease of all subsets. The investigators hypothesize that an increased rate of spontaneous apoptosis was responsible for the decreased lymphocyte numbers.

2. The response of lymphocytes to the nonspecific mitogen PHA is significantly lower in HLA-B8 and/or DR3-positive individuals than in those who possess neither HLA marker. There are no significant differences between those subjects possessing both HLA markers or one of them (Amer et al, 1986).

3. Production of IL-1 and IL-2 by peripheral blood mononuclear cells upon stimulation with PHA is significantly lower in normal subjects who are HLA-B8 or DR3 positive, or both (Hashimoto et al, 1989, 1990). It is possible that this is a partial explanation for the reduced proliferative response to PHA.

Interestingly, there is an increased frequency of the HLA B8 and DR3 antigens in patients with some autoimmune diseases (eg, Graves' disease, myasthenia gravis, insulin-dependent diabetes mellitus [IDDM], and systemic lupus erythematosus [SLE]). The obvious question relates to whether individuals who have reduced immune function due to the presence of these HLA antigens will then have a further reduction of immune function by stress that will significantly increase their susceptibility to a viral infection that then initiates an autoimmune disease. For our purpose, the concern is in regard to whether individuals who are HLA-B8 or HLA-DR3 positive, or positive for both, have a different response to stressor-induced immune alteration than do those who do not possess one or both of these HLA antigens. Unfortunately, no data are available to make this determination.

PERSONALITY, STRESS HORMONES, AND THE IMMUNE SYSTEM

Behavioral characteristics in individuals may influence their hormonal or immune response to stress. To put it another way, hormonal responses to stress within individuals may influence behavioral characteristics.

I am suggesting the possibility that characteristics of the hormonal response to stress will be associated with different personality characteristics. For example, studies have shown that individuals who view themselves as not being attractive to others and as having low self-esteem and frequent depression have a different cortisol response to a repetitive stressor than that of individuals who view themselves as attractive, who have high self-esteem, and who are rarely depressed (Kirschbaum et al, 1995). Individuals who fall within the first category have large cortisol increases when exposed to the same psychological stressor on each of 5 consecutive days. The second group of individuals have an increased cortisol response the first day they experience the stressor (which had a lower maximum concentration than the other group), followed by only a slight elevation on all subsequent days. Is this a chicken and egg situation? Does the characteristic of the hormonal response influence personality, or does personality influence the hormonal response?

Baseline cortisol concentrations have been reported to differ in individuals with different personality characteristics. Those who experience more anxiety and distress have higher baseline cortisol levels than the levels in individuals who do not have these traits (Kagan et al, 1988; Bell et al, 1993). Individuals who repress anxiety or who experience high levels of anxiety have higher baseline cortisol levels than those of individuals who experience low levels of anxiety (Brown et al, 1996).

Interestingly, baseline cortisol levels can influence stressor-induced immune alterations. Individuals with higher cortisol levels will have more glucocorticoid receptors occupied than will individuals with low cortisol levels. A stressor-induced increase in cortisol will have fewer glucocorticoid receptors to bind to in individuals with higher baseline cortisol levels and would be expected to have less of an immune alteration caused by stress.

Stress hormones may show variable changes in response to stress. In one of our studies, subjects were exposed to a psychological stressor. Some of the individuals exhibited elevations of norepinephrine and epinephrine, elevation of heart rate and systolic blood pressure, and alteration of some immune parameters (Manuck et al, 1991). Other individuals did not have the biochemical, physiological, or immune alterations. An explanation for the differences has not been determined. However, the data indicate that the uniqueness of an individual response to stress must be experimentally determined rather than assuming that a particular individual will have a characteristic response to any given stressor.

Children have been studied and characterized as having personality characteristics of being very inhibited or very uninhibited. The inhibited children were found to have higher baseline heart rates and higher heart rates when stressed (Kagan et al, 1988) and higher levels of catecholamines (Kagan et al, 1987). What happens to their immune systems when they are stressed? The concentration of catecholamine receptors changes when lymphocytes are exposed to high concentrations of catecholamines. Therefore, it may be hypothesized that greater stress-induced immune system changes will be found in individuals with lower resting baseline catecholamine concentrations. Indeed, there are experimental data to support this likelihood (Mills et al, 1995).

Children who display higher levels of cortisol in the morning have been found to display behaviors suggestive of an increased fearfulness manifested as shyness (Schmidt et al, 1997). A study of children beginning a school year found some children to maintain high cortisol levels after the initial settling-in period and in others whose cortisol levels became lower once familiarity with the environment developed (Gunnar et al, 1997). Those whose cortisol levels decreased were outgoing, more competent and well-liked in comparison with the other children who were solitary and who had a negative affect. Although I cannot be unequivocally certain, assume that these children will grow to be adults and will have behaviors and immune functions that differ from other adults based on these findings when they were children. This will create a mixed population of subjects when studies of stressor-induced immune alteration are conducted. Variability of results from studies of stressor-induced immune alteration may be related to a variety of undetermined factors, such as the one just described, which are not definable at the time human studies are performed.

In a study of monkeys, our research group found that when monkeys were stressed by living in an unstable housing condition, the lymphocytes of monkeys that had the characteristic of affiliating with other monkeys had greater responsiveness to nonspecific mitogenic stimulation than did lymphocytes from monkeys that did not affiliate with other monkeys (Kaplan et al, 1991). However, affiliation was only important as a modifier of lymphocyte function in monkeys that were low in aggressive characteristics. Interestingly, natural killer (NK) cell activity was highest in affiliative monkeys, regardless of whether they were aggressive. Hormone measurements were not performed. However, the data raise the question of whether the personality characteristics of affiliation and aggression can influence the effect of stress on immune function. Studies of stressor-induced immune alteration do not take these behavioral characteristics into consideration.

Monkey studies have also indicated that social rank may be a factor in increased risk of infection. Using experimental infection of monkeys with a virus that induces a "common cold," monkeys of the lowest social rank had a significantly greater likelihood of being infected (Cohen et al, 1997). This finding suggests a less efficient immune system. Whether there is a hormonal basis that contributes to behavioral patterns that promote dominance or submissiveness and, in addition, contribute to the regulation of the function of the immune system, has not been determined. Clearly, many of the cited studies raise the question regarding whether some patterns of behavior are associated with particular neurohormonal environments that are capable of regulating immune function.

Behavior can be developed in experimental animals by selective breeding of animals with specific behavioral characteristics. Two populations of rats that differed in their behavior after receiving an electric shock to their tails were established (Scott et al, 1996). The two groups were then studied for differences in several CNS activities. Differences were found in the electrical activity and catecholamine content and metabolism in the locus coeruleus and parts of the hypothalamus. Unfortunately, no immune studies or studies of stressor-induced immune function were performed. However, the study suggests a possible genetic regulatory mechanism over CNS function with a possible associated effect on behavior.

Differences in immune function and susceptibility to experimentally induced autoimmune disease have been associated with different functional activities of the HPA axis. The National Institutes of Health (NIH)-derived strain of Lewis rats (LEW/N) is highly susceptible to the development of experimentally induced autoimmune disease. The Fischer strain of rats from which the LEW/N were derived is resistant to autoimmune disease development. The LEW/N rats have decreased activity of the HPA axis in comparison with the Fischer rats (Derijk and Sternberg, 1994). As corticosterone participates in down regulation of the immune and inflammatory response, increased immune and inflammatory activity would be anticipated in the LEW/N rat. Thus, this data supports the likelihood that differences within the function of the CNS are likely to be associated with differences in immune function and possibly, the course of immune mediated disease.

Another interesting question is whether an individual has to be aware of their being stressed for physiological changes to occur. For fun, I performed the color-word confounding stress task (Stroop test) that is used in many of our research studies. I did the test and never felt stressed, as I knew all aspects of the procedure and was not doing it for anything other than to gain an understanding of the procedure. To my surprise, both my heart rate and systolic blood pressure increased. This makes one wonder whether the brain can react to a stressor without the individual perceiving that something is activating the brain. This is likely to occur, as changes in cerebral blood flow have been found when subjects experience a change in a learned procedure but are not aware of the change (Berns et al, 1997). Blood flow decreased in the prefrontal cortex (associated with abstract thinking, decision making, and social behavior) and parietal areas (involved with the appreciation of spatial relationships and initiation of movement). If changes in CNS function and physiological activities can occur without awareness that events in one's environment are inducing such change, self-report information that one is currently experiencing, or not experiencing, a situation that is a stressor will not be entirely reliable and will introduce another source of variability into studies of stressor-induced immune alteration. The individual may not consciously perceive a situation as being stressful, but the brain may be reacting to the situation.

Clearly, the study of stressor-induced immune alterations is complex. Variability in the function of the HPA axis, the association of different behavioral characteristics with differences in CNS activities, as well as not knowing how meaningful a stressor is to an experimental subject introduce considerable variability into the studies that will be reported. Even with this variability, however, there are consistent stressor-induced alterations in both the quantitative and qualitative aspects of immune function. Assuming that any particular individual, such as yourself, will experience these alterations when exposed to a stressor is inappropriate and beyond the scope of the experimental data.

STUDIES OF STRESSOR-INDUCED IMMUNE ALTERATION

Numerous experimental approaches have been used to create stress in study subjects. Jumping out of an airplane with a parachute, having to prepare and deliver a short speech, lack of sleep, or being presented with a difficult mental task have been studied as acute stressors. Stress effects on the immune system that are associated with events in an individuals life, such as taking examinations, natural environmental disasters, marital difficulties, or caring for a mentally demented spouse have also been studied. Experimental animals have been studied in situations in which they are restrained, shocked, forced to swim, or housed under variable conditions.

> It is possible to summarize the data succinctly. Yes, stress is associated with an alteration in the functional capabilities of the immune system. Is this a simple relationship? It is not.
>
> Will every individual who experiences stressor-induced immune alteration develop a change in health? Probably not.
>
> Can a particular individual who will experience health alterations due to stressor-induced immune alteration be predicted? Probably not.
>
> If an individual can develop behaviors that prevent stress form altering immune system function, will a better quality of health be achieved in comparison with what would occur if stress were to alter the function of their immune system? No one knows for sure.

Studies will be presented that exemplify relevant aspects of the interaction between stress and immune function. As will be described, there are both suppressing and enhancing responses of the immune system to stress. The what, why, and how of these variable outcomes are not well defined. Indeed, the outcome is often a surprise. However, that should not be surprising.

The final function of the immune system is dependent on a group of subcontractors (APCs, T cells, B cells, cytokines), each of which must have their input in a well-defined and properly sequenced manner. Too much or too little of the activities of a subcontractor will disrupt the final assembly. Different qualities of function of the final product (the effective immune response) will be related to alteration of the activity of a component of the immune system.

White Blood Cell Numbers

A logical starting point for evaluating the effect of stress on the immune system is determining whether stress alters the numbers of different peripheral blood leukocyte populations. In humans, an acute stressor causes an increase in the total number of leukocytes in blood (Herbert and Cohen, 1993; Kiecolt-Glaser et al, 1993). Possible sources of the increased number of leukocytes are leukocytes released from the spleen or detaching from endothelial cells lining blood vessels.

In humans, cortisol causes an efflux of granulocytes from the spleen and bone marrow (Toft et al, 1994). Epinephrine induces an initial increase in the number of lymphocytes in blood, followed by an increase in the number of granulocytes (Samuels, 1951).

In rats, corticosterone produces a decrease in the number of peripheral blood lymphocytes (Dhabhar et al, 1996b). The decrease of lymphocytes in the blood may be due to a redistribution of the lymphocytes to tissue. If this occurs in humans as well, it would suggest that during different phases of the circadian rhythm of cortisol, there are effects on lymphocyte numbers both in the blood and on immune function. Of course, if high levels of glucocorticoids produce an alteration of lymphocyte trafficking patterns and the redistribution of lymphocytes, it is possible that the lymphocytes will have an inhibited function as a result of glucocorticoid receptors being occupied.

Lymphocytes bearing the CD8 marker and markers for natural killer (NK) cells have the largest numerical increase in blood in response to acute stress (Benschop et al, 1996). The increase of NK cell numbers is likely due to an effect of catecholamines binding to β-adrenergic receptors on the NK cells with a subsequent alteration of adhesion molecules, decreasing NK cell binding to endothelial cells (Benschop et al, 1993, 1994). One research group has reported that the increased numbers of CD8 cells in blood may be due to a population of NK cells which bear the CD8 marker (Schedlowski et al, 1996).

Stress-induced changes in CD4 and B lymphocyte numbers are much less in magnitude than that of NK cells. However, in vitro studies indicate that adhesion of T cells to IL-1-activated endothelial cells is decreased by catecholamines (Carlson et al, 1996).

Both acute stress and chronic stress produce similar alterations of lymphocyte populations for all subsets other than the CD8 population (Herbert and Cohen, 1993). Acute stress increases the number of CD8 cells, while chronic stress decreases CD8 numbers.

There are important implications to the above observations. The most important relates to the function of the leukocytes that are counted when blood is collected through a needle placed into a vein. These leukocytes are not adherent to endothelial cells; therefore, it is unlikely that they are the cells that will be involved in the inflammatory response mediated by cells rolling along endothelial cells and that respond to increased concentrations of adhesion molecules and chemotactic stimuli as they move into tissue. Thus, an increase of a leukocyte population in blood, if the cells are derived from cells that demarginate from endothelial cells, would suggest that there is a decreased capability for mediating an inflammatory response. This would be true regardless of whether the decreased adhesiveness were due to changes on endothelial cells or leukocytes. A decrease of cell numbers in the blood that occurred secondary to a redistribution of the leukocytes, raises the question of whether the leukocytes would have a normal function when acted upon by the high levels of glucocorticoids or catecholamines that induced their redistribution.

White Blood Cell Function

Suppression. It is both easy and difficult to discuss stressor-induced changes in the function of populations of white blood cells. Information was presented in Chapter 2 regarding stress-induced changes in neutrophil function. With regard to lymphocytes, numerous studies have found a decreased proliferation to stimulation with nonspecific mitogens. That's the easy part. The hard part is determining what that means with regard to maintaining a functional immune system.

What does a decrease in lymphocyte nonspecific mitogenic responsiveness mean? If there is no response it mean that the lymphocytes are not able to participate in activating an effector immune response. If there is a response that is below the normal range for the laboratory performing the assay it may mean that there will not be an effective immune response. Maybe! The problem is that with a low response, even a very low response, there is no accurate way to interpret the relationship between the mitogenic response and what the lymphocytes can do to facilitate or participate in an immune response.

With the lack of ability to properly interpret a nonspecific mitogenic response, why are these assays used in so many psychoneuroimmunology studies? I believe that the proper answer is that nonspecific mitogenic assays provide a marker that is an indication of the hormonal alterations induced by stress. Decreased nonspecific mitogenic function has been reported when human subjects were exposed to a laboratory stressor (Manuck et al, 1991; Naliboff et al, 1991; Bachen et al, 1992), an acute stress occurring in an individual's life (Schleifer et al, 1983; Kiecolt-Glaser et al, 1986; Taylor et al, 1989), or a chronic stress (Bartrop et al, 1977; Kiecolt-Glaser et al, 1987a, 1988, 1991). Studies of stress in nonhuman primates and rodents also show decreased nonspecific mitogenic function with stress. Thus, it appears to be a fairly uniform finding that stress suppresses the ability of lymphocytes to respond to stimulation with nonspecific mitogens.

An appropriate approach to determine which hormones are modifying mitogenic responsiveness is to use specific antagonists. When this has been done, catecholamines are found capable of suppressing nonspecific mitogenic function of human peripheral blood lymphocytes (Maisel et al, 1991; Bachen et al, 1995). In rats, peripheral blood lymphocyte nonspecific mitogenic function is influenced by corticosterone (Cunnick et al, 1988).

What are the implications of this? Do the data from human and animal studies indicate that stress hormones have a direct effect on lymphocytes? They would if nonspecific mitogens acted on lymphocytes without the need of participation from any other cell. Unfortunately, that is unlikely as nonspecific mitogenic stimulation of lymphocytes requires an accessory cell (Lipsky et al, 1976). Thus, these studies do not allow a distinction to be made between a stress hormone effect on accessory cells (macrophages and/or monocytes) or lymphocytes.

An in vitro experiment designed to resolve whether stress hormones acted directly on lymphocytes or on accessory cells provided useful data (Elliott et al, 1992). Purified T lymphocytes were isolated from the blood of healthy individuals. A monoclonal antibody to CD3 was bound to the wells of a plastic microculture plate. This antibody will bind to the CD3 molecule that is present on all T lymphocytes. If the lymphocytes are cultured in a high density of antibody to CD3, the antibody will provide costimulation signals between the lymphocytes and mitosis will be induced. Accessory cells are not required using this approach.

Dexamethasone binds to the glucocorticoid receptor, isoproterenol binds to the β-adrenergic receptor, and prostaglandin E_2 binds to the prostaglandin receptor. The addition of any of the three chemicals, in a physiological concentration, inhibited lymphocyte mitosis induced by the CD3 antibody. Thus, in vitro, when the lymphocytes were cultured with stress hormones, a direct effect on lymphocytes could be demonstrated as a reduction of mitosis.

When an antibody to the CD28 molecule on T lymphocytes was added to the cultures along with the antibody to CD3, the amount of mitosis of the T lymphocytes doubled. CD28 is a costimulatory molecule that binds to the B7 molecule on dendritic cells (see Chapter 2). The antibody to CD28 activates the costimulation pathway without the presence of a dendritic cell. The combination of antibodies to CD3 and CD28 completely reversed the suppression of mitosis induced by isoproterenol and produced an approximate 50% reduction in the suppression of mitosis caused by prostaglandin E_2. There was no effect on the suppression of dexamethasone except at the highest concentration of dexamethasone used (10^{-8} M).

This straightforward experiment indicates the complexity of stressor-related functional modification of lymphocyte function. The following lessons emerge from this experiment:

1. In vivo, primary activation of naive lymphocytes requires the costimulation molecules. Thus, an inhibitory effect of catecholamines, or prostaglandin, on lymphocyte function may be reversed by the interaction between costimulatory molecules on T lymphocytes and dendritic cells. The alteration of lymphocyte mitosis by binding of glucocorticoid to the glucocorticoid receptor may, or may not, be altered by activation of the costimulatory molecule.

2. In vivo, activation of effector (memory) lymphocytes is independent of costimulatory molecules. Indeed, activation of effector lymphocytes often takes place in parenchymal tissues at the site of a tissue cell presenting antigenic peptides in its surface MHC molecules, but that lack costimulatory molecules. Without the effect of buffering from the costimulation molecules, it can be hypothe-

sized that stress hormone suppression of effector lymphocyte mitosis would be more efficient due to the lack of buffering by costimulatory molecules

3. Until the influence of a direct effect of stress hormones on isolated populations of naive and effector lymphocytes can be studied experimentally we do not know whether each population is altered under the identical hormonal influences. Indeed, antigen specific activation of lymphocyte mitosis may have different parameters than does the induction of nonspecific mitosis in lymphocytes.

Enhancement. There are reports showing that stress may actually enhance, rather than suppress, components of the host defense system. For example, the ability of phagocytic cells in the spleen to phagocytose was enhanced by the stress of social conflict (Lyte et al, 1990). The number of leukocytes infiltrating the skin in a delayed hypersensitivity skin reaction to an iummunogenic chemical, a manifestation of CD4 T-cell immunity, have been found to be increased by stress (Dhabhar and McEwen, 1996a). It is hypothesized that the enhanced response in the skin was due to low concentrations of glucocorticoids or catecholamines increasing the movement of lymphocytes from the blood into tissues. This may occur if the adhesion interactions between lymphocytes and vascular endothelial cells is increased, so that there are more lymphocytes available to respond to chemotactic stimuli.

Our research group studied the alteration of antigen-specific responses in rats that had been stressed by a mild electrical footshock (Wood et al, 1993). Rats were stressed 1 day before, on the day of, 1 day after, and 3 days after being immunized with the T-cell-dependent antigen, hemocyanin, obtained from the keyhole limpet. Seventeen days after being immunized, several immune parameters were measured. The results from animals that were not stressed were compared with the results from animals that had been stressed. The data are presented in Table 4.1.

There are interesting aspects to the data:

1. Lymphocyte transformation to nonspecific mitogen was the same in all groups of rats. Thus, it is unlikely that the stressor produced a longlasting "generalized" increase in immune function. It is likely that the enhancement of immune function is antigen specific.

2. When stressed 1 day before immunization there is no effect on the immune response. This suggests that the hormonal response to the stressor does not produce a longlasting effect on antigen-specific immune function. When stressed 3 days after immunization, there was also no effect on the immune response. This suggests that 3 days after immunization, all immune interactions that are susceptible to modification by stress hormones have been completed. It is likely that there must be a temporal association of the stressor-induced hormonal changes and immune activation and the early components of immune activation (APC function and APC–T-cell interaction) are most susceptible to stressor-induced augmentation.

Other research groups have also studied the antibody response to keyhole limpet hemocyanin (KLH) in rats or mice that had been stressed. In each case, the stressed unclear. It could be related to different hormonal responses with age due to ╍ns in the nervous system, or it could be due to different background stress ╍3-month-old mice as compared with 9-month-old mice. Or, more likely, it ╍ due to something that I can't think of.

╍vestigators conducted a further study to determine whether a mild stressor ╍ame effect as did a more extreme stressor. Mice were immunized with sheep ╍ytes and, 72 hours later, they experienced a mild stressor of being placed into ╍k boxes, but they were not shocked. Electrical shock suppressed the number ╍phocytes producing antibody to sheep erythrocytes when delivered 72 hours ╍igen injection. However, the mild stressor at 72 hours produced an enhance-╍ the number of antibody producing B lymphocytes. Thus, the particular mix ╍ones or the concentration of hormones produced in response to either a se-╍ssor or a mild stressor may produce different effects on an antigen specific ╍ response. The above series of experiments point to the complexities of the ╍al interactions on cells of the immune system and strengthen the importance ╍utions against generalizations.

╍ht into the mechanism of enhancement is provided by severing the splenic ╍ pretreatment of animals with a β-adrenergic antagonist prior to exposure of ╍ mild stressor that enhances the splenic B cell antibody response to sheep ╍cytes (Croiset et al, 1990). Rats were exposed to a novel environment and im-╍ly immunized with sheep erythrocytes. Five days later, the number of B lym-╍s producing antibody to sheep erythrocytes was measured. The rats exposed ╍ovel environment had significantly more antibody-producing cells than did ╍ t had not been exposed to the stressor. However, if their splenic nerve had ╍vered to prevent catecholamine release in the spleen, or if the rats were pre-╍ with a β-adrenergic antagonist before exposure to the novel environment, ╍as no enhancement of the B-cell response. The enhanced response was not ╍n rats exposed to a severe stressor. Thus, this study suggests that a certain ╍ catecholamines, at the time of immunization, may enhance an antigen-spe-╍mune response. However, there is also a report that indicates that an antibody ╍cotropin-releasing factor (CRF) inhibited the mild stressor-induced enhance-

╍GESTION: Can a little stress enhance immunity and larger amounts of ╍s suppress immunity? Is a little stress good and more stress bad? This is not ╍common question. Indeed, an argument can be made for a little stress being ╍. Consider what you do when you have to write a paper, write a grant, or just ╍ a deadline. Most people wait until the last minute before completing the ╍ even though they had adequate time to complete it earlier. Last-minute acti-╍n of mental capabilities seems to be associated with the stress of meeting the ╍line. It suggests that productivity and mental focus may increase with stress. ╍ess, at a specific time (when mental creativity must be heightened), can be ╍ficial, is it possible that stress at a specific time during immune activation ╍ also be beneficial to immune activation.

TABLE 4.1 Stress-Induced Alteration of an Antigen-Specific Ir

	Day Of Stre		
Assay	1 Day Before Immunization	Day of Immunization	1 D Imi
Antibody to the antigen	Same as control rats	Significantly increased in comparison with control rats	Sig i c v r
Lymphocyte mitosis to the antigen	Same as control rats	Significantly increased in comparison with control rats	Sig ir c w ra
Infiltration of delayed hypersensitivity skin-test reactivity	Same as control rats	Significantly increased in comparison with control rats	Sigr in co w ra
Nonspecific lymphocyte transformation	Same as control rats	Same as control rats	Sam co

rodents produced lower amounts of antibody to KLH thai stressed controls (Laudenslager et al, 1988; Fleshner et a 1990). The explanation for the different response is not evi the standard factors, such as sex, species, strain, age, prior unknown characteristic of the antigen used. However, the re

There are studies that enumerate the number of B lymph to the antigen to which they were immunized. In these stu usually sheep erythrocytes. Use of this antigen permits the u the actual number of lymphocytes producing antibody to the

When 9-month-old mice were immunized with sheep er electrical shock stress immediately after, or 24 hours after, i a significant increase in the number of spleen B lymphocyte sheep erythrocytes in comparison to control animals (Zalcn cal shock delivered 72 hours after antigen injection produce in the number of antibody-producing lymphocytes in comp mals. This suggests that timing of the stressor to a componen immune response is important. It is likely that, at the early sta take and processing. This process may have been enhance hours, B-cell proliferation or T cells providing help to B c function reduced by stress hormones.

The use of the same protocol of electric footshock immed after, immunization in 3-month-old mice did not enhance th producing B lymphocytes. The reason for different outcom

ences is
alteratio
levels i
could b
The
had the
erythro
the sho
of B ly
after a
ment i
of hor
vere st
immur
hormo
of prec
Insi
nerve
rats to
erythr
media
phocy
to the
rats th
been s
treate
there
found
level
cific i
to cor

SU
stre
an u
goo
mee
task
vati
dea
If s
ber
ma

ment of the antibody response to sheep erythrocytes (Berkenbosch et al, 1991). Thus, the relative importance of glucocorticoids or catecholamines in stressor-induced immune enhancement needs further study.

In vitro studies have been used to identify the participation of the β-adrenergic receptor in enhancing a primary immune response. Incubation of sheep erythrocytes with mouse spleen lymphocytes in vitro stimulates antibody production by the mouse B lymphocytes (Sanders and Munson et al,, 1984). Inclusion of norepinephrine in the culture medium increases the number of antibody-producing B lymphocytes. There has been the suggestion that the enhanced response may be due to a catecholamine-induced increased responsiveness to IL-2 (Zalcman et al, 1994).

NK Lymphocytes

Acute stressors have been reported to increase the number of NK cells in blood (Landmann et al, 1984; Naliboff et al, 1991; Bachen et al, 1992; Schedlowski et al, 1993; Herbert et al, 1994). There are also reports in which NK numbers do not change after an acute stressor (Ironson et al, 1990; Sieber et al, 1992). NK numbers have been reported to remain normal when a stressor becomes chronic (Kiecolt-Glaser et al, 1988, 1991) and have also been reported to be decreased by chronic stress (Kiecolt-Glaser et al, 1987b).

Thus, the data suggest that stress is often associated with an initial increase of NK cells in the blood, with the numbers becoming normal as the stressor becomes chronic. The initial increase is likely due to catecholamines altering the adhesion molecule interaction between NK cells and the vascular endothelial molecules (Benschop et al, 1993, 1994). However, with continued stress, several changes may occur that allow the NK cells to return to normal numbers. Possible factors include reduction of catecholamine concentrations, decreased receptor concentration for catecholamines on NK cells, increased synthesis of adhesion molecules by NK cells, increased synthesis of adhesion molecules by endothelial cells, or release of new NK cells from the bone marrow that have matured in the presence of high concentrations of catecholamines and therefore have different parameters of responsiveness to catecholamines than do NK cells that had matured when catecholamine concentrations were low.

With regard to NK functions there are studies which suggest that regardless of whether the stressor is acute or chronic, NK cell function does not change (Kiecolt-Glaser et al, 1984; Moss et al, 1989; Knapp et al, 1992). There are also studies that report a decrease of NK function with acute and chronic stress (Kiecolt-Glaser et al, 1984, 1985; Irwin et al, 1990; Esterling et al, 1994). Finally, there are studies that report an increase of NK function by acute stress (Naliboff et al,, 1991; Antoni et al, 1990), but not in chronic stress.

The direction of alteration of NK function by stress may be related to the concentration of hormones in the blood, or the combination of hormones that are altered by stress. This is suggested by studies that report different alterations of NK function in individuals experiencing different types of emotional states (Kiecolt-Glaser et al, 1984; Irwin et al, 1986, 1991) or when studies are done at different times in relationship to a stressor (Tonnesen et al, 1987). Even sleep deprivation has been reported to alter NK function (Irwin et al, 1996).

There are lessons suggested by the response of NK cells to stress. Clearly, a dynamic process is taking place that produces different alterations based on parameters such as the duration and intensity of the stressor and how long after the stress event the assay is performed. The coping skills of the individual are also likely to be important.

It is important to remember that stress does not alter NK function out of the range of normal values. If there is an association of stress with disease susceptibility and altered NK function, the effect of stress hormones on physiologic processes other than on NK function, may be responsible for the alteration of disease susceptibility. The altered NK function may be a marker for hormonal alterations but may not be linked to disease alterations.

This latter point raises the question of association and linkage. How does anyone know when a stressor-induced alteration of immune function is responsible for an alteration of disease susceptibility? An increased susceptibility to upper respiratory infection in a subject with a lowered response of lymphocytes to stimulation with nonspecific mitogens is an association. Is the increased susceptibility to an upper respiratory infection linked to the change of lymphocyte function? That is unknown. However, if research programs establish a linkage between stress, alteration of immune function, and disease, a powerful component of preventive medicine will have been identified.

Cytokines

Appropriate cytokine production (both the mix of cytokines and their concentration) is essential for the activation of an immune response that will provide resistance to infectious diseases and that will minimize the likelihood of the development of autoimmune disease. Stress hormones may exert some of their effects on altering immune function by altering the production of cytokines by mononuclear phagocytes and lymphocytes. Different immune alterations would be expected if the cytokines produced by Th1 or Th2 cells were preferentially altered.

Peripheral blood lymphocytes of medical students undergoing the stress of examinations have been studied for the number of cells expressing the receptor for IL-2 (IL-2R) and for IL-2R mRNA. Comparison of low stress and high stress conditions found fewer cells expressing IL-2R and lower amounts of IL-2R mRNA during times of high stress (Glaser et al, 1990). Production of IL-2 by phytohemagglutinin (PHA) stimulated lymphocytes was increased during times of high stress. However, without adequate numbers of IL-2 receptors to bind to, the net effect of IL-2 on lymphocyte function would be expected to be decreased.

Lymphocyte production of interferon-γ (IFN-γ) has also been reported to be decreased by stress in humans (Glaser et al, 1987; Dobbin et al, 1991). However, IL-1 production by monocytes stimulated with lipopolysaccharide, in vitro, was increased when cells from students undergoing a stressor were studied (Dobbin et al, 1991).

Physical exercise produces hormonal changes similar to those produced by a psychological stressor with elevations of plasma concentrations of glucocorticoids and catecholamines. Exercise also produces alterations of several parameters of immune function (Moyna et al, 1996). Of course, the mechanism of induction of the hormonal and immune changes associated with exercise can not be considered equivalent to those induced by a psychological stressor due to the physiological processes activated by exercise. However, there are interesting effects on cytokines that are induced by exercise and that indicate that cytokine production is altered when the hormonal composition of blood is altered.

The advantage of referring to studies of cytokine alterations related to exercise is that some studies have measured the concentration of cytokines in plasma, rather than the release of cytokines from lymphocytes and mononuclear phagocytic cells in vitro. The plasma studies indicate that exercise produces an increase of (1) IL-6; (2) IL-1 receptor antagonist (IL-1ra), the naturally occurring inhibitor of IL-1 (Drenth et al, 1995); (3) TNF-α (Espersen et al, 1990) (TNF-α is released by activated macrophages and has the biological properties of increasing vascular permeability, which enhances the localized inflammatory reaction by facilitating the egress of inflammatory cells, antibodies, and complement, into tissues); and (4) soluble IL 2R (an indication that lymphoid cell turnover was increased) (Weinstock et al, 1997). Plasma concentrations of IFN-γ were not increased by exercise (Weinstock et al, 1997). Unfortunately, the measurement of cytokines in plasma that would allow a differentiation of an effect of exercise on the functional activity of Th1 and Th2 lymphocytes has not been done. However, the effect of exercise on Th1 and Th2 cytokine production by stimulated lymphocytes in vitro, has been reported.

An indication of the functional alteration of Th1 and Th2 lymphocytes is indicated by measuring, for example, IFN-γ as an indication of Th1 function and IL-4 as an indication of Th2 function. Exercise has been reported to increase the in vitro production of IFN-γ while leaving IL-4 production undisturbed (Moyna et al, 1996). If this reflects an in vivo enhancement of cell mediated immunity, it could be hypothesized that exercise would enhance resistance to viral infections by promoting a cytotoxic response to infected cells.

Another important question relates to the technical aspects of determining cytokine production in vitro. If the procedures used to generate the cytokines are not optimal, data may be obtained that do not accurately reflect the functional activity of Th1 and Th2 cells. Indeed, the kinetics of production of IFN-γ and IL-4 differ and technical factors such as the nature of the stimulating agent, whether whole blood or isolated lymphocytes are stimulated, and the density of the cytokine-producing cells placed in culture all can influence cytokine production (Gonzalez et al, 1994).

Whole blood cultures and isolated T cells frequently differ in the amount of IFN-γ or IL-4 produced per T cell placed into culture. In different subjects, whole blood cultures produced either more or less cytokine than did the isolated T cells. This raises the question of what information an assay is supposed to provide. If the assay for cytokine production were being asked to provide information regarding what is likely to be occurring in vivo, a whole blood assay may be appropriate. If the assay were being asked to provide information regarding the capability of a lymphocyte to produce cytokine, the isolated lymphocyte assay may be appropriate. Thus, when studying the effect of stress on cytokine production by T cells, the lack of proper attention to technical procedures and experimental design may lead to the publication of data that do not accurately reflect either the biological condition in vivo or the true function of a T cell.

An effect of stress on altering cytokine production from Th1 and Th2 lymphocytes with a resultant effect on class switching of immunoglobulin production from IgM to different subtypes of IgG has been reported (Fleshner et al, 1996). Stress reduced the production of antibodies dependent on cytokines released from Th1 lymphocytes, while antibody classes dependent on cytokines released from Th2 lymphocytes remained intact. Thus, there are stressor-induced alterations of cytokine production, which by influencing the classes of immunoglobulin produced by B lymphocytes may contribute to an increased susceptibility to infectious disease by decreasing the concentration of Th1-dependent complement-fixing antibodies produced.

Immunoglobulins

There are two ways to evaluate the effect of stress on immunoglobulins. One approach is to determine whether stress alters the total concentration of each class of immunoglobulin (IgG, IgA, IgM, IgE) or whether stress alters the concentration of a specific antibody. Immunoglobulins are proteins, and their synthesis would be expected to be altered by factors that alter protein synthesis. For example, decreased nutrition subsequent to chronic stress may reduce protein synthesis and therefore concentrations of immunoglobulin.

IgM immunoglobulin is almost entirely found within the vascular system, while IgG is equally distributed both intra- and extravascularly. During stress, when blood pressure and heart rate are elevated, fluid leaves the intravascular space and enters the extravascular space. This increases the concentration of large molecules in plasma (Jern et al, 1989). Thus, hemoconcentration would be expected to increase the concentration of IgM in plasma making interpretation of the mechanism of stress related IgM increase difficult. Is the IgM increased due to increased synthesis or hemoconcentration?

A review of reports of the alteration of total concentrations of plasma IgG, IgA, or IgM provides variable results, with increases, decreases, and no changes reported. This is not surprising. Arguments for stress decreasing the production of total immunoglobulin can be formulated based on stress decreasing the function of helper T lymphocytes that stimulate antibody-producing B lymphocytes. However, stress effects on decreasing protein synthesis and inducing hemoconcentration may also contribute to the quantitative immunoglobulin alterations.

A better assessment of stress on antibody production can be obtained by evaluating specific antibody responses. When evaluating specific antibody responses, a concern relates to whether a primary or a secondary immune response is being measured. A secondary antibody response occurs when both B and T lymphocytes have previously been activated by specific antigen. Thus, the parameters of activation differ in comparison with those of the primary antibody response, which involves activation of naive lymphocytes. Studies designed to detect different effects of stress in modifying a primary or a secondary immune response have not been carefully conducted.

There is a report that the secondary immune response of monkeys that had been separated from their mothers did not differ in comparison with the secondary response of monkeys that had not been separated from their mothers (Laudenslager et al, 1986). We obtained different results when we studied the secondary immune response in monkeys to immunization with tetanus toxoid (Cunnick et al, 1991). Monkeys that were stressed by repeated reorganization of their social group produced significantly more antibody in response to a secondary immunization than did monkeys that were not stressed.

Measurement of the effect of stress on the secondary antibody response presents many questions. For example, was the primary immunization given at a time of stress? Was stress continuous between the primary and secondary immunization? Was the same stressor experienced during the primary and secondary immunization? Do different concentrations of injected antigen produce the same results? Does secondary challenge at different times after the primary response produce the same results?

A single study that does help clarify some of these concerns gave three immunizations to medical students with hepatitis vaccine, each at a time of examination stress (Glaser et al, 1992). Those students reporting higher levels of stress and loneliness had lower levels of antibody after the first two immunizations. However, after the third immunization, there were no significant differences between the students with regard to the amount of antibody produced, hence the suggestion that stress has the capability of suppressing the primary immune response to a greater degree than the secondary antibody response.

If the primary immune response is effected by stress, there are numerous questions regarding, for example, which phase of the immune response is altered, whether the alterations of cell function lead to suppression or enhancement of the antibody response, and when during the immune response the stressor has to be experienced. These parameters have been discussed earlier in this chapter in the section on white blood cell function.

The amount of antibody produced in response to primary immunization has been reported to be decreased when subjects experience higher versus lower levels of stress (Glaser et al, 1992; Kiecolt-Glaser et al, 1996). Lower primary antibody responses have also been reported in monkeys experiencing stress at the time of immunization (Coe et al, 1988). However, there are also reports that stress may be associated with higher antibody responses to a primary immunization (Cunnick et al, 1991; Petry et al, 1991; Wood et al, 1993).

If stress interferes with a primary antibody response, consideration may need to be given to adjusting the protocols for immunization. Possibly the number of booster immunizations given may need to be increased.

Stress is associated with activation of latent viral infections. Synthesis of viral proteins occurs when there is activation of latent viral infections. Decreased T-cell function which is responsible for latent viral reactivation suggests that antibody production would be decreased as T cell help to B lymphocytes is decreased. However, there are several studies which indicate that antibody production to latent viral antigens increases during stress (Glaser et al, 1985, 1993; Kiecolt-Glaser et al, 1987a,b). As these are secondary antibody responses, it is suggested that the hormonal response to stress and their effect on the function of the immune system is different during a primary response than during a secondary response.

Adhesion Molecules

Stressor-induced alteration of adhesion molecules, either on lymphocytes or on endothelial cells, would be expected to alter the trafficking patterns of lymphocytes and granulocytes and prevent the proper accumulation of leukocytes at tissue sites where inflammatory responses were occurring. An adrenal hormone-induced decrease of adhesion molecules on CD4 lymphocytes in mice has been reported (Tarcic et al, 1995). Cortisol has also been shown to decrease the expression of adhesion molecules for neutrophils on endothelial cells (Cronstein et al, 1992). If granulocytes and lymphocytes are unable to properly accumulate at tissue sites where they are needed, it is likely that there will be an increased susceptibility to infectious diseases.

Secretory IgA

The secretory IgA (sIgA) immune system coats the mucosal surfaces of the body and prevents the attachment of infectious agents to epithelial cells. Decreased production of sIgA is associated with an increased susceptibility to gastrointestinal and upper and lower respiratory infections. Stress, loneliness, and depression are even associated with periodontal disease, although whether this is due to decreased sIgA production has not been established (Bosch et al, 1996; Breivik et al, 1996). If stress is associated with a decrease in the concentration of sIgA on mucosal surfaces, an increased susceptibility to periodontal disease may occur.

Studies have been performed to determine whether an individual's mood or undesirable events occurring in their lives has an effect on the amount of antigen specific sIgA present in saliva. The experimental subjects included dental students and married men. Indeed, the amount of antigen-specific sIgA antibody was decreased when the experimental subjects experienced stress in comparison with times when they had a high positive mood (Stone et al, 1996). The reduced sIgA production may be due to the release of neuropeptides in the mucosa and reducing protein synthesis by B lymphocytes or neuropeptides effecting the release of sIgA from B lymphocytes. Further studies should clarify the role of stress and stress hormones in altering sIgA production (Valdimarsdottir and Stone, 1997)

Delayed Hypersensitivity

The mechanisms and cells involved in the delayed-type hypersensitivity (DTH) skin-test response were described in Chapter 2 (Figure 2.38A–C). Primary sensitization involves Langerhan's cells and CD4 Th1 lymphocytes. The effector response involves activated CD4 Th1 lymphocytes interacting with the peptide to which they were sensitized being presented in MHC II molecules of an APC, most likely a Langerhan's cell in the skin. Thus, there are two stages (sensitization and effector) in which the

DTH can be modified by stress. Studies evaluating the effect of stress on the DTH response report both enhancement and suppression of the response (Wood et al, 1993; Dhabhar and McEwen, 1996a; Kawaguchi et al, 1997; Tingate et al, 1997). This is not surprising in view of the many different processes that could be altered by stress related hormones.

However, the implications of an altered DTH skin test response go beyond what is measured in the skin. The cell-mediated immune mechanism that produces the DTH response is also responsible for providing resistance against infection caused by intracellular pathogens. It would be of benefit to the maintenance of resistance to infectious disease and health to know what hormonal alterations are associated with an enhancement of DTH responses. Whether behaviors or emotions, or both could be used to create the hormonal environment where DTH responses are enhanced would be of potential importance.

SUMMARY

Yes, stress does alter immune function if the subject experiencing the stressor has activation of the stress responsive areas of the brain, which then modify the neurohormonal content of plasma and within lymphoid tissues. Whether the immune alteration enhances or diminishes the ability of the immune system to eliminate infectious agents can not be accurately evaluated by measurements of selected quantitative or qualitative components of the immune system. Why enhancement or suppression of immune function occurs subsequent to a stressor is unclear. However, given the difficulties of interpreting the biological significance of studies of altered immune function, there is ample evidence that the alterations are biologically significant. This information is presented in Chapter 6.

REFERENCES

Amer A, Singh G, Darke C, Dolby AE. Impaired lymphocyte responsiveness to phytohemagglutinin associated with the possession of HLA-B8/DR3. Tissue Antigens. 28: 193–198, 1986.

Antoni MH, August S, LaPerriere A, Baggett HL, Klimas N, Ironson G, Schneiderman N, Fletcher MA. Psychological and neuroendocrine measures related to functional immune changes in anticipation of HIV-1 serostatus notification. Psychosomatic Medicine. 52: 496–510, 1990.

Bachen EA, Manuck SB, Marsland AL, Cohen S, Malkoff SB, Muldoon MF, Rabin BS. Lymphocyte subset and cellular immune responses to a brief experimental stressor. Psychosomatic Medicine. 54: 673–679, 1992.

Bachen EA, Manuck SB, Cohen S, Muldoon MF, Raibel R, Herbert TB, Rabin BS. Adrenergic blockade ameliorates cellular immune responses to mental stress in humans. Psychosomatic Medicine. 57: 366–372, 1995.

Bartrop RW, Luckhurst E, Lazarus L, Kiloh LG, Penny R. Depressed lymphocyte function after bereavement. Lancet. 1: 834–836, 1977.

Bell IR, Martino GM, Meredith KE, Schwartz GE, Siani MM, Morrow FD. Vascular disease factors, urinary free cortisol, and health histories in older adults: Shyness and gender interactions. Biological Psychology. 35: 37–49, 1993.

Benschop RJ, Oostveen FG, Heijnen CJ, Ballieux RE. Beta-2 adrenergic stimulation causes detachment of natural killer cells from cultured endothelium. European Journal of Immunology. 23: 3242–3247, 1993.

Benschop RJ, Nieuwenhuis EES, Tromp EAM, Godaert GLR, Ballieux RE, vanDoornen LJP. Beta adrenergic blockade: Effects of beta-adrenergic blockade on immunologic and cardiovascular changes induced by mental stress. Circulation. 89: 762–769, 1994.

Benschop RJ, Rodriguez-Feuerhahn M, Schedlowski M. Catecholamine-induced leukocytosis: Early observations, current research, and future directions. Brain, Behavior, and Immunity. 10: 77–91, 1996.

Berkenbosch F, Wolvers DAW, Derijk R. Neuroendocrine and immunological mechanisms in stress induced immunomodulation. Journal of Steroid Biochemistry and Molecular Biology. 40: 639–647, 1991.

Berns GS, Cohen JD, Mintun MA. Brain regions responsive to novelty in the absence of awareness. Science. 276: 1272–1275, 1997.

Bosch JA, Brand HS, Ligtenberg TJM, Bermond B, Hoogstraten J, Amerongen AVN. Psychological stress as a determinant of protein levels and salivary-induced aggregation of Streptococus gordonii in human whole saliva. Psychosomatic Medicine. 58: 374–382, 1996.

Breivik T, Thrane PS, Murison R, Gjermo P. Emotional stress effects on immunity, gingivitis and periodontitis. European Journal of Oral Sciences. 104: 327–334, 1996.

Brown LL, Tomarken AJ, Orth DN, Loosen PT, Kalin NH, Davidson RJ. Individual differences in repressive-defensiveness predict basal salivary cortisol levels. Journal of Personality and Social Psychology. 70: 362–371, 1996.

Carlson SL, Beiting DJ, Kiani CA, Abell KM, McGillis JP. Catecholamines decrease lymphocyte adhesion to cytokine-activated endothelial cells. Brain, Behavior, and Immunity. 10: 55–67, 1996.

Caruso C, Bongiardina C, Candore G, Cigna D, Romano GC, Colucci T, DiLorenzo G, Gervasi F, Manno M, Potestio M, Tantillo G. HLA-B8,DR3 haplotype affects lymphocyte blood levels. Immunological Investigations. 26: 333–340, 1997.

Coe CL, Rosenberg LT, Levine S. Effect of maternal separation on the complement system and antibody responses in infant primates. International Journal of Neuroscience. 40: 289–302, 1988.

Cohen S, Line S, Manuck SB, Rabin BS, Heise ER, Kaplan JR. Chronic social stress, social status, and susceptibility to upper respiratory infections in nonhuman primates. Psychosomatic Medicine. 59: 213–221, 1997.

Croiset G, Heijnen CJ, van der Wal WE, deBoer SF, deWied D. A role for the autonomic nervous system in modulating the immune response during mild emotional stimuli. Life Sciences. 46: 419–425, 1990.

Cronstein BN, Kimmel SC, Levin RI, Martiniuk F, Weissmann G. A mechanism for the antiinflammatory effects of corticosteroids: The glucocorticoid receptor regulates leukocyte adhesion to endothelial cells and expression of endothelial-leukocyte adhesion molecule 1 and intercellular adhesion molecule 1. Proceedings of the National Academy of Sciences USA. 89: 9991–9995, 1992.

Cunnick JE, Lysle DT, Armfield A, Rabin BS. Shock-induced modulation of lymphocyte responsiveness and natural killer activity: Differential mechanisms of induction. Brain, Behavior, and Immunity. 2: 102–110, l988.

Cunnick JE, Cohen S, Rabin BS, Carpenter AB, Manuck SB, Kaplan JR. Alterations in specific antibody production due to rank and social instability. Brain, Behavior, and Immunity. 5: 357–369, 1991.

Derijk R, Sternberg EM. Corticosteroid action and neuroendocrine-immune interactions. Annals of the New York Academy of Sciences. 746: 33–41, 1994.

Dhabhar FS, McEwen BS. Stress induced enhancement of antigen-specific cell-mediated immunity. Journal of Immunology. 156: 2608–2615, 1996a.

Dhabhar FS, Miller AH, McEwen BS, Spencer RL. Stress-induced changes in blood leukocyte distribution. Journal of Immunology. 157: 1638–1644, 1996b.

Dobbin JP, Harth M, McCain GA, Martin RA, Cousin K. Cytokine production and lymphocyte transformation during stress. Brain, Behavior, and Immunity. 5: 339–348, 1991.

Drenth JPH, Van Uum SHM, Van Deuren M, Pesman GJ, van der Ven-jongekrijg J, van der Meer, J. Endurance run increases circulating IL-6 and IL-1ra but downregulates ex vivo TNF-α and IL-1β production. Journal of Applied Physiology. 79: 1497–1503, 1995.

Elliott L, Brooks W, Roszman T. Inhibition of anti-CD3 monoclonal antibody-induced T-cell proliferation by dexamethosone, isoproterenol, or prostaglandin E2 either alone or in combination. Cellular and Molecular Neurobiology. 12: 411–427, 1992.

Espersen GT, Elbaek A, Ernst E, Toft E, Kaalund S, Jersild C, Grunnet N. Effect of physical exercise on cytokines and lymphocyte subpopulations in human peripheral blood. Acta Pathology Microbiology and Immunology Scandinavia. 98: 395–400, 1990.

Esterling BA, Kiecolt-Glaser JK, Bodnar JC, Glaser R. Chronic stress, social support, and persistent alterations in the natural killer cell response to cytokines in older adults. Health Psychology. 13: 291–298, 1994.

Fleshner M, Laudenslager ML, Simons L, Maier S. Reduced serum antibodies associated with social defeat in rats. Physiology and Behavior. 45: 1183–1187, 1989.

Fleshner M, Brennan FX, Nguyen K, Watkins LR, Maier SF. RU486 blocks differentially suppressive effects of stress on in vivo anti-KLH immunoglobulin response. American Journal of Physiology. 40: R1344–R1352, 1996.

Glaser R, Kiecolt-Glaser JK, Speicher CE, Holliday JE. Stress, loneliness, and changes in herpesvirus latency. Journal of Behavioral Medicine. 8: 249–260, 1985a.

Glaser R, Kiecolt-Glaser JK, Stout JC, Tarr KL, Speicher CE, Holliday JE. Stress-related impairments in cellular immunity. Psychiatry Research. 16: 233–239, 1985b.

Glaser R, Rice J, Sheridan J, Fertel R, Stout J, Speicher C, Pinsky D, Kotur M, Post A, Beck M, Kiecolt-Glaser JK. Stress related immune suppression: Health implications. Brain, Behavior, and Immunity. 1: 7–20, 1987.

Glaser R, Kennedy S, Lafuse WP, Bonneau RH, Speicher CE, Hillhouse J, Kiecolt-Glaser JK. Psychological stress-induced modulation of interleukin 2 receptor gene expression and interleukin 2 production in peripheral blood leukocytes. Archives of General Psychiatry. 47: 707–712, 1990.

Glaser R, Kiecolt-Glaser JK, Bonneau RH, Malarkey W, Kennedy S, Hughes J. Stress-induced modulation of the immune response to recombinant hepatitis B vaccine. Psychosomatic Medicine. 54: 22–29, 1992.

Glaser R, Pearson GR, Bonneau RH, Esterling BA, Atkinson C, Kiecolt-Glaser JK. Stress and the memory T-cell response to the Epstein-Barr virus in healthy medical students. Health Psychology. 12: 435–442, 1993.

Gonzalez S, Beck L, Wilson N, Spiegelberg HL. Comparison of interferon-γ and interleukin-4 production by peripheral blood mononuclear cells and isolated T cells after activation with polyclonal T cell activators. Journal of Clinical Laboratory Analysis. 8: 277–283, 1994.

Gunnar MR, Tout K, deHaan M, Piece S, Stansbury K. Temperament, social competence, and adrenocortical activity in preschoolers. Developmental Psychobiology. 31: 65–85, 1997.

Hashimoto S, McCombs CC, Michalski JP. Mechanism of a lymphocyte abnormality associated with HLA-B8/DR3 in clinically healthy individuals. Clinical and Experimental Immunology. 76: 317–323, 1989.

Hashimoto S, Michalski JP, Berman MA, McCombs C. Mechanism of a lymphocyte abnormality associated with HLA-B8/DR3: Role of interleukin-1. Clinical and Experimental Immunology. 79: 227–232, 1990.

Herbert TB, Cohen S. Stress and immunity in humans: A meta-analytic review. Psychosomatic Medicine. 55: 364–379, 1993.

Herbert TB, Cohen S, Marsland AL, Bachen EA, Rabin BS, Muldoon MF, Manuck SB. Cardiovascular reactivity and the course of immune response to an acute psychological stressor. Psychosomatic Medicine. 56: 337–344, 1994.

Ironson G, LaPerriere A, Antoni MH, O'Hearn P, Schneiderman N, Klimas N, Fletcher MA. Changes in immune and psychological measures as a function of anticipation and reaction to news of HIV-1 antibody status. Psychosomatic Medicine. 52: 247–270, 1990.

Irwin M, Daniels M, Bloom ET, Weiner H. Life events, depression, and natural killer cell activity. Psychopharmacology Bulletin. 22: 1093–1096, 1986.

Irwin M, Patterson T, Smith TL, Caldwell C, Brown SA, Gillin JC, Grant I. Reduction of immune function in life stress and depression. Biological Psychiatry. 27: 22–30, 1990.

Irwin M, Brown M, Patterson T, Hauger R, Mascovich A, Grant I. Neuropeptide Y and natural killer cell activity: Findings in depression and Alzheimer caregiver stress. FASEB Journal. 5: 3100–3107, 1991.

Irwin M, McClintick J, Costlow C, Fortner M, White J, Gillin JC. Partial night sleep deprivation reduces natural killer and cellular immune responses in humans. Journal of the Federation for the Advancement of Science and Experimental Biology. 10: 643–653, 1996.

Jern C, Wadenvik H, Mark H, Hallgren J, Jern S. Hematological changes during acute mental stress. British Journal of Hematology. 71: 153–156, 1989.

Kagan J, Reznick JS, Snidman N. The physiology and psychology of behavioral inhibition in children. Child Development. 58: 1459–1473, 1987.

Kagan J, Reznick JS, Snidman N. Biological basis of childhood shyness. Science. 240: 167–171, 1988.

Kaplan JR, Heise ER, Manuck SB, Shively CA, Cohen S, Rabin BS, Kasprowics AL. The relationship of agonistic and affiliative behavior patterns to cellular immune function among Cynomolgus monkeys (*Macaca fascicularis*) living in stable and unstable social groups. American Journal of Primatology. 25: 157–173, 1991.

Kawaguchi Y, Okada T, Konishi H, Fujino M, Asai J, Ito M. Reduction of the DTH response is related to morphological changes of Langerhans cells in mice exposed to acute immobilization stress. Clinical and Experimental Immunology. 109: 397-401, 1997.

Kiecolt-Glaser JK, Garner W, Speicher C, Penn GM, Holliday G, Glaser R. Psychosocial modifiers of immunocompetence in medical students. Psychosomatic Medicine. 46: 7–14, 1984.

Kiecolt-Glaser JK, Glaser R, Strain EC, Stout JC, Tarr KL, Holliday JE, Speicher CE. Modulation of cellular immunity in medical students. Journal of Behavioral Medicine. 9: 5–21, 1986.

Kiecolt-Glaser JK, Fisher LD, Ogrocki P, Stout JC, Speicher CE, Glaser R. Marital quality, marital disruption, and immune function. Psychosomatic Medicine. 49: 13–34, 1987a.

Kiecolt-Glaser JK, Glaser R, Shuttleworth EC, Dyer CS, Ogrocki P, Speicher CE. Chronic stress and immunity in family caregivers of Alzheimer's disease victims. Psychosomatic Medicine. 49: 523–525, 1987b.

Kiecolt-Glaser JK, Kennedy S, Malkoff S, Fisher L, Speicher CE, Glaser R. Marital discord and immunity in males. Psychosomtic Medicine. 50: 213–229, 1988.

Kiecolt-Glaser JK, Dura JR, Speicher CE, Track OJ, Glaser R. Spousal caregivers of dementia victims: Longitudinal changes in immunity and health. Psychosomatic Medicine. 53: 345–362, 1991.

Kiecolt-Glaser JK, Malarkey WB, Chee MA, Newton T, Cacioppo TJ, Mao H-Y, Glaser R. Negative behavior during marital conflict is associated with immunological down-regulation. Psychosomatic Medicine. 55: 410–412, 1993.

Kiecolt-Glaser JK, Glaser R, Gravenstein S, Malarkey W, Sheridan J. Chronic stress alters the immune response to influenza virus vaccine in older adults. Proceedings of the National Academy of Sciences USA. 93: 3043–3047, 1996.

Kirschbaum C, Prussner JC, Stone AA, Federenko I, Gaab J, Lintz D, Schommer N, Hellhammer DH. Persistent high cortisol responses to repeated psychological stress in a subpopulation of healthy men. Psychosomatic Medicine. 57: 468–474, 1995.

Knapp PH, Levy EM, Giorgi RG, Black PH, Fox BH, Heeren TC. Short-term immunological effects of induced emotion. Psychosomatic Medicine. 54: 133–148, 1992.

Landmann RMA, Muller FB, Perini CH, Wesp ME, Wrne P, Buhler FR. Changes of immunoregulatory cells induced by psychological and physical stress: Relationship to plasma catecholamines. Clinical and Experimental Immunology. 58: 127–135, 1984.

Laudenslager ML, Reite M, Held PE. Early mother/infant separation experiences impair the primary but not the secondary antibody response to a novel antigen in young pigtail monkeys. Psychosomatic Medicine. 48: 304, 1986.

Laudenslager ML, Fleshner M, Hofstadter P, Held PE, Simons L, Maier S. Suppression of specific antibody production by inescapable shock: Stability under varying conditions. Brain, Behavior, and Immunity. 2: 92–101, 1988.

Lipsky PE, Ellner JJ, Rosenthal AL. Phytohemagglutinin-induced proliferation of guinea pig thymus-derived lymphocytes. I. Accessory cell dependence. Journal of Immunology. 116: 868–875, 1976.

Lyte M, Nelson SG, Thompson ML. Innate and adaptive immune responses in a social conflict paradigm. Clinical Immunology and Immunopathology. 57: 137–147, 1990.

Maisel AS, Murray D, Lotz M, Rearden A, Irwin M, Michel MC. Propranolol treatment affects parameters of human immunity. Immunopharmacology. 22: 157–164, 1991.

Manuck SB, Cohen S, Rabin BS, Muldoon MF, Bachen EA. Individual differences in cellular immune response to stress. Psychological Science. 2: 1–5, 1991.

Mills PJ, Berry CC, Dimsdale JE, Ziegler MG, Nelesen RA, Kennedy BP. Lymphocyte subset redistribution in response to acute experimental stress: Effects of gender, ethnicity, hypertension, and the sympathetic nervous system. Brain, Behavior, and Immunity. 9: 61–69, 1995.

Moss RB, Moss HB, Peterson R. Microstress, mood and natural killer cell activity. Psychosomatics. 30: 279–283, 1989.

Moyna NM, Acker GR, Fulton JR, Weber K, Goss FL, Robertson RJ, Tollerud DJ, Rabin BS. Lymphocyte function and cytokine production during incremental exercise in active and sedentary males and females. International Journal of Sports Medicine. 17: 585–591, 1996.

Moynihan JA, Ader R, Grota LJ, Schachtman TR, Cohen N. The effects of stress on the development of immunological memory following low dose antigen priming. Brain, Behavior, and Immunity. 4: 1–12, 1990.

Naliboff BD, Benton D, Solomon GF, Morley J, Fahey JL, Bloom E, Makinodan T, Gilmore S. Immunological changes in young and old adults during brief laboratory stress. Psychosomatic Medicine. 53: 121–132, 1991.

Petry LJ, Weems LB, Livingstone JN. Relationship of stress, distress, and the immunologic response to a recombinant hepatitis vaccine. The Journal of Family Practice. 32: 481–486, 1991.

Samuels AJ. Primary and secondary leukocyte changes following intramuscular injection of epinephrine hydrochloride. Journal of Clinical Investigation. 30: 941–947, 1951.

Sanders VM, Munson AE. Beta adrenoceptor mediation of the enhancing effect of norepinephrine on the murine primary antibody response in vitro. Journal of Pharmacology and Experimental Therapeutics. 230: 183–191, 1984.

Schedlowski M, Jacobs R, Stratmann G, Richter S, Hadicke A, Tewes U, Wagner TOF, Schmidt RE. Changes of natural killer cells during acute psychological stress. Journal of Clinical Immunology. 13: 119–126, 1993.

Schedlowski M, Hosch W, Oberbeck R, Benschop RJ, Benschop RJ, Jacobs R, Raab HR, Schmidt RE. Catecholamines modulate human natural killer (NK) cell circulation and function via spleen independent β2-adrenergic mechanisms. Journal of Immunology. 156: 93–99, 1996.

Schleifer SJ, Keller SE, Camerino M, Thornton JC, Stein M. Suppression of lymphocyte stimulation following bereavement. Journal of the American Medical Association. 250: 374–377, 1983.

Schmidt LA, Fox NA, Rubin KH, Sternberg EM, Gold PW, Smith CC, Schulkin J. Behavioral and neuroendocrine responses in shy children. Developmental Psychobiology. 30: 127–140, 1997.

Scott PA, Cierpial MA, Kilts CD, Weiss JM. Susceptibility and resistance of rats to stress–induced decreases in swim-test activity: A selective breeding study. Brain Research. 725: 217–230, 1996.

Sieber WJ, Rodin J, Larson L, Ortega S, Cummings N. Modulation of human natural killer cell activity by exposure to uncontrollable stress. Brain, Behavior, and Immunity. 6: 141–156, 1992.

Stone AA, Marco CA, Cruise CE, Cox DS, Neale JM. Are stress-induced immunological changes mediated by mood? A closer look at how both desirable and undesirable daily events influence sIgA antibody. International Journal of Behavioral Medicine. 3: 1–13, 1996.

Tarcic N, Levitan G, Ben-Yosef D, Prous D, Ovadia H, Weiss DW. Restraint stress-induced changes in lymphocyte subsets and the expression of adhesion molecules. Neuroimmunomodulation. 2: 249–257, 1995.

Tingate TR, Lugg D,. Muller HK, Stowe RP, Pierson DL. Antarctic isolation: Immune and viral studies. Immunology and Cell Biology. 75: 275-283, 1997

Taylor GR, Neale LS, Dardano B. Immunological analysis of US space shuttle crew members. Aviation and Space Medicine. 57: 213–217, 1989.

Toft P, Helbo-Hansen HS, Tonnesen E, Lillevang ST, Rasmussen JW, Christensen NJ. Redistribution of granulocytes during adrenaline infusion and following administration of cortisol in healthy volunteers. Acta Anaesthesiologica Scandinavica. 38: 254–258, 1994.

Tonnesen E, Brinklov MM, Christensen NJ, Olesen AS, Madsen T. Natural killer cell activity and lymphocyte function during and after coronary artery bypass grafting in relation to the endocrine stress response. Anesthesiology. 67: 526–533, 1987.

Valdimarsdottir HB, Stone AA. Psychosocial factors and secretory immunoglobulin A. Critical Reviews in Oral Biology and Medicine. 8: 461–474, 1997.

Weinstock C, Konig D, Harnischmacher R, Keul J, Berg A, Northoff H. Effect of exhaustive exercise stress on the cytokine response. Medicine and Science in Sports and Exercise. 29: 345–354, 1997.

Wood PG, Karol MH, Kusnecov AW, Rabin BS. Enhancement of antigen-specific humoral and cell-mediated immunity by electric footshock stress in rats. Brain, Behavior, and Immunity. 7: 121–134, 1993.

Zalcman S, Henderson N, Richter M, Anisman H. Age-related enhancement and suppression of a T-cell dependent antibody response following stressor exposure. Behavioral Neuroscience. 105: 669–676, 1991.

Zalcman S, Green-Johnson JM, Murry L, Wan W, Nance DM, Greenberg AH. Interleukin-2 induced enhancement of an antigen specific IgM plaque forming cell response is mediated by the sympathetic nervous system. Journal of Pharmacology and Experimental Therapeutics. 271: 977–982, 1994.

5

How Does the Hormonal Response Induced by Stress Alter the Immune System?

The link between the brain and the immune system must be mediated through soluble factors whose concentration increases as a result of psychological or physical stress or whose synthesis is initiated as a result of stress. Specific receptors must be present on the membrane or in the cytoplasm of the cells that are effected by stress. Because a variety of different cells comprise the immune system, and these cells are at various stages of maturity as the bone marrow and thymus continue to discharge new cells daily, and the cells have different molecules on their membrane depending on whether they are naive or memory cells, it is unlikely that the influence of stress hormones on modulating immune function will be a simple phenomenon. For example, although there is overwhelming evidence for the suppression of components of the immune response by stress, there are also reports of stressor-induced enhancement of the immune response (Wood et al, 1993; Dhabhar et al, 1996).

A limitation to studies regarding the hormonal modulation of immune function is that data are only available for what is studied. Stressing an experimental subject and studying and reporting changes of natural killer (NK) cell function does not let the research team know of other immune system changes that were also induced. With the vast complexity of the immune system, a change in one component can have an impact on the function of many other components. Performing in vitro studies that reveal altered mitosis or cytokine production does not provide information regarding functional changes in cell mediated immunity or antibody production that would occur in vivo. If a particular hormone is found to decrease cytokine production by Th1 cells, and the hormone is not tested for altering the function of dendritic cells or B lymphocytes or the antigen-presenting capabilities of macrophages, only a limited idea of the hormones effect on the immune system will be revealed. Whether the in vitro changes induced when studying a single hormone are reflective of the changes induced by that hormone in vivo where multiple hormones are simultaneously acting on lymphoid cells is also unclear. It is important to remember this background when reading this chapter.

To reliably determine the effect a neuropeptide or hormone has on the function of a cell of the immune system would require:

Isolation of each type of cell (Th1, Th2, CD8, NK, B), at different stages of maturation and as antigen naive cells and memory/effector cells

Incubation with a range of concentrations of hormones that may be found in plasma or at synapses where sympathetic nerves terminate at lymphocytes or dendritic cells in secondary lymphoid tissues

Incubation with combinations of hormones that may be found in plasma or at synapses where sympathetic nerves terminate at lymphocytes or dendritic cells in secondary lymphoid tissues

Measurement of hormone induced changes in the concentration of antigen receptors, costimulation molecules, cytokine production, and functions such as antibody production, cell-mediated immunity, antigen presentation

Stressor-induced enhancement of cell-mediated immune function could occur because of hormone-induced increases in cytokine production, increases of antigen-processing cells, and their function or increases of specific cell numbers that mediate cellular reactions. Does stressor-induced enhancement of immunity occur because lymphoid cells are working twice as hard, or because there are twice as many cells? Decreased immune function could occur for the opposite reasons.

As stressor-induced hormones are reviewed in this chapter, a repetition will emerge. There are only a finite number of types of lymphoid cells upon which a hormone can work. However, the cells that contain receptors for each hormone, the number of receptors, the concentration of hormone, the maturity of the lymphoid cell, the functional status of the cell when it binds the hormone, the presence of multiple hormones with enhancing or suppressing properties, and the lymphoid tissue where the hormone is binding to lymphoid cells, can each influence the final effect on immune function. As will become apparent in this chapter, there no unequivocal answers regarding the biological changes induced by stress hormones on the immune system. Regardless of the current state of knowledge, stress does modulate resistance to infectious agents (Cohen et al, 1991, 1997a,b).

There is extensive information regarding the effect of stress hormones on immune function both in vivo and in vitro. Yet, because of the complexity of the immune system, there is still a lack of in-depth understanding regarding the mechanisms and characteristics of how the immune alterations are brought about. Part of the problem relates to the continuing evolution of out understanding of how the immune system components (both cellular and soluble molecules) interact with each other to develop an effective immune response. In addition, a stressor elicits changes in the concentration of many hormones, each of which may act on a single lymphoid cell, provided the cell has receptors for each hormone. Given this complexity, it is impressive that we know as much as we do regarding mechanisms of stressor-induced immune alteration.

The following discussion is an example of what is known and unknown about the effect of stress related hormones on cells of the immune system.

CATECHOLAMINES

Effects on Lymphocyte Numbers

There are several neuropeptides and hormones that, upon binding to their receptors, can modify the numbers of cells of the immune system circulating in the blood. An example is provided by injecting epinephrine and then following quantitative and qualitative changes of lymphocytes in the blood (in humans, lymphocyte changes in the spleen and lymph nodes cannot be measured). Injection of epinephrine into healthy human subjects is associated with a transient increase of the number of lymphocytes in the peripheral blood (Crary et al, 1983). The mitogenic responses to nonspecific stimulation of T and B lymphocytes is reduced and returns to the pre-injection level by 120 minutes after injection. Other studies have reported similar findings, with increases of CD8 and NK cells consistently reported after the injection of catecholamine agonists into humans (Landmann et al, 1984; Maisel et al, 1989; van Tits et al, 1991). Similar quantitative and qualitative changes are detected 5–6 minutes after initiation of a psychological or physical stressor (Herbert et al, 1994; Moyna et al, 1996).

A concern relates to how an injection of epinephrine increases the number of lymphocytes in the blood, with the major increase being of CD8 and NK lymphocytes along with a decrease of lymphocyte responsiveness to nonspecific stimulation with mitogen. For simplicity, let us assume that the increase of lymphocyte numbers is due to the increase of CD8 and NK lymphocytes. Where can these cells come from?

Bone Marrow. The bone marrow is the source of all lymphocytes. There are no studies which can clarify the importance of the marrow as a source of stressor-induced increased numbers of CD8 and NK cells in the blood. Catecholamines may alter the adhesion properties of lymphocytes by decreasing adhesion molecules on lymphocytes or on stromal cells in the marrow, causing a release of cells from the marrow. However, an argument can be made against the marrow on the basis of the increased number of CD8 cells in blood following stress. The marrow contains immature T cells that do not have the CD4 or CD8 markers on their membrane. Therefore, it is unlikely that if the marrow were induced to discharge T lymphocytes into the blood that the observed changes of more CD8 cells would be seen. A similar argument is not applicable for B lymphocytes or NK lymphocytes.

A study performed with rabbits suggests the bone marrow may contribute to the increased lymphocytes in the blood (Toft et al, 1992). Lymphocytes were isolated from 24 rabbits and radioactively labeled before being reinjected into the rabbits.

Twenty-four hours later, the rabbits received injections of epinephrine or saline. The activity of the labeled cells was imaged with a gamma counter. The results showed that after epinephrine injection, the radioactivity in the spleen and bone marrow decreased approximately 90%, while the radioactivity in the heart, lung, and liver each approximately doubled. In peripheral blood, there was an increase of approximately 10%. Thus, in this rabbit model, epinephrine produces a significant redistribution of lymphocytes from the spleen and bone marrow to the peripheral blood, lungs, and liver. However, as the lymphocytes were obtained from the blood and were manipulated in the laboratory prior to being reinjected into the rabbits, they may not have behaved as would lymphocytes that are maturing in the marrow.

Secondary Lymphoid Tissue. The spleen and lymph nodes contain naive T and B lymphocytes and T and B memory lymphocytes. However, the flow of blood through each of these tissues differs with the spleen being placed directly in the blood stream and lymph nodes releasing lymphocytes into the efferent lymphatic vessel which then enter the bloodstream through the thoracic duct. Owing to these anatomical considerations and the rapid alteration of lymphocyte numbers in the blood, the spleen would be a likely source of the cells. However, that is not supported by experimental data, as splenectomized subjects showed the same changes in stress-induced peripheral blood lymphocytes as spleen intact subjects (Grazzi et al, 1993; Schedlowski et al, 1996).

Demargination from Endothelial Cells. Naive lymphocytes adhere to specialized high endothelial cells that are present in the postcapillary venules of lymph nodes. This adherence is associated with the ability of naive lymphocytes to cross the endothelial cells and enter the nodes. The naive lymphocytes have an L-selectin molecule that binds to receptors (CD34) on the high endothelial cells. Memory/effector lymphocytes do not synthesize the L-selectin and cannot bind to high endothelial cells. Rather, they display the integrin adhesion molecules VLA-4 and LFA-1 which bind to receptors on endothelial cells in tissues, particularly where the expression of the VLA-4 and LFA-1 have been upregulated by cytokines released as part of an inflammatory response.

Thus, it is possible that there are lymphocytes that are rolling along and traversing endothelial cells throughout the body. However, if catecholamine concentrations are increased, these cells may demarginate from the endothelial cells and be measured in the blood. An increased migration of lymphocytes into secondary lymphoid tissues was found in animals that had been sympathectomized (Madden et al, 1994). This suggests that a decrease of catecholamines was associated with an increase of adhesion molecules for receptors in secondary lymphoid tissue. When a needle is placed into a vein, the cells in the collected blood are those cells that are in the center of the flow, rather than the cells attached to the blood vessel wall.

Increased catecholamine concentrations would be expected to be associated with decreased adhesion. When lymphocytes were collected from mice that had been sympathectomized (which results in an increase of β-adrenergic receptors on the lymphocytes) and transferred to normal mice, there was a decreased migration into lymphoid tissues. This suggests that increased responsivity to catecholamines (assuming that the lymphocytes from the sympathectomized mice had increased numbers of adrenergic receptors) is associated with less adherence to endothelial cells. The increase of lymphocytes in the blood of subjects injected with catecholamine is compatible with decreased endothelial adhesion caused by catecholamine binding to adrenergic receptors.

Infusion of the adrenergic agonist, isoproterenol, into humans alters the concentration of adhesion molecules on peripheral blood lymphocytes (Mills et al, 1997). Isoproterenol (an adrenergic agonist) caused an increase in the total number of CD8 lymphocytes in the blood. The CD8 cells that increased in the blood had reduced concentrations of L-selectin on their membranes. This suggests several possibilities; (1) CD8 cells with fewer selectin molecules are released from rolling along the vascular endothelial cells and enter the blood stream with the mechanical effects of an increase in heart rate and blood pressure, (2) isoproterenol inhibited the production of L-selectin by CD8 cells and they were released from the endothelial cells without mechanical effects, (3) CD8 cells with lowered concentrations of L-selectin were released from secondary lymphoid tissues.

A release of the ICAM-1 adhesion molecule from vascular endothelial cells by vigorous exercise has been reported (Rehman et al, 1997). This is prevented by pretreatment of the subjects with a β-adrenergic antagonist, suggesting a catecholamine dependent mechanism that may decrease the adhesion molecule concentration on endothelial cells. ICAM-1 binds to the LFA-1 adhesion molecule that is on T lymphocytes.

Other in vitro studies of lymphocyte attachment to endothelial cells show catecholamine-induced effects (Benschop et al, 1993, 1994c). The effect of catecholamine on altering adhesion to endothelial cells is primarily on the lymphocyte rather than on the endothelial cell. The effect on catecholamines on adhesion of NK cells was duplicated by incubation of the cells with forskolin, which elevates the intracellular concentration of cAMP, as does catecholamine. Thus, the loss of adhesion may be due to a cAMP-dependent mechanism.

A study that reported an increase of NK lymphocyte numbers in peripheral blood after catecholamine injection did not find a change in the concentration of adhesion molecules on the NK cells (Schedlowski et al, 1996). Thus, as the alterations of immune and cardiovascular parameters are correlated (NK numbers and heart rate increase) (Benschop et al, 1995) the mechanism of catecholamine induced increases of NK cell numbers may have a mechanical component to it. Increased blood flow may knock lymphoid cells off the endothelial cells or dislodge them from other tissues.

A consideration for the alteration of lymphocyte populations in blood by stress is related to alterations of the flow characteristics of blood. Is it possible that the increase of heart rate and systolic blood pressure induced by stress is what is responsible for dislodging lymphocytes from endothelial cells? Indeed, we found that the greatest change in lymphocyte subset numbers were in those subjects who we exposed to a psychological stressor and who had the greatest elevation of systolic blood pressure and heart rate (Manuck et al, 1991). However, as those subjects also had the highest elevation of catecholamines, it could be that a combination of a hemodynamic processes and direct effects of catecholamines on lymphocytes were responsible for the observed changes. Pretreatment of subjects prior to their being stressed with an adrenergic antagonist to block catecholamine binding abolished the cardiovascular and changes in immune cells in the blood (Benschop et al, 1994b; Bachen et al, 1995).

A comparison of the effects of an acute psychological stressor on cardiovascular and immune parameters in individuals with low or high levels of daily stress in their lives evaluated the effect of baseline stress levels on stressor-induced changes of lymphocyte numbers in the blood (Benschop et al, 1994a). Acute stressor-induced elevations of heart rate and blood pressure were the same regardless of daily stress levels. However, there was an increase in the number of blood NK cells only in those individuals with low levels of daily stress. The high chronic stress group had a higher baseline number of NK cells. This study contributes to the likelihood that catecholamines are responsible for the increase of the number of blood NK cells and that in subjects with high levels of chronic stress the cells are already circulating in the blood with no further increment by additional stress.

Experimental conditions that dissociated NK cells from endothelial cells in vitro did not have an effect on T cell adhesion to endothelial cells (Benschop et al, 1993). Thus, an explanation for the observation of stressor-induced increases of NK and CD8 cells in the blood is not apparent. However, a possible explanation has been suggested as a subpopulation of NK cells may have the CD8 marker on their membrane (Benschop et al, 1994c). As there are NK cells which weakly express the CD8 marker, this is a possible explanation of the experimental findings and would indicate that the only lymphocyte population that increases with stress are the NK cells. Careful replication of studies which report an increase of CD8 cells in the blood by stress (Manuck et al, 1991; Naliboff et al, 1991), exercise (Moyna et al, 1996), or isoproterenol infusion (van Tits et al, 1990), would be helpful to clarify the actual cell populations which become altered.

Epinephrine reduced the attachment of lymphocytes to human umbilical vein endothelial cells grown in tissue culture and incubated with IL-1 (Carlson et al, 1996). The concentration of adhesion molecules on the lymphocytes and endothelial cells did not appear to be altered. Affinity measurements for the tightness of binding of the lymphocytes to the endothelial cells were not made. As the endothelial cells used in the in vitro studies had to be grown in tissue culture, it is uncertain that the observations regarding changes in adhesion induced by catecholamines relate to in vivo conditions. The same array of adhesion molecules present in vivo may not have been present when the endothelial cells were grown in culture. Also, modulation of adhesion molecules on the lymphocytes by catecholamine may not reproduce changes that occur in vivo where other hormones are simultaneously present and whose concentration may also be altered by stress.

In addition to changes in the blood, alteration of lymphocyte migration patterns by catecholamines may occur in tissue. Mouse lymph node lymphocytes labeled with a fluorescent dye have been traced when injected intravenously into mice syngeneic (identical twins) with the lymphocyte donor (Carlson et al, 1997). The lymphocytes migrated to the T-cell areas of the nodes and spleen (paracortex and white pulp). When the lymphocytes were pretreated with a β-adrenergic agonist, increased numbers of lymphocytes, which were predominantly T cells, migrated to the T-cell areas of the secondary lymphoid tissues. Thus, this study suggests that activation of the adrenergic receptor may generate adhesion molecules on T lymphocytes that increase their accumulation in the secondary lymphoid tissues.

What cell populations are increased in the blood by stress? Are they NK and CD8, or are they NK with a CD8 marker on them? How much of the increase is due to hemodynamic alterations induced by an increased heart rate and how much is due to changes in the adhesion molecule concentration or affinity on lymphocytes and endothelial cells? If there is an increase of CD8 cells, where do they come from if they do not marginate on endothelial cells? Is the increase of NK cell numbers solely due to demargination?

Why is the main change found in the NK population? Possibly because the number of adrenergic receptors on NK cells is more than the number on other lymphocyte populations and therefore there is a greater effect on NK cells. Indeed, different populations of lymphocytes have different numbers of adrenergic receptors (Khan et al, 1986; Maisel, et al, 1989; van Tits et al, 1991). As might be predicted, the NK cell population has the largest number of adrenergic receptors, B lymphocytes have the next highest number. The CD8+ lymphocytes have fewer adrenergic receptors than B lymphocytes, but a greater number of receptors than the CD4+ lymphocyte population, which has the fewest number of receptors. Therefore, to be consistent there should also be an increase of the number of B lymphocytes in the blood after stress or catecholamine injection. Yet the B-lymphocyte population, which has the second highest number of adrenergic receptors after the NK cells, shows little change in numbers in the peripheral blood after stress, exercise, or the infusion of catecholamines. Interestingly B lymphocytes do not show a stressor-induced alteration of their responsiveness to the nonspecific pokeweed mitogen. T lymphocytes do show a stress-induced reduction of responsiveness to the T-cell mitogen, phytohemagglutinin (PHA). It is possible that the second messenger systems in T and B lymphocytes differ with the β-adrenergic receptor not being coupled to a second messenger that can alter the function of B lymphocytes. In T lymphocytes, the adrenergic receptor may be coupled to a second messenger that can alter mitogenic function. Monocytes have been reported to contain high numbers of β-adrenergic receptors (Maisel et al, 1989). No data are available for adrenergic receptors on dendritic cells, although these cells play a central role in immune activation.

Incubating lymphocytes, in vitro, with catecholamines, leads to an elevation of cyclic adenosine monophosphate (cAMP) and decreased mitogenic function. However, different lymphocyte subsets, in humans, when incubated with a β-adrenergic agonist, isoproterenol, accumulate different amounts of cAMP (Maisel et al, 1989). Basal cAMP levels are similar in all lymphocyte subsets but following incubation with isoproterenol, little elevation of cAMP was found in B lymphocytes. CD8 and NK lymphocytes accumulated much larger amounts of cAMP than B lymphocytes, indicating that the number of β-adrenergic receptors is not associated with accumulation of cAMP. Thus, if the alteration of lymphocyte numbers in blood following stress is due to cAMP formation, NK lymphocytes would be expected to show the largest increase, as they do.

The cell population that accumulated the least amount of cAMP after incubation with isoproterenol was the CD4 lymphocytes. Yet, this is the population that has decreased responsiveness following stress and stimulation with PHA. Therefore, the evidence and logic that support a direct role of catecholamines having an effect on CD4 lymphocyte function, in vivo, is not strong.

Effects on Lymphocyte Function

Stress-induced decreased mitosis of lymphocytes in response to nonspecific mitogens may be mediated by catecholamines as an adrenergic antagonist prevented stressor-induced suppression of lymphocyte mitosis (Benschop et al, 1994b; Bachen et al, 1995). However, it is uncertain whether this is a direct effect of catecholamines on cell division, a reduction of the production of cytokines that stimulate cell division, or the induction of modulators such as nitric oxide, which inhibits lymphocyte mitosis (Kizaki et al, 1996). However, as with most aspects of immune system function, nothing is as clear as we would like it to be. For example, there are studies that report that catecholamines are capable of inducing an increase of mitosis in a variety of cell types (Merten et al, 1993; deBlois et al, 1996; Saito et al, 1997). Catecholamines have also been reported to decrease mitosis and increase or decrease IL-6 production, depending on the stage of maturation of the target cell (Frediani et al, 1996), and protein synthesis has also been reported to be increased by catecholamines (Decker et al, 1993).

The effect of catecholamines on the alteration of lymphocyte function is short lived (Crary et al, 1983; van Tits et al, 1991), lasting only about 2 hours. Infusion of catecholamines, for as long as 6 hours, is reported to have a short duration of effect on blood pressure and heart rate (Tulen et al, 1993). Acute episodes of stress and catecholamine elevation may not be able to sustain a prolonged effect on immune function that would have biological significance as within 2 hours of termination of a psychological stressor or the stress of severe exercise, immune function returns to normal (Moyna et al, 1996). This suggests that for catecholamines to have an effect on immune function that can predispose to illness, catecholamine levels must be chronically elevated. This is supported by a study of stress duration and susceptibility to infection (Cohen et al, 1998)

Of course this implies that chronic catecholamine elevation will alter lymphocyte function in the same way as does acute catecholamine elevation. Whether this actually occurs is unknown. Remember that millions of new lymphocytes are being produced daily. Whether lymphocytes that have resided in blood for 1, 2, 3, or 14 days, respond to the effects of high concentrations of catecholamines in identical manners needs to be determined. It is possible that decreasing numbers of adrenergic receptors will be present depending on the duration of time that the lymphocytes are exposed to high catecholamine concentrations. Fewer catecholamine receptors may be associated with decreased responsiveness to the effects of catecholamines.

Another concern in studying the effect of catecholamines on the function of immune cells relates to the concentration of catecholamine that is present at the cell membrane. Different concentrations of catecholamine will be present at nerve terminals, in the blood, or in parenchymal tissues. As the number of adrenergic receptors decreases in the presence of high concentrations of catecholamines, the responsivity of different lymphocytes to subsequent catecholamine exposure may differ (Mills et al, 1997b). Even catecholamine elevation due to congestive heart failure will decrease the number of adrenergic receptors on lymphocytes (Wu et al, 1996). If the alteration of immune function when a lymphocyte binds catecholamine to adrenergic receptors is related to the number of adrenergic receptors present, the prior interaction of the lymphocyte with catecholamines in different compartments of the body may influence how lymphocyte function will be altered.

Within the spleen, there is close contact between the sympathetic nerve terminal and lymphoid cells. However, in the blood or tissue there will be lower concentrations of catecholamines. In addition, lymphocytes are mobile cells, moving through secondary lymphatic tissue and parenchymal tissues. The concentration of catecholamine they are exposed to will likely fluctuate as they move. It is possible that different concentrations of catecholamines will either exert a positive or negative influence on the function of a single cell. It is also possible that low concentrations of catecholamines may activate one type of cell and higher concentrations may activate another type of cell. Until studies are done with isolated cell populations, it will not be possible to determine why different catecholamine concentrations may have different effects on lymphoid cell function.

It is reliably established that lymphocytes can change the molecules on their membrane at different stages of function. Examples include the change in trafficking of naive and effector/memory lymphocytes which is related to the change of a selectin molecule when a naive lymphocyte is activated and a change of the form of the CD45 molecule on naive (CD45RA) and activated lymphocytes (CD45RO). There is no information regarding hormonal receptors on lymphocytes other than approximation of numbers present on different classes of lymphocytes. Examples of different classes of lymphocytes include (1) naive CD4, (2) effector/memory CD4 that have not reacted with their specific antigen, (3) effector/memory CD4 that have reacted to their specific antigen, (4) naive CD4 that have migrated from the thymus within a few hours of being collected for study, and (5) naive CD4 that have migrated from the thymus 2 weeks ago. In addition, there are CD4 lymphocytes in the lymph nodes, spleen, bronchial associated lymphoid tissues, gut-associated lymphoid tissues, and parenchymal tissues.

When different classes of lymphocytes are studied, they must be separated from other lymphocytes. This usually involves collection of blood and isolation of the population that will be studied by a selection procedure that may or may not change the number of molecules on the cell membrane. Thus, we must be careful in interpreting data regarding numbers of adrenergic receptors on lymphocytes. Not only is it unlikely that we know the actual numbers because of the diversity of each lymphocyte population, but it is equally difficult to assign biological effects related to receptor number.

Each individual has epinephrine and norepinephrine present in the plasma and tissue fluids at all times. Throughout the day, related to mental stress and physical activity, the concentration of catecholamines will change. Some increases may be of short duration and others of long duration. Every day tens of millions of mature but naive lymphocytes are released into the blood. The concentration of catecholamine during the maturation of the lymphoid cells may or may not permanently alter the number of adrenergic receptors on the lymphocyte membrane while the cell is naive.

An in vitro study has been reported that indicates that incubating human peripheral blood derived monocytes with epinephrine, insulin, or somatostatin, decreases the ability of the mononuclear phagocytic cells to kill mycobacterium avium when the monocytes are simultaneously incubated with tumor necrosis factor (TNF) (Bermudz et al, 1990). This study suggests that the mononuclear phagocytic cells may be a target of stressor-induced hormones. As stress has also been shown capable of modifying macrophage function in rodents, (Zwilling et al, 1991), it is likely that if additional studies of mononuclear phagocyte function are performed in humans after stress, alterations of function may be detected. Based on the limited data available, stress would be expected to decrease the ability of macrophages to kill ingested microorganisms and therefore, increase susceptibility to diseases caused by intracellular bacteria or mycobacterium.

Immunization of individuals at times of stress in their lives results in lower amounts of antibody production than does immunization of individuals who are not under stress. There is increased susceptibility to infection with viruses causing the common cold when an individual is under high, rather than low, levels of stress. Reactivation of latent viral infections occurs at times of stress. It is therefore likely that catecholamines do alter immune function. A goal would be to understand how this occurs so that strategies could be devised to prevent stressor-induced immune suppression and to enhance the function of the immune system, especially in older individuals.

GLUCOCORTICOIDS

Cortisol can be bought at any drug store or supermarket as an over-the-counter medication for application to the skin for the treatment of a wide variety of skin rashes. Often, a beneficial effect is achieved as the cortisol cream will reduce the amount of inflammation in skin (an accumulation of neutrophils, macrophages, and lymphocytes in the skin). Glucocorticoids (cortisol in humans and corticosterone in rodents) also modify the function of cells of the immune system, although short-term studies of stress on immune function are often terminated before cortisol becomes elevated, and studies in adrenalectomized animals still result in stressor-induced immune alteration (Keller et al, 1983; Manuck et al, 1991). However, the data are not entirely definitive, as it has also been demonstrated in rats that stressor-induced alteration of peripheral blood mitogenic function is dependent on glucocorticoids (Cunnick et al, 1990). Thus, it will be important to consider the type of immune function, the compartment of the body in which the immune system is being studied (blood, spleen, lymph nodes, parenchymal tissue), the characteristics of the immune cells, and the characteristics of the stressor with regard to its intensity and duration,when considering the importance and contribution of glucocorticoids to stressor-induced immune alteration.

There are several modulating factors regarding glucocorticoids and their effects on the immune system:

1. The physical state of the glucocorticoid than can bind to specific receptors in the cytoplasm of cells is unbound to the plasma carrier of glucocorticoids, corticosterone binding globulin (CBG). Standard assays that measure glucocorticoids report both the free and the bound hormone. Thus, the biologically available hormone concentration cannot be determined unless the concentration of CBG is measured. As the concentration of CBG decreases with stress, an increase of total glucocorticoid may be associated with greater numbers of glucocorticoid receptors becoming occupied than occurs when CBG levels are not decreased (Fleshner et al, 1995; Spencer et al, 1996). This may lead to an accentuation of the glucocorticoid modifying capabilities on the immune system.

2. If all the glucocorticoid receptors in a cell are occupied, elevations of free plasma glucocorticoid concentrations will not have an effect on metabolic processes in the cell. As there is a circadian rhythm to glucocorticoid concentrations, different numbers of hormone receptors may be available at different times of the day.

3. The immune systems of different species respond differently to glucocorticoids. The rat, mouse, hamster, and rabbit are very sensitive to glucocorticoids with the thymus, spleen, lymph nodes, and peripheral blood showing marked reduction of viable lymphocytes subsequent to low-level (10^{-7} M) glucocorticoid administration. Lymphoid cell death is primarily through apoptosis (Cohen et al, 1989). Lymphoid cells of humans, monkeys, and guinea pigs are more resistant to glucocorticoids, with concentrations of 10^{-4} M–10^{-6} M having little effect on lymphocyte viability (Claman, 1972). Whether the sensitivity of steroid sensitive species is actually due to cell death or, in addition, whether changes in leukocyte trafficking patterns change the numbers of cells in the blood has not been determined (Moorhead and Claman, 1972). Thus, it is important to consider the species in which studies of glucocorticoid effects on the immune system are performed. Extrapolation of alterations of immune function from a steroid sensitive to a steroid-resistant species, or vice versa, should be avoided. There may also be different effects of glucocorticoids when bound by dividing cells in comparison with nondividing cells.

4. Different numbers of glucocorticoid receptors may be available to bind when an acute stressor is invoked on an individual who has low levels of life stress in comparison with an individual who has high levels of life stress.

Unoccupied glucocorticoid receptors are located in the cytoplasm of cells. When the receptor binds to glucocorticoid it changes its shape and moves to the nucleus where a site on the receptor binds to DNA. The production of proteins increases or decreases as a result. Obviously, depending on which proteins undergo alteration of their synthesis, essential immune processes such as adhesion molecules or cytokine production may become altered.

There are 2 receptors for adrenal steroids. Type I adrenal steroid receptor is primarily mineralocorticoid binding but also has a high binding affinity for glucocorticoids. The type II adrenal steroid receptor binds dexamethasone, a synthetic glucocorticoid, with a greater affinity than natural glucocorticoids, while type I receptors bind glucocorticoids more efficiently than they bind dexamethasone (Spencer et al, 1990). Because the synthetic and naturally occurring glucocorticoids have different affinities for the two different glucocorticoid receptors, it is possible that studies of the effect of dexamethasone, which is frequently used in studies of immune modulation, on immune function do not entirely reflect the changes caused by the naturally occurring hormone.

A hormone can have no effect unless a receptor for the hormone is present on or in a cell. The type II receptors are present in higher concentration than type I receptors in all tissues of the rat. Cells of the immune system contain higher concentrations of type II receptors than other tissues. Both T and B lymphocytes isolated from human spleen are reported to have the same number of available type I and II receptors (Armannini et al, 1988). However, consideration of the source of the cell populations studied is needed in order to properly evaluate these observations. The cells were obtained from the spleens of cadaveric kidney donors. Cadaveric donors usually suffer a traumatic death, receive extensive amounts of medication to maintain their blood pressure and cardiac output, and frequently receive glucocorticoid injections. It is likely that the spleen lymphoid cells were exposed to high concentrations of glucocorticoids before assay for glucocorticoid receptors. This places the reliability of the observation in question with regard to the actual number of available receptors present in a resting state.

Different effects of binding of specific agonists to the type I or type II receptor have been reported for circulating leukocyte numbers in rats (Miller et al, 1994). Aldosterone, which selectively binds to the type I receptor decreased NK cell numbers in the blood. RU28362, a type II agonist increased NK numbers. Whether increases and decreases of adhesion molecules on the NK cells accounted for these changes was not determined. As alterations of protein synthesis are associated with adrenal steroid binding, this may have been a factor in inducing the changes in NK numbers in the blood with either more or fewer NK cells marginating along the endothelial cells. Dexamethasone and cortisol injection also increased the number of NK cells and CD8 cells in the blood (Singh et al, 1996).

In humans there is a glucocorticoid-dependent decrease of the total number of lymphocytes in the blood (Fauci and Dale, 1975). Changes in trafficking patterns or cell death may cause this change. The characteristics of the change can have significant implications. For example, if the lymphocytes increase their adherence to endothelial cells (resulting in fewer cells available for collection through a needle inserted into a vein), there may be enhanced migration of the lymphocytes into parenchymal tissues and increased resistance to infectious agents (Dhabhar and McEwen, 1996).

If effector cells were to migrate into parenchymal tissues, it would be anticipated that they would soon reenter the blood from the thoracic duct. Similarly, if naive cells were to migrate more efficiently into secondary lymphoid tissues, it would be anticipated that they would soon reenter the blood from the thoracic duct. Indeed, as the lymphocyte count is usually depressed for approximately 24 hours after a bolus injection of glucocorticoid, the glucocorticoid-modulated cells may remain in parenchymal or lymphoid tissue for as long as 24 hours. However, as new lymphocytes are normally released from the marrow and thymus, glucocorticoid-induced cell death remains a possible explanation for the decreased lymphocyte numbers. As lymphoid cells age and die, they would not be replaced in adequate numbers.

In addition to changing cell numbers in the blood, there are indications that glucocorticoids can modify the ability of lymphocytes to divide. Dexamethasone binding to type II receptors decreases the ability of rat spleen lymphocytes to divide when incubated with Concanavalin A (Con A) (Miller et al, 1991). Whether the reduction of mitosis is due to inhibition of cytokine production or other pathways necessary for cell division has not been determined. Regardless of the mechanism, in rodents there is an indication that lymphocyte function may be altered and that NK numbers in the blood may be altered.

Chronic elevation of cortisol occurs in subjects who have Cushing's syndrome. Thus, they are an interesting population for study, although caution must be used in interpreting the data relating to chronic stressor-induced alterations of the immune system. In Cushing's syndrome, the plasma cortisol level is elevated and often does not undergo circadian changes. The maturing lymphoid cells are exposed to higher concentrations of cortisol than when they mature in normal individuals. Adrenocorticotropic hormone (ACTH) production is elevated in many subjects with Cushing's syndrome (often this is the cause of the Cushing's syndrome). Thus, ACTH may also have an effect on the lymphoid cells.

Lymphocyte subpopulation numbers are altered in patients with Cushing's syndrome. The number of CD8 cells is increased and NK function decreased (Kronfol et al, 1996). Functionally, IL-2 production by nonspecific mitogen stimulated lymphocytes is decreased and concentrations of the soluble IL-2 receptor in plasma were decreased (Sauer et al, 1994). It has not been determined whether these changes reflected a decrease in CD4 lymphocytes and an increase in CD8 lymphocyte numbers or an altered metabolic function of T lymphocytes by glucocorticoids. However, the data indicate that glucocorticoid elevation is Cushing's syndrome produces immune alterations often found in association with stress.

An important alteration of Th1 and Th2 lymphocyte biological function is induced by glucocorticoids. When human blood lymphocytes are incubated with low concentrations of cortisol (0.1–10 μM) and IL-4, the concentration of IgE that is released is markedly increased in comparison to the amount released without added cortisol (Wu et al, 1991). IgE production is dependent on IL-4 produced by Th2 lymphocytes that induce B lymphocytes to switch the class of heavy chain from μ to ε. Thus, glucocorticoids may favor Th2 activity.

Physiologically low concentrations of glucocorticoids are known to enhance cytokine production by Th2 cells while inhibiting cytokine production by Th1 cells

(Daynes et al, 1989). Decreased Th1 activity would reduce cell-mediated immunity (delayed-type hypersensitivity reactions). This would be expected to produce an amelioration of diseases associated with a cell-mediated immune pathogenesis. High concentrations of glucocorticoids would inhibit both Th1- and Th2-derived cytokines, producing a suppression of all T-cell-mediated immune responses. A casual review of the effects of glucocorticoids on diseases that have an inflammatory component or that are mediated by cellular immune mechanisms readily attests to the ability of glucocorticoids to ameliorate an inflammatory response and a cellular immune response.

Glucocorticoids can have a pharmacological effect, when used in high concentrations, by suppressing immune reactions. This is the basis of many therapeutic strategies for the management of immune-mediated diseases, such as rheumatoid arthritis or multiple sclerosis, or medical situations such as organ transplants. However, the elevation of glucocorticoid concentrations associated with psychological stress or physical exercise is not as high as that achieved by pharmacological means. As stress will produce an elevation of hormones other than glucocorticoids, the interaction of the various hormones in modifying immune function must always be considered. Unfortunately, few studies have been done to evaluate multiple hormones simultaneously acting on cells of the immune system.

Determination of habituation of catecholamine and glucocorticoid production with repeated or chronic stress has been evaluated. These data are reported here because they relate to the magnitude of the immune altering hormonal response induced by stress. Parachute jumping was used as a stressor in humans to evaluate whether habituation of cortisol production occurred with repeated jumping (Deinzer et al, 1997). After the third jump, some of the subjects had significantly lower cortisol responses than after the first and second jump. However, there were subjects who maintained a high response after the third jump. Thus, habituation does occur in some individuals at a time when it does not occur in others. This suggests a lack of uniformity of glucocorticoid responses in different individuals when experiencing repeated stress.

Most studies of the hormones and neuropeptides that modulate immune function evaluate catecholamines and glucocorticoids. Possibly, these are the most important stress-induced immune modulating factors. However, they are not the only hormones that can affect the immune system and whose concentration is increased by stress. The following sections will discuss several other hormones and some of the ways in which they can alter immune function. Whether they actually do so in vivo and how multiple hormones interact to alter immune function has not been determined. Thus, even though each hormone can elicit changes in components of the immune system, these changes should be considered as the potential capability of each individual hormone to alter immune function. Actual effects can only be determined through careful studies using specific antagonists that either evaluate end stage immune function in vivo (eg, antibody production or cell-mediated immune reactions) or look at discrete components in vitro (eg, cytokine release or NK cytotoxicity).

The following list is comprehensive but not complete. The discussion of each hormone will develop an understanding of the various aspects of the immune system that are susceptible to modification.

SUBSTANCE P

Substance P (SP) is a neuropeptide of 11 amino acids that is classified as a tachykinin (ie, elicits an increased heart rate subsequent to lowering of blood pressure). SP is found in many areas of the brain as well as in nerves innervating secondary lymphoid tissues and has a wide distribution in tissues. SP is stored in nerve endings. Receptors for SP are found on the membranes of both T and B cells, mononuclear phagocytic cells, and mast cells. It is released from sensory nerve fibers and contributes to the induction of localized inflammatory reactions. In this regard SP can be said to have a proinflammatory (preceding inflammation) activity, similar to some of the cytokines (IL-1, IL-6, TNF).

Receptors for SP are present on lymphoid cells, although whether all subpopulations of lymphocytes have SP receptors remains undetermined (Kaltreider et al, 1997). SP receptors are also located on endothelial cells, possibly mediating alterations of adhesion molecules (Tang et al, 1993).

The activities of SP on the immune system include:

1. Functions as a chemoattractant factor for inflammatory cells (Payan, 1989; Schratzberger et al, 1997).

2. Induces the release of histamine from mast cells (Shanahan et al, 1985). The release of mediators from mast cells can be caused by a conditioned stress response and is mediated by SP (MacQueen et al, 1989).

3. Causes smooth muscle contraction. This property of SP may contribute to the ability of SP to enhance inflammation by increasing the permeability of small blood vessels. SP also is a chemoattractant for T and B lymphocytes, a property which would further enhance its ability to contribute to an inflammatory response (Herzberg et al, 1995; Schratzberger et al, 1997). Although the migration of lymphocytes into tissue may be affected by SP, the migration of lymphocytes into lymph nodes may not be influenced by SP (Heerwagen et al, 1995). Thus, a principal role of SP may be as a mediator of tissue inflammation, rather than directing the traffic of lymphocytes into secondary lymphatic tissue. Indeed, if SP enhanced the migration of memory/effector lymphocytes into secondary lymphoid tissue there may be a diminished ability of these cells to enter inflammatory reaction sites in parenchymal tissues.

4. Can increase the rate of mitotic division of activated lymphocytes (Covas et al, 1995, 1997). This is an interesting observation as denervation of joints has an ameliorating effect on inflammation of arthritic conditions. The modulation of lymphocyte mitogenic responsiveness is influenced by the concentration of SP to which the cells are exposed. Thus, experimental conditions can be established where SP will either enhance or decrease the response of lymphocytes responding to nonspecific mitogens (Argo et al, 1995). This is important to bear in mind, as the concentrations of neuropeptides that lymphocytes are exposed to will vary greatly at synaptic sites in the spleen between nerve endings and lymphocytes, or in the blood where dilution of neuropeptides released from nerve terminals occurs.

5. May alter the ability of dendritic cells to present antigen to T lymphocytes (Staniek et al, 1997).

6. Mononuclear phagocytic cells and T lymphocytes are induced to release cytokines by SP (Wagner et al, 1987; Lotz et al, 1988; Remeshwar et al, 1993; Goafa et al, 1996).

7. Increases the expression of adhesion molecules of vascular endothelial cells and on lymphocytes (Vishwanath et al, 1996). However, this finding needs to be further evaluated as an earlier report did not find that SP could enhance adhesion of lymphocytes to endothelial cells (Smart et al, 1994).

8. Increases immunoglobulin production by B lymphocytes (Hart et al, 1990).

SP has the capability of influencing many phases of the immune response, as described above. Nonspecific acute inflammation and specific immune-mediated responses appear to be susceptible to SP influence. However, catecholamines and glucocorticoids may also influence the same responses. How do the alterations induced by SP interact with the alterations produced by the other hormones? That is unexplored. An appreciation that the immune alterations produced by hormones whose concentration increases in response to stress reflects the summation of the enhancing and suppressing components of the various hormonal modifications should be emerging.

NEUROPEPTIDE Y

Neuropeptide Y (NPY) is present in the neurons of the central nervous system (CNS) and in the neurons in numerous tissues throughout the body, including the mucosa. NPY is co-localized in nerve terminals in lymphatic tissues with norepinephrine. In the rat NPY nerve terminals are located primarily in the macrophage rich areas of the spleen (Meltzer et al, 1997). Whether there are antigen-presenting dendritic cells in the same location as these neurons has not been determined.

Lymphocytes have receptors for NPY and therefore NPY may modulate their function (Petitto et al, 1994). It is likely that macrophages and/or dendritic cells also have NPY receptors.

NPY mRNA is detected in human peripheral blood monocytes, B lymphocytes, and T lymphocytes when the cells are activated (Schwarz et al, 1994). The physiological role of lymphocyte or monocyte-derived NPY is unknown. If NPY synthesis is inducible, and NPY inhibits immune reactions, as has been suggested (Friedman et al, 1995), its synthesis may serve as a negative control preventing excessive immune activation. NPY-induced decreased antibody production to a T-dependent antigen may occur because of NPY effects on dendritic cells, T lymphocytes, or B lymphocytes, or on all these cells.

Incubation of NK cells with NPY decreases their function (Nair et al, 1993) and NPY plasma levels are negatively correlated with NK activity (Irwin et al, 1991). NPY has not been reported to induce vasodilation or increase the adhesion of endothelial cells for leukocytes (Kim et al, 1994).

Although there are studies indicating that NPY has a suppressive role on immune function, NPY has been reported to increase mitosis of lymphocytes in the gastrointestinal mucosa (Elitsur et al, 1994). In this study, removal of monocytes from in vitro cultures ameliorated the enhancing effect of NPY, suggesting that NPY exerts its enhancement of mitosis of GI lymphocytes through a mononuclear phagocytic cell pathway.

CALCITONIN GENE-RELATED PEPTIDE

The hormone called calcitonin gene-related peptide (CGRP) was originally believed to be derived from the genome that produces calcitonin, a product of the thyroid gland that increases the urinary excretion of calcium. CGRP, consisting of 37 amino acids, is found in spinal cord motor neurons and in sensory neurons terminating near dendritic cells of the skin and in primary and secondary lymphatic tissues. Many, but not all, of the sensory nerves that contain CGRP also contain SP. CGRP receptors, which are present on T and B lymphocytes (McGillis et al, 1993a), when bound by CGRP result in increases of intracellular cAMP (McGillis et al, 1993b). Because of its anatomical location in and near cells that are essential for immune function, and the presence of receptors on lymphocytes, it is likely that CGRP is another neurohormone that can modulate immune function.

Some of the immune modulating activities of CGRP are:

1. Vasodilation is an important component of the inflammatory response as there is an increase of fluid leakage and the ability of cells to migrate out of the vasculature. CGRP, located in nerves terminating near or in the walls of blood vessels, may enhance the acute inflammatory response due to its effect as a vasodilator.

2. Maturation of immature B lymphocytes is inhibited by CGRP (McGillis et al, 1995).

3. An early aspect of immune activation is the uptake, processing, and presentation of antigen by dendritic cells. CGRP has been found localized in nerves in the skin which are closely associated with dendritic cells and the dendritic cells have CGRP at their surface (Asahina et al, 1995a). CGRP reduces the ability of dendritic cells to present antigen to T lymphocytes (Hosoi et al, 1993). Antigen presentation by dendritic cells to T cells involves recognition of the antigenic peptide in major histocompatibility complex (MHC) presentation molecules and the interaction of costimulatory molecules (B7 on dendritic cells with CD28 on T cells). CGRP has been shown to interfere with B7 production on the membrane of dendritic cells (Asahina et al, 1995b). IL-1 production by dendritic cells, which is important for the activation of T cells, is inhibited by CGRP (Torii et al, 1997).

4. Dendritic cells in the skin have two functions. One is as part of the system leading to immune activation. This involves dendritic cells ingesting, processing,

and presenting antigen to the appropriate T lymphocyte while the proper co-stimulation reactions are occurring. As described above, there is evidence that CGRP can interfere with many of these steps. The other important of dendritic cells is to present antigen to effector/memory T lymphocytes to mediate a delayed hypersensitivity reaction. This reaction does not require costimulation. CGRP may interfere with the stress-modified manifestation of the delayed hypersensitivity reaction (Asahina et al, 1995c; Kawaguchi et al, 1997). However, it must be remembered that catecholamines, glucocorticoids, SP and NPY are also increased and may be modulating the delayed hypersensitivity response.

5. In vitro studies of human T lymphocytes have shown that CGRP can inhibit the production of the B7.2 costimulatory molecule on human monocytes and decrease the antigen-specific reactivity of T lymphocytes obtained from individuals immunized to tetanus toxoid (Fox et al, 1997). Finally, the mitogenic response of lymphocytes to nonspecific mitogens of T cells is suppressed by CGRP (Boudard and Bastide, 1991), while responses of B cells may be less suppressed (Umeda et al, 1988).

Thus, CGRP meets the criteria that would be required to identify it as an immune modulator. It is in the nerves that are located where they should be located to affect immune function. There are receptors on lymphocytes and antigen-presenting cells (APCs). It modifies cytokine production, costimulator molecule production, lymphocyte maturation, lymphocyte activation, and in vivo immune reactions. Thus, it can join the list of molecules that are important regulators of immune function.

Of course, it would be ideal if all studies of neuropeptides and hormone modification were done in a single species. However, the trends indicating the immune functions which are susceptible to alteration by neuropeptides are likely to cross species lines provided that receptors for the hormones are present on lymphoid cells.

VASOACTIVE INTESTINAL PEPTIDE

Vasoactive intestinal peptide (VIP) is a 28-amino acid peptide that is present in neurons of the CNS and in peripheral nerves. VIP-containing nerves are located in both primary and secondary lymphoid tissues, around blood vessels (appropriate for a neuropeptide containing the term "vasoactive"), and in the gastrointestinal tract. As would be required for VIP's ability to modulate the function of lymphoid cells, there are VIP receptors on both T and B lymphocytes (Danek et al, 1983; Ottaway and Greenberg, 1984; Johnson et al, 1996). Binding of VIP to its receptor on lymphocytes increases cAMP production (O'Dorisio et al, 1985) and, as would be anticipated in conjunction with increased cAMP levels, decreases the responsiveness of lymphocytes to stimulation with nonspecific mitogens (Ottaway and Greenberg, 1984).

Some of the immune modulating activities of VIP are:

1. VIP may influence lymphocyte maturation. In the bone marrow B-cell maturation is promoted by IL-7 which is produced by bone marrow stromal cells. VIP

can inhibit this process of B-cell maturation (Shimozato and Kincade, 1997). Thymus-residing immature lymphocytes are sensitive to glucocorticoid induced cell death. VIP has been found to protect thymocytes from this process (Ernstrom et al, 1995). The thymus is rich in VIP-containing neurons.

2. Cytokine production by T lymphocytes is modified by VIP. The results vary and may depend on whether cell lines or primary cultures of spleen, lymph node, or blood lymphocytes are studied (Nio et al, 1993; Wang et al, 1996). Both Th1-derived (IL-2) and Th2-derived (IL-4 and IL-10) cytokine production can be modified by VIP, with the concentration of VIP possibly influencing whether enhancement (low VIP concentrations) or inhibition (high VIP concentrations) will occur.

3. Modulation of cytokine production may influence the class of immunoglobulin produced by B lymphocytes. Th1-derived cytokines promote the complement-activating classes of immunoglobulin, while Th2-derived cytokines promote IgA and IgE production by B lymphocytes. Immunoglobulin production by B lymphocytes is modified by VIP. In vitro cultures of human peripheral blood lymphocytes with VIP enhanced IL-4 induced IgE synthesis (Hassner et al, 1993). Lymphocytes obtained form the lamina propria of the colon, which is rich in IgA synthesizing B lymphocytes, increase the amount of IgA they produce when VIP is added to the tissue culture medium they are growing in. Whether the modification of immunoglobulin production by B lymphocytes is related to alterations of cytokine production by T lymphocytes or a direct effect of VIP on B lymphocytes by binding to VIP receptors on B cells has not been determined.

4. VIP has been reported to have a variety of influences of the interactions between lymphocytes and endothelial cells. The adherence of rat peritoneal lymphocytes is increased by VIP (de la Fuente et al, 1994) or is not altered by VIP (Miura et al, 1997). Adhesion of resting human T lymphocytes to integrins and fibronectin on the extracellular matrix is enhanced by VIP (Johnston et al, 1994). However, adhesion to fibronectin was decreased in activated T cells. Thus, the state of the cell (naive or effector) may influence the characteristics of the response to neuropeptides. Another possible explanation for the variable effects of VIP is the presence of different receptors or different concentrations of VIP receptors on different populations of lymphoid cells.

5. Chemotaxis of lymphocytes was studied with variable findings. Human T lymphocytes had an enhancement of chemotactic migration, while rat lymphocytes either had less responsiveness or no response. There is no way to generalize the effects of VIP on adherence or chemotactic properties, other than to suggest that VIP may alter these properties. Obviously, this can be of benefit as a supplemental mediator of an inflammatory response.

VIP, like the other neuropeptides, may participate in the modulation of immune function. As described above, there is no clear consensus as to the specific types of modulation that VIP can induce. Indeed, there probably is not a single type of change induced by VIP. Rather the concentration of VIP, the concentration of VIP receptor, the type of cell being acted upon, and the characteristics of the cell being acted on, as well as the influence of other neuropeptides, will determine the actual characteristics of function of any particular immune response.

SOMATOSTATIN

Somatostatin (SOM) is a 28-amino acid peptide found in, and released from, sensory nerve terminals, many of which are in nerves terminating in lymphoid follicles of the gastrointestinal tract. SOM is also found in and released from lymphoid cells (Teitelbaum et al, 1996).

There are SOM receptors on lymphoid cells (Sreedharan et al, 1989). Comparison of resting thymus-derived lymphocytes with nonspecific mitogen-activated thymus-derived lymphocytes revealed the appearance of a SOM receptor on the activated lymphocytes that was not present on the resting cells (Sedqi et al, 1996).

There may be biological significance for the appearance of SOM receptors on activated lymphocytes. For example, during activation of T lymphocytes, interaction between the CD28 molecule on the T cell and B7 molecules on the APC occurs. Activation of the T cell elicits a new costimulatory molecule, the CTLA-4 molecule, on the membrane of the T cell. Binding of the CTLA-4 to the B7 inhibits the activation of the T cell and may serve as a regulator of immune proliferation. Whether different subtypes of hormonal receptors appear at different stages of activation of lymphocytes and have an enhancing or inhibiting effect on lymphocyte function needs to be determined. This may help in understanding some of the variability of lymphocytic responses to hormone binding.

The effect of SOM on lymphocyte mitosis has been found to be concentration dependent with low concentrations of SOM reducing mitogen induced mitosis (Payan et al, 1984), but at high SOM concentrations mitosis is enhanced (Pawlikowski et al, 1987). Inhibition of SOM synthesis by anti-sense oligonucleotides, in mitogen stimulated cultures of rat spleen lymphocytes resulted in an enhanced rate of cell proliferation (Aguila et al, 1996). This suggests that endogenous production of SOM by activated lymphocytes contributes to the regulation of mitosis of the lymphocytes. The inhibiting effects of SOM were also identified in vivo where neutralization of SOM by an antibody significantly increased the immune response to a parasite (Yun et al, 1996).

NK function and immunoglobulin synthesis is decreased by SOM (Stanisz et al, 1986; Eglezos et al, 1993). Whether the decreased immunoglobulin synthesis is due to a direct effect of SOM on dendritic cell uptake and processing of antigen (Johannson et al, 1993), a direct effect on B lymphocytes, or is mediated by T lymphocytes, has not been defined. However, as SOM has been reported to increase cytokine release from both macrophages and T lymphocytes, consideration of a direct effect of SOM on B lymphocytes or dendritic cells is the more likely possibility (Nio et al, 1993; Komorowski and Stepien, 1995). Other studies indicate that the effect of SOM on macrophage function is dependent on the concentration of SOM (Chao et al, 1995).

Other immune function-modifying effects of SOM may exist and may be found if looked for. However, it must be continually remembered that concentrations of the hormone, the presence of different numbers or subtypes of receptors, the presence of multiple hormones, and studies in different species, will all contribute to variability of the effect of SOM on the immune response.

GROWTH HORMONE

Growth hormone (GH) is a 191-amino acid protein that is synthesized by cells of the anterior lobe of the pituitary and is also produced by lymphocytes and mononuclear phagocytic cells (Hattori et al, 1990; Weigent et al, 1991b). GH participates in the regulation of growth of the body, tissue metabolism and tissue repair. GH may also participate in the regulation of the growth and function of the immune system.

Receptors for GH are present on lymphoid cells (Kelly et al, 1991). A study of GH receptors in chickens found the highest concentration of GH receptors on macrophages and possibly, dendritic cells. This suggests a role for GH in regulating phagocytic function and possibly antigen presentation.

Another hormone, insulin like growth factor (IGF-I), is produced by the liver and other tissues in response to GH and interacts with GH to promote the growth enhancing effects of GH on tissues. IGF-I has autocrine, paracrine, and endocrine activity. IGF-I and GH may not have a complete overlap in regard to the tissues which they effect. The various components of the immune system may be effected to different degrees by GH or IGF-I, depending on the presence of receptors for the hormones on lymphoid cells.

GH may be a stress related modulator of immune function as psychological and physical stress increase the production of GH. Running on a treadmill produced a marked elevation of the concentration of GH excreted in urine (Flanagan et al, 1997). Restraint stress in monkeys produced a ten fold increase of urinary GH (Gauquelin-Koch et al, 1996). Marital conflict in association with hostile behavior produced a significant elevation of plasma GH (Malarkey et al, 1994). Thus, GH is a hormone whose concentration is elevated at times of stress.

GH may be a hormone that is required for normal maturation and function of the immune system (Clark et al, 1993). GH and IGF-I contribute to the maturation of lymphoid cells in the marrow (Merchav et al, 1988) and in the thymus (Berschorner et al, 1991). This function would be unrelated to the biological function of GH as an immune modifier at a time of stress.

GH alters several parameters of the immune system. The amount of antibody produced in response to tetanus toxoid was positively related to the plasma GH concentration in captured free-ranging rhesus monkeys (Laudenslager et al, 1993). Children with GH deficiency, when treated with exogenous GH, had a significant increase of phagocytic function of neutrophils and monocytes but did not have a change in the numbers of lymphocyte subpopulations (Manfredi et al, 1994). The lack of an effect on lymphocytes may be due to a loss of GH receptors in children with GH deficiency. The opposite of GH deficiency is the excessive production of GH associated with acromegaly. Acromegalic patients had elevated phagocytic cell functions, while numbers of lymphocyte subpopulations and mitogenic responses were normal (Kotzmann et al, 1994). Thus, the GH-deficient and acromegalic patient studies suggest that GH can increase phagocytosis. Studies of GH deficiency in adults found a significant decrease in the number of NK lymphocytes (Span et al, 1996).

The effect of GH on lymphocyte function appears to be enhancing. There is a report that exogenous GH enhances the mitosis of B cells and immunoglobulin synthesis in vitro (Rapaport et al, 1987). An indirect evaluation of GH having an effect on lymphocyte mitogenic function was done by using an antibody to GH to neutralize GH in tissue culture supernatants (Lattuada et al, 1996). The proliferation of lymphocytes was significantly suppressed when the antibody was added to the supernatants. This suggests a role for GH in lymphocyte mitosis. GH may be produced by lymphocytes in culture, consistent with an autocrine role for GH.

IGF-I receptors are found on various cells of the immune system (Stuart et al, 1991; Kooijman et al, 1992). Binding of IGF-I to its receptor on lymphocytes increases the mitogenic response of lymphocytes to mitogenic stimulation (Schillaci et al, 1994). IGF-I may also have a significant enhancing influence on the amount of antibody produced by B lymphocytes (Kimata et al, 1994)

Another interesting aspect of GH, but not related to stress, is the indication that the age associated reduction of GH production reduces immune function. In this regard infusion of GH and IGF-1 into aged monkeys or humans reverses age associated alterations of lymphoid histology, increases the numbers of T lymphocytes in blood and spleen, increases the mitogenic responsiveness of T lymphocytes and the function of NK lymphocytes, increases cytokine production, and increases the amount of antibody produced in response to immunization with antigen (LeRoith et al, 1996; Khorram et al, 1997).

GH is a hormone that appears to have enhancing effects on immune function. GH participates in the normal development of the immune system and, as an enhancer of immune function, may counteract some of the immune inhibiting aspects of other hormones. In addition, GH concentration decreases may contribute to the decrease of immune function found in aging.

PROLACTIN

Prolactin (PRL) is produced by cells of the anterior pituitary and its primary function is in lactation, although PRL receptors are present in many different tissues, including liver, kidney, intestine, and adrenals. In addition to being produced by the pituitary, PRL is produced by lymphoid cells (Pellegrini et al, 1992), and there are PRL receptors on lymphoid cells (Russell et al, 1985). PRL receptors may be increased on lymphocytes of experimental animals which spontaneously develop autoimmune disease (Berczi, 1993; Gagnerault et al, 1993). Removal of the pituitary in rats is associated with involution of the thymus which is reversed by treatment with PRL (Nagy et al, 1983).

The concentration of PRL increases in plasma at times of stress (Larsen and Mau, 1994; Malarkey et al, 1994). Therefore, PRL may contribute to the modulation of immune function both at times of stress (when PRL concentrations increase in serum) and during immune reactions to antigens (when lymphoid cells may release PRL, which will have an autocrine or a paracrine influence).

There is a possible scenario in which PRL may function as a suppressor of immune function. Adding PRL in superphysiological concentrations (5- to 10-fold) suppressed in vitro lymphocyte proliferation and IL-2 production (Matera et al, 1992). If these concentrations are reached in localized accumulations of lymphocytes engaged in mediating an immune response, inhibition of an activated immune response may occur.

Functional influences of PRL on the immune system can be evaluated by procedures that interfere with PRL binding to its receptor on lymphoid cells or that inhibit PRL production. For example, bromocriptine, which prevents secretion of PRL by the pituitary, decreased immune function. Restoration of immune function by PRL replacement occurs.

There are clinical conditions in which there is chronic elevation of PRL. The immune systems of patients with prolactinomas were found to be similar to those of control subjects other than the number of CD4 lymphocytes, which was significantly increased in the patients with chronic elevated PRL (Koller et al, 1997). Of course, chronic elevation of PRL may have altered the number of PRL receptors on cells resulting in decreased responsiveness to PRL.

PRL may also have the capability of counteracting the immune-modulating effect of other hormones. For example, suppression of immune function is characteristic of spontaneously hypertensive rats. The mechanism of suppression is through a catecholamine-activated pathway. The suppressed lymphocyte function is reversed by PRL, suggesting that PRL can activate metabolic pathways that ameliorate the suppressive actions of catecholamines (Purcell et al, 1993).

MELATONIN

Melatonin is produced by the pineal gland, an endocrine gland located in the brain. The release of melatonin from the pineal is suppressed by light and increased in the dark. Melatonin is associated with sleep induction and sexual maturation. Melatonin receptors have been found on lymphoid cells which suggests that it may contribute to immune function alteration (Gonzalez-Haba et al, 1995; Garcia-Perganeda et al, 1997).

It is unclear whether all lymphocyte populations contain a melatonin receptor or whether T lymphocytes have greater receptor concentrations than found on B lymphocytes. However, an influence of melatonin on the immune response to T-dependent antigen (Maestroni et al, 1986), and the lack of an effect of melatonin on the antibody response to T-independent antigens (Maestroni et al, 1988) suggests that melatonin primarily effects T lymphocyte function.

In vivo treatment of animals with melatonin produces an immune-enhancing effect on both cell-mediated immunity and antibody production (Maestroni et al, 1988). The immune enhancing activity was confined to the secondary immune response. Thus, effector/memory lymphocytes, rather than naive lymphocytes, may be more susceptible to the influence of melatonin. Long term treatment of mice with melatonin did not alter the function of lymphocytes to nonspecific mitogen or the function of NK cells (Provinciali et al, 1997). Melatonin may therefore primarily alter the function of effector/memory antigen specific cells.

It is possible that melatonin could have an effect on immune function that has been altered by stress. Suppression of nonspecific lymphocyte function by trauma was found to be reversible by melatonin (Wichmann et al, 1996).

In vitro effects of melatonin on lymphocyte responsiveness to stimulation with nonspecific mitogen have failed to suggest a direct role of melatonin on altering lymphocyte function (Pahlavani et al, 1997; Rogers et al, 1997). Thus, it is likely that even though there are melatonin receptors on lymphocytes, that melatonin mediates its effects through activation of another mediator pathway, possibly the opioid system (Maestroni et al, 1987).

As melatonin concentrations undergo a circadian rhythm, and the effect of melatonin on immune function may be indirect and not fully characterized, a precise role for melatonin in stressor-induced immune alteration or in immune regulation cannot be defined. However, it is likely that melatonin is one of the hormones capable of influencing immune function.

ENKEPHALINS AND ENDORPHINS

Enkephalins and endorphins are naturally occurring proteins found in the brain with pain relieving capabilities. Three endogenous substances are lumped together under the term "opioid". They are β-endorphin, enkephalin, and dynorphin. The opioids are split from large molecule synthesized in the pituitary and adrenals, the "proopiomelanocortin" molecule (source of ACTH and β-endorphin), "proenkephalin A"; (source of met-enkephalin and leu-enkephalin), and "proenkephalin B" (source of dynorphin). Proopiomelanocortin is derived from the anterior and intermediate lobe of the pituitary. Proenkephalin is found in the adrenal, central, and peripheral nervous system.

The opioids have characteristics that are associated with their being modulators of immune function. T and B lymphocytes and mononuclear phagocytic cells have receptors for opioids (Hazum et al, 1979; Wybran et al, 1979; Carr et al, 1989). Their presence on dendritic cells has not been determined. Alteration of cell function by opioid receptors may involve reduction of cAMP activation, reduction of calcium efflux, and reduction of activation of inositol-triphosphate, all pathways associated with cell activation (Mazumder et al, 1993; P.S. Johnson, 1994; Kojima et al, 1997). However, there is also evidence that opioid binding can increase calcium mobilization, suggesting that different types of opioid receptors may mediate different intracellular changes (Shahabi et al, 1996). As there are at least three different classes of opioid receptors, μ, δ, κ, different concentrations of ligands and receptors may induce variable effects in different lymphoid cells. Receptor measurement on the different classes, ages, and naive or activated cells would be needed to help to fully understand the possible range of effects of the opioids on the immune system.

There is evidence that opioid agonists can alter the effect of catecholamine binding to catecholamine receptors (Pepe et al, 1997). Opioid binding ameliorated the elevation of cAMP induced by catecholamines. Obviously, as we have been emphasizing, the in vitro studies provide information regarding potential alterations that can be induced by hormones, but in vivo conditions in which there are multiple hormonal interactions occurring in the same cell at a point in time may markedly differ in their effects when compared with what is measured in vitro.

Opioids are produced and released in response to stress and/or pain. Stress activates the HPA axis with a release of ACTH and β-endorphin from the pituitary. There is release of enkephalin from the adrenal medulla. Thus the plasma concentration of opioids increases with stress. In addition, cells of the immune system synthesize and release opioids when the lymphoid cells are activated (Zurawski et al, 1986; Harbour et al, 1987; DeBold et al, 1988; Cabot et al, 1997).

Opioids as Modulators of Immune Function

Opioids produce analgesia (Terman et al, 1984). There are two possible functions for the opioids that are produced by lymphoid cells. The opioids may help to relieve pain at localized sites of tissue inflammation and they may function to modulate the activity of the immune system, either enhancing or suppressing function.

In vitro studies of opioids influencing lymphocyte responses to nonspecific mitogen have indicated that both enhancement and suppression can occur (Gilman et al, 1982; Heijnen et al, 1987). A variability of responses is not surprising. Consider what a test of nonspecific mitogen responsiveness does. A large proportion of lymphocytes will respond to PHA or Con A, possibly more than 50% of T cells collected in a blood specimen. The proportion of naive versus effector/memory cells will differ between individuals, as will the state of activation of T cells, depending on whether an infection or other immune stimulating event is occurring. If the individual is experiencing high levels or low levels of stress in their lives the concentration of various stress related hormones present will vary, including the opioids. The concentration of opioids present will influence the number of opioid receptors present and the ability of the cells to respond to nonspecific mitogen.

Consideration of opioid binding to nonopioid receptors is also an important consideration in opioid induced immune modulation as opioid binding to nonopioid receptors can have different effects on lymphocyte function than does opioid binding to opioid receptors (Heijnen et al, 1985). Even the strength of an antibody response may be differentially susceptible to opioid modulation with low responses augmented and high responses suppressed by opioids (Williamson et al, 1988; Heijnen et al, 1991).

The effects of opioids on cytokine production is no less variable than are the other immune modulating effects of opioids. Reports of both increased and decreased cytokine production can be found (Morgan, 1996; Bajpai et al, 1997).

Thus, the opioids are capable of modulating several aspects of immune function. However, the alterations they induce will be variable and dependent on numerous parameters present at the time the opioids increase in concentration.

SEROTONIN

Serotonin (5-hydroxytryptamine; [5-HT]) is produced by neurons located primarily in the pons and upper brain stem and also by platelets outside the CNS. Stress can induce an elevation of 5-HT levels in plasma (Takada et al, 1995; Fuller, 1996). There are serotonin receptors on lymphoid cells which may allow 5-HT to contribute to immune modulation. However, 5-HT may increase activation of the HPA axis, making in vivo assessment of immunomdulatory effects of 5-HT difficult due to increased plasma concentrations of glucocorticoids and endorphin.

5-HT increases the intracellular concentration of cAMP and produces a variable effect of enhanced or diminished function of lymphocytes (Aune et al, 1993, 1994; Iken et al, 1995). In human immunodeficiency virus (HIV)-positive individuals 5-HT has been found to increase lymphocyte mitogenic function (Hofmann et al, 1996; Eugen-Olsen et al, 1997).

As with all hormone-induced modulation of the immune system, there are the recurring concerns regarding the specific influence of 5-HT in vivo. Although 5-HT can be shown to influence the function of lymphoid cells, the ability of 5-HT to produce functional changes within the hormonal milieu that is present at a given point in time is undetermined.

LYMPHOCYTE PRODUCTION OF HORMONES

The traditional view of hormone production has focused on tissues such as the pituitary, adrenal, thyroid, or endocrine pancreas. Hormone production by these tissues influences the physiological activity of other tissues at various sites of the body. However, cytokines produced by lymphoid cells also function as hormones. For example, cytokine production by a Th1 lymphocyte will induce an alteration of function of a B lymphocyte inducing the B lymphocyte to stop producing IgM antibody and switch to producing IgG antibody. The cytokine acts at the short distance between the two cells.

What can be the biological purpose of lymphocyte production of hormones? First, to maintain homeostasis it can be hypothesized that there must be control mechanisms that prevent excessive activation of the immune system. One of the primary purposes of the immune system is to eliminate foreign materials from the body. Excessive activation of these pathways may produce damage to self-tissue. For example, tumor necrosis factor (TNF) is produced by mononuclear phagocytic cells and lymphoid cells. At low concentrations, where its effects are of an autocrine or paracrine nature (having its biological effects on the cells producing it or within a few cells from where it is produced) TNF increases adhesion molecule presentation of vascular endothelial cells, activates phagocytic cell activity, and stimulates mononuclear phagocytic cells to release cytokines which enhance the local inflammatory response. In higher concentration TNF enters the bloodstream (similar to a hormone) and has the systemic effects of stimulating prostaglandin synthesis in the hypothalamus, which elevates temperature and causes mononuclear phagocytic cells to release large quantities of IL-1 and IL-6 into the circulation, which causes the liver to release acute-phase reactants (C-reactive protein, C3 complement, α2-macroglobulin, fibrinogen), which may enhance bacterial removal. However, large quantities of TNF decrease myocardial output and perfusion of tissues and cause vasodilation and intravascular thrombus formation. The disseminated intravascular coagulation (DIC) and circulatory collapse may lead to death.

One possible regulatory pathway is for the local production of hormones which down-regulate cytokine production by cells of the immune system while the lymphoid cells are working to eliminate infectious agents. Of course this has to be a balancing act where too much suppression of the immune response would be detrimental as the infection would not be eliminated and too little suppression may allow harmful tissue changes associated with excessive TNF production.

Second, the hormones produced by the lymphocytes in a local immune reaction may enter the circulation and influence the central nervous system to produce hormones that down-regulate the immune reaction. An example would be the passage of IL-1 to the brain, where the pituitary would respond with ACTH production, inducing the adrenal to produce glucocorticoid to decrease immune activity. Possibly ACTH production by lymphoid cells may activate the adrenal to produce glucocorticoids.

There are many examples of the systemic regulatory effect of cytokines. There is an increase in plasma catecholamines at the peak of the antibody response when a T-dependent antigen is injected into an experimental animal (Besedovsky and Sorkin, 1977a,b). As part of a regulatory mechanism, it is likely that plasma levels of catecholamines and lymphoid tissue concentrations of catecholamines increase when the immune system signals the brain that the immune system is activated.

Cytokine released from mononuclear phagocytic cells are capable of activating the HPA axis as the injection of purified IL-1 into rodents results in an increase of plasma ACTH and corticosterone. The effect of IL-1 is not directly on adrenal cells as neutralization of CRH prevents the IL-1-induced increase in corticosterone, and the effect of IL-1 is primarily on cells which produce CRH as IL-1 did not increase plasma concentrations of prolactin, melanocyte-stimulating hormone, or growth hormone (Besedovsky et al, 1986, 1991).

Some of the hormones that have been identified as products of either lymphocytes or mononuclear phagocytic cells are ACTH, CRH, follicle-stimulating hormone (FSH), thyroid-stimulating hormone (TSH), VIP, and growth hormone (GH). Some of the hormones are not constitutively produced, but rather are induced when there is activation of the immune response (Smith et al, 1990; Blalock, 1992). However, there is also constitutive presence of some of the hormones (Leceta et al, 1996). Receptors for many of the hormones have been identified in or on lymphocytes. It is possible that some of the hormones are involved with increasing and maintaining the activity of the immune response, while others may decrease immune function.

Some of the hormones produced by lymphocytes are not produced intact but rather as fragments of the intact molecule (Harbour et al, 1987; Smith et al, 1990). The biological effects of the immune derived hormone fragments may differ from the biological effects of intact molecules. A critical factor would be the characteristics and location of the receptors for the various hormones. It is possible that there is an

interaction between antigen, cytokines, and hormones that promote the immune reaction and maintain the viability and function of the activated immune cells. For example, TSH increases antibody production by B cells (Kruger et al, 1989) and
growth hormone promotes lymphocyte mitosis (Weigent et al, 1991a). Other hormones act to dampen the immune reaction to prevent the systemic leakage of cytokines that will have deleterious systemic effects.

If it is assumed that the production of hormones by cells of the immune system is
a normal component of immune regulation, our concern relates to the biological implications of psychological or physical stress disrupting this normal regulatory pathway. Stress increases the production of hormones such as glucocorticoids and
catecholamines, which suppress immune function. But, stress may also decrease the
production of hormones by immune cells which stimulate the brain to increase glucocorticoid and catecholamine production. If the hormones locally produced by lymphoid cells are important for immune regulation by signaling the brain that an
immune response is occurring, the brain may not receive this signal at a time of
stress. This disruption of the lymphoid contribution may result in less production of
catecholamines and glucocorticoids, which would attenuate suppression of the immune response. Thus, it is possible that although stress is associated with decreased
immune function, the suppression of immune function is partially ameliorated by
having less signaling to the brain of hormones from lymphoid cells that dampen the
immune response.

OTHER HORMONES

A long list of hormones can be generated that have been shown to produce in vitro alterations of immune cell function. Examples would include TSH (Peele et al, 1993;
Raiden et al, 1995), vasopressin (Bell et al, 1993; Jessop et al, 1995; Gauquelin-Koch
et al, 1996), chorionic gonadotropin (Athreya et al, 1993; Lin et al, 1995), and luteiniz-
ing hormone (Wilson et al, 1995).

As has been emphasized at the beginning of this chapter, numerous factors make
interpretation of in vitro and in vivo alterations of immune function by individual
hormones difficult. Little can be added by extending the discussion of individual
hormones.

The basic considerations are: Does stress increase the concentration of the hormone in plasma or its release from nerve terminals? Are there receptors for the hormone on cells of the immune system?

If the answer to both questions is "yes," the hormone may participate in stressor-
induced immune alteration. However, when multiple hormones are interacting with
their specific receptor on the same lymphoid cell, the effects of each individual hormone may not be the same as compared with when the hormone is acting alone.

Another aspect is: Do lymphocytes synthesize immune function modulating hormones? Are there receptors for the hormones on cells of the immune system?

If the answer to both questions is "yes," the hormone may participate in immune
regulation at sites of effector lymphocyte activation. This would be an autocrine or
paracrine effect of the hormones.

REFERENCES

Aguila MC, Rodriguez AM, Aguila-Mansilla HN, Lee WT. Somatostatin antisense oligo-deoxynucleotide mediated stimulation of lymphocyte proliferation in culture. Endocrinology. 137: 1585–1590, 1996.

Argo A, Stanisz AM. Neuroimmunomodulation: Classical and non-classical cellular activation. Advances in Neuroimmunology. 5: 311–319, 1995.

Armannini D, Endres S, Kuhnle U, Weber PC. Parallel determination of mineralocorticoid and glucocorticoid receptors in T- and B-lymphocytes of human spleen. Acta Endocrinologica. 118: 479–482, 1988.

Asahina A, Hosoi J, Grabbe S, Granstein RD. Modulation of Langerhans cell function by epidermal nerves. Journal of Allergy and Clinical Immunology. 96: 1178–1182, 1995a.

Asahina A, Moro O, Hosoi J, Lerner EA, Xu S, Takashima A, Granstein RD. Specific induction of cAMP in Langerhans cells by calcitonin gene related peptide: Relevance to functional effects. Proceedings of the National Academy of Sciences USA. 92: 8323–8327, 1995b.

Asahina A, Hosoi J, Beissert S, Stratigos A, Granstein RD. Inhibition of the induction of delayed-type and contact hypersensitivity by calcitonin-gene related peptide. Journal of Immunology. 154: 3056–3061, 1995c.

Athreya BH, Pletcher J, Zulin F, Weiner DB, Willimas WV. Subset specific effects of sex hormones and pituitary gonadotropins on human lymphocyte proliferation in vitro. Clinical Immunology and Immunopathology. 66: 201–211, 1993.

Aune TM, McGrath KM, Sarr T, Bombara MP, Kelley KA. Expression of 5HT1a receptors on activated human T cells. Regulation of cyclic AMP levels and T cell proliferation by 5-hydroxytryptamine. Journal of Immunology. 151: 1175–1183, 1993.

Aune TM, Golden HW, McGrath KM. Inhibitors of serotonin synthesis and antagonists of serotonin 1A receptors inhibit lymphocyte function in vitro and cell mediated immunity in vivo. Journal of Immunology. 153: 489–498, 1994.

Bachen EA, Manuck SB, Cohen S, Muldoon MF, Raible R, Herbert TB, Rabin BS. Adrenergic blockade ameliorates cellular immune responses to mental stress in humans. Psychosomatic Medicine. 57: 366–372, 1995.

Bajpai K, Singh VK, Dhawan VC, Haq W, Mathur KB, Agarwal SS. Immunomodulation by two potent analogs of met-enkephalin. Immunopharmacology. 35: 213–220, 1997.

Bell J, Adler MW, Greenstein JI, Liu-Chen LY. Identification and characterization of I125 arginine vasopressin binding sites on human peripheral blood mononuclear cells. Life Sciences. 52: 95–105, 1993.

Benschop RJ, Oostveen FG, Heijnen CJ, Ballieux RE. Beta 2-adrenergic stimulation causes detachment of natural killer cells from cultured endothelium. European Journal of Immunology. 23: 3242–3247, 1993.

Benschop RJ, Brosschot JF, Godaert GL, DeSmet MB, Geenen R, Olff M, Heijnen CJ, Ballieux RE. Chronic stress affects immunologic but not cardiovascular responsiveness to acute psychological stress in humans. American Journal of Physiology. 266: R75–R80, 1994a.

Benschop RJ, Nieuwenhuis EE, Tromp EA, Godaert GL, Ballieux RE, van Doornen LJ. Effects of beta-adrenergic blockade on immunologic and cardiovascular changes induced by mental stress. Circulation. 89: 762–769, 1994b.

Benschop RJ, Nijkamp FP, Ballieux RE, Heijnen CJ. The effects of beta-adrenoceptor stimulation on adhesion of human natural killer cells to cultured endothelium. British Journal of Pharmacology. 113: 1311–1316, 1994c.

Benschop RJ, Godaert GL, Geenen R, Brosschot JF, De Smet MB, Olff M, Heijnen CJ, Ballieux RE. Relationships between cardiovascular and immunological changes in an experimental stress model. Psychological Medicine. 25: 323–327, 1995.

Berczi I. The role of prolactin in the pathogenesis of autoimmune disease. Endocrine Pathology. 4: 178–195, 1993.

Bermudz LE, Wu M, Young LS. Effect of stress-related hormones on macrophage receptors and response to tumor necrosis factor. Lymphokine Research. 9: 137–145, 1990.

Berschorner WE, Divic J, Pulido H, Yao X, Kenworthy P, Bruce G. Enhancement of thymic recovery after cyclosporine by recombinant human growth hormone and insulin like growth factor I. Transplantation. 52: 879–884, 1991.

Besedovsky HO, Sorkin E. Hormonal control of immune processes. Endocrinology. 2: 504–513, 1977a.

Besedovsky HO, Sorkin E. Network of immune–neuroendocrine interactions. Clinical and Experimental Immunology. 27: 1–12, 1977b.

Besedovsky H, Del Rey A, Sorkin E, Dinarello CA. Immunoregulatory feedback between interleukin-1 and glucocorticoid hormones. Science. 233: 652–654, 1986.

Besedovsky HO, Del Rey A, Klusman I, Furukawa H, ArditiGM, Kabiersch A. Cytokines as modulators of the hypothalamus–pituitary–adrenal axis. Journal of Steroid Biochemistry and Molecular Biology. 40: 613–618, 1991.

Blalock JE. Production of peptide hormones and neurotransmitters by the immune system. Chemical Immunology. 52: 1–24, 1992.

Boudard F, Bastide M. Inhbition of mouse T cell proliferation by CGRP and VIP: Effects of these neuropeptides on IL-2 production and cAMP synthesis. Journal of Neuroscience Research. 29: 29–41, 1991.

Cabot PJ, Carter L, Gaiddon C, Zhang Q, Schafer M, Loeffler JP, Stein C. Immune cell derived beta-endorphin. Production, release, and control of inflammatory pain in rats. Journal of Clinical Investigation. 100: 142–148, 1997.

Carlson SL, Beiting DJ, Kiani CA, Abell KM, McGillis JP. Catecholamines decrease lymphocyte adhesion to cytokine-activated endothelial cells. Brain, Behavior, and Immunity. 10: 55–67, 1996.

Carlson SL, Fox S, Abell KM. Catecholamine modulation of lymphocyte homing to lymphoid tissues. Brain, Behavior, and Immunity. 11: 307–320, 1997.

Carr DJJ, DeCosta BR, Kim CH, Jacobson AE, Guarcello V, Rice KC, Blalock JE. Opioid receptors on cells of the immune system: Evidence for O and K classes. Journal of Endocrinology. 122: 161–168, 1989.

Chao TC, Cheng HP, Walter RJ. Somatostatin and macrophage function: modulation of hydrogen peroxide, nitric oxide and tumor necrosis factor release. Regulatory Peptides. 58: 1–10, 1995.

Claman HN. Corticosteroids and lymphoid cells. New England Journal of Medicine. 287: 388–397, 1972.

Clark R, Strasser J, McCabe S, Robbins K, Jardieu P. Insulin-like growth factor-I stimulation of lymphopoiesis. Journal of Clinical Investigation. 92: 540–548, 1993.

Cohen JJ. Lymphocyte death induced by glucocorticoids. In Anti-Inflammatory Steroid Action: Basic and Clinical Aspects. Schleimer RP, Claman HN, Oronsky AL (eds). Academic Press, San Diego, 1989, pp 110–131.

Cohen S, Tyrrell DAJ, Smith AP. Psychological stress and susceptibility to the common cold. New England Journal of Medicine. 325: 606–612, 1991.

Cohen S, Line S, Manuck SB, Rabin BS, Heise ER, Kaplan JR. Chronic social stress, social status, and susceptibility to upper respiratory infections in nonhuman primates. Psychosomatic Medicine. 59: 213–221, 1997a.

Cohen S, Doyle WJ, Skoner DP, Rabin BS, Gwaltney JM. Social ties and susceptibility to the common cold. Journal of the American Medical Association. 277: 1940–1944, 1997b.

Cohen S, Frank E, Doyle WJ, Skoner DP, Rabin BS, Gwaltney JM. Types of stressor that increase susceptibility to the common cold in healthy adults. Health Psychology. 17: 214–223, 1998.

Covas MJ, Pinto LA, Pereira JA, Victorino RM. Effects of neuropeptide, supstance P, on lymphocyte proliferation in rheumatoid arthritis. Journal of International Medical Research. 23: 431–238, 1995.

Covas MJ, Pinto LA, Victorino RM. Effects of substance P on human T cell function and the modulatory role of peptidase inhibitors. International Journal of Clinical and Laboratory Research. 27: 129–134, 1997.

Crary B, Borysenko M, Sutherland DC, Kutz I, Borysenko J.Z, Benson H. Decrease in mitogen responsiveness of mononuclear cells from peripheral blood after epinephrine administration in humans. Journal of Immunology. 130: 694–697, 1983.

Cunnick J, Lysle DT, Kucinski BJ, Rabin BS. Evidence that shock induced immune suppression is mediated by adrenal hormones and peripheral beta-adrenergic receptors. Pharmacology, Biochemistry, and Behavior. 36: 645–651, 1990.

Danek A, O'Dorisio MS, O'Dorisio TM, George JM. Specific binding sites for vasoactive intestinal polypeptide on nonadherent peripheral blood lymphocytes. Journal of Immunology. 131: 1173–1177, 1983.

Daynes RA, Araneo BA. Contrasting effects of glucocorticoids on the capacity of T cells to produce the growth factors interleukin 2 and interleukin 4. European Journal of Immunology. 19: 2319–2325, 1989.

deBlois D, Schwartz SM, van Kleef EM, Su JE, Griffin KA, Bidani AK, Daemen MJ, Lombardi DM. Chronic alpha 1-adrenoreceptor stimulation increases DNA synthesis in rat arterial wall. Modulation of responsiveness after vascular injury. Arteriosclerosis, Thrombosis, and Vascular Biology. 16: 1122–1129, 1996.

DeBold CR, Menefee JK, Nicholson WE, Orth DN. Proopiomelanocortin gene is expressed in many normal human tissues and in tumors not associated with ectopic adrenocorticotropin syndrome. Molecular Endocrinology. 2: 862–870, 1988.

Decker RS, Cook MG, Behnke-Barclay MM, Decker ML, Lesch M, Samarel AM. Catecholamines modulate protein turnover in cultured, quiescent rabbit cardiac myocytes. American Journal of Physiology. 265: H329–H339, 1993.

Deinzer R, Kirschbaum C, Gresele C, Hellhammer DH. Adrenocortical responses to repeated parachute jumping and subsequent h-CRH challenge in inexperienced healthy subjects. Physiology and Behavior. 61: 507–511, 1997.

de la Fuente M, Delgado M, del Rio M, Garrido E, Leceta J, Gomariz RP. Vasoactive intestinal peptide modulation of adherence and mobility in rat peritoneal lymphocytes and macrophages. Peptides. 15: 1157–1163, 1994.

Dhabhar FS, McEwen BS. Stress-induced enhancement of antigen-specific cell-mediated immunity. Journal of Immunology. 156: 2608–2615, 1996.

Eglezos A, Andrews PV, Helme RD. In vivo inhibition of the rat primary antibody response to antigenic stimulation by somatostatin. Immunology and Cell Biology. 71: 125–129, 1993.

Elitsur Y, Luk GD, Colberg M, Gesell MS, Dosescu J, Moshier JA. Neuropeptide Y (NPY) enhances proliferation of human colonic lamina propria lymphocytes. Neuropeptides. 26: 289–295, 1994.

Ernstrom U, Gafvelin G, Mutt V. Rescue of thymocytes from cell death by vasoactive intestinal peptide. Regulatory Peptides. 57: 99–104, 1995.

Eugen-Olsen J, Afzelius P, Andreses L, Iversen J, Kronborg G, Aabech P, Nielsen JO, Hofmann B. Serotonin modulates immune function in T cells from HIV seropositive subjects. Clinical Immunology and Immunopathology. 84: 115–121, 1997.

Fauci AS, Dale DC. The effect of hydrocortisone on the kinetics of normal human lymphocytes. Blood. 46: 235–243, 1975.

Flanagan DE, Taylor MC, Parfitt V, Mardell R, Wood PJ, Leatherdqle BA. Urinary growth hormone following exercise to assess growth hormone production in adults. Clinical Endocrinology. 46: 425–429, 1997.

Fleshner M, Deak T, Spencer RL, Laudenslager ML, Watkins LR, Maier SF. A long-term increase in basal levels of corticosterone and a decrease in corticosteroid-binding globulin after acute stressor exposure. Endocrinology. 136: 5336–5342, 1995.

Fox FE, Kubin M, Cassin M, Niu Z, Hosoi J, Torii H, Granstein RD, Trinchieri G, Rookj AH. Calcitonin gene related peptide inhibits proliferation and antigen presentation by human peripheral blood mononuclear cells: Effects of B7, interleukin 10, and interleukin 12. Journal of Investigative Dermatology. 108: 43–48, 1997.

Frediani U, Becherini L, Lasagni L, Tanini A, Brandi ML. Catecholamines modulate growth and differentiation of preosteoclastic cells. Osteoporosis International. 6: 14–21, 1996.

Friedman EM, Irwin MR, Nonogaki K. Neuropeptide Y inhibits in vivo specific antibody production in rats. Brain, Behavior, and Immunity. 9: 182–189, 1995.

Fuller RW. Serotonin receptors involved in regulation of pituitary–adrenocortical function in rats. Behavioural Brain Research. 73: 215–219, 1996.

Gagnerault MC, Touraine P, Savino W, Kelly PA, Dardeene M. Expression of prolactin receptors in murine lymphoid cells in normal and autoimmune situations. Journal of Immunology. 150: 5673–5681, 1993.

Garcia-Perganeda A, Pozo D, Guerrero JM, Calvo JR. Signal transduction for melatonin in human lymphocytes: Involvement of a pertussis toxin-sensitive G protein. Journal of Immunology. 159: 3774–3781, 1997.

Gauquelin-Koch G, Blanquie JP, Viso M, Florence G, Milhaud C, Gharib C. Hormonal response to restraint in rhesus monkeys. Journal of Medical Primatology. 25: 387–396, 1996.

Gilman SC, Schwartz JM, Milner RJ, Bloom FE, Feldman JD. β-endorphin enhances lymphocyte proliferative responses. Proceedings of the National Academy of Sciences USA. 79: 4226–4230, 1982.

Goafa FZ, Chancellor-Freeland C, Berman AS, Kage R, Leeman SE, Beller DI, Black PH. Endogenous substance P mediates cold water stress-induced increase in interleukin-6 secretion from peritoneal macrophages. Journal of Neuroscience. 16: 3745–3752, 1996.

Goetzl EJ, Grotmol T, VanDyke RW, Turck CW, Wershil B, Galli SJ, Sreedharan SP. Generation and recognition of vasoactive intestinal peptide by cells of the immune system. Annals of the New York Academy of Sciences. 594: 34–44, 1990.

Gonzalez-Haba MG, Gaarcia-Maurino S, Calvo JR, Goberna R, Guerrero JM. High-affinity binding of melatonin by human circulating T lymphocytes (CD4$^+$). FASEB Journal. 9: 1331–1335, 1995.

Grazzi L, Salmaggi A, Dufour A, Ariano C, Colangelo AM, Parati E, Lazzaroni M, Nespolo A, Bordin G, Castellazzi C. Physical effort-induced changes in immune parameters. International Journal of Neuroscience. 68: 133–40, 1993.

Harbour DV, Smith EM, Blalock JE. A novel processing pathway for proopiomelanocortin in lymphocytes: Endotoxin induction of a new pro-hormone cleaving enzyme. Journal of Neuroscience Research. 18: 95–101, 1987.

Hart R, Dancygier H, Wagner F, Lersch C, Classen M. Effect of substance P on immunoglobulin and interferon-gamma secretion by cultured human duodenal mucosa. Immunology Letters. 23: 199–204, 1990.

Hassner A, Lau MS, Goetzl EJ, Adelamn DC. Isotype specific regulation of human lymphocyte production of immunoglobulins by sustained exposure to vasoactive intestinal peptide. Journal of Allergy and Clinical Immunology. 92: 891–901, 1993.

Hattori N, Shimatsu A, Sugita M, Kumagai S, Imura H. Immunoreactive growth hormone(GH) secrction by human lymphocytes. Augmented release by exogenous GH. Biochemical and Biophysical Research Communication. 168: 396–401, 1990.

Hazum E, Chang KJ, Cuatrecasas P. Specific nonopiate receptors for β-endorphin. Science. 205: 1033–1035, 1979.

Heerwagen C, Pabst R, Westermann J. The neuropeptide substance P does not influence the migration of B, CD8$^+$ and CD4$^+$ (naive and memory) lymphocytes from blood to lymph in the normal rat. Scandinavian Journal of Immunology. 42: 480–486, 1995.

Heijnen CJ, Bevers C, Kavelaars A, Ballieux RE. Effect of α-endorphin on the antigen induced primary antbody response of human blood B cells in vitro. Journal of Immunology. 136: 213–216, 1985.

Heijnen CJ, Zijlstra J, Kavelaars A, Croiset G, Ballieux RE. Modulation of the immune response by POMC derived peptides. I. Influence on proliferation of human lymphocytes. Brain, Behavior, and Immunity. 1: 284–291, 1987.

Heijnen CJ, Kavelaars A, Ballieux RE. Corticotropin-releasing hormone and proopiomelanocortin-derived peptides in the modulation of immune function. In Psychoneuroimmunology. Ader R, Felten DL, Cohen N (eds). Academic Press, San Diego, 1991, pp 429–446.

Herbert TB, Cohen S, Marsland AL, Bachen EA, Rabin BS, Muldoon MF, Manuck SB. Cardiovascular reactivity and the course of immune response to an acute psychological stressor. Psychosomatic Medicine. 56: 337–344, 1994.

Herzberg U, Murtaugh MP, Mullet MA, Beitz AJ. Electrical stimulation of the sciatic nerve alters neuropeptide content and lymphocyte migration in the subcutaneous tissue of the rat hind paw. Neuroreport. 6: 1773–1777, 1995.

Hofmann B, Afzelius P, Iversen J, Kronborg G, Aabech P, Benfield T, Dybkjaer E, Nielsen JO. Buspirone, a serotonin receptor agonist increases CD4 cell counts and modulates the immune system in HIV-seropositive subjects. AIDS. 10: 1339–1347, 1996.

Hosoi J, Murphy GF, Egan CL, Lerner EA, Grabbe S, Asahina A, Granstein RD. Regulatipon of Langerhans cell function by nerves containing calcitonin gene related peptide. Nature. 363: 159–163, 1993.

Iken K, Chheng S, Fargin A, Goulet AC, Kouassi E. Serotonin upregulates mitogen-stimulated B lymphocytes through 5-HT1A receptors. Cellular Immunology. 163: 1–9, 1995.

Irwin MR, Brown M, Patterson T, Hauger R, Mascovich A, Grant I. Neuropeptide Y and natural killer cell activity: Findings in depression and Alzheimer caregiver stress. FASEB Journal. 5: 3100–3107, 1991.

Jessop DS, Chowdrey HS, Lightman SL, Larsen PJ. Vasopressin is located within lymphocytes in the rat spleen. Journal of Neuroimmunology. 56: 219–223, 1995.

Johannson O, Hilliges M, Wang L. Somatostatin like immunoreactivity is found in dendritic guard cells of human sweat glands. Peptides. 14: 401–403, 1993.

Johnson MC, McCormack RJ, Delgado M, Martinez C, Ganea D. Murine T lymphocytes express vasoactive intestinal receptor 1 (VIP R1) mRNA. Journal of Neuroimmunology. 68: 109–119, 1996.

Johnson PS, Wang JB, Wang WF, Uhl GR. Expressed mu opiate receptor couples to adenylate cyclase and phophatidyl inositol turnover. Neuroreport. 5: 507–509, 1994.

Johnston JA, Taub DD, Lloyd AR, Conlon K, Oppenheim JJ, Kevlin DJ. Human T lymphocyte chemotaxis and adhesion induced by vasoactive intestinal peptide. Journal of Immunology. 153: 1762–1768, 1994.

Kaltreider HB, Ichikawa S, Byrd PK, Ingram DA, Kishiyama JL, Sreedharan SP, Warnock ML, Beck JM, Goetzel EJ. Upregulation of neuropeptides and neuropeptide receptors in a murine model of immune inflammation in lung parenchyma. American Journal of Respiratory Cell and Molecular Biology. 16: 133–144, 1997.

Kawaguchi Y, Okada T, Konishi H, Fujino M, Asai J, Ito M. Reduction of the DTH response is related to morphological changes of Langerhans cells in mice exposed to acute immobilization stress. Clinical and Experimental Immunology. 109: 397–401, 1997.

Keller SE, Weiss JM, Schleifer SJ, Miller NE, Stein M. Stress-induced suppression of immunity in adrenalectomized rats. Science. 221: 1301–1304, 1983.

Kelly PA, Djiane J, Postel-Vinay MC, Edery M. The prolactin/growth hormone receptor family. Endocrine Reviews. 12: 235–251, 1991.

Khan MM, Sansoni P, Silverman ED, Engleman G, Melmon KL. Beta-adrenergic receptors on human suppressor, helper, and cytolytic lymphocytes. Biochemical Pharmacology. 35: 1137–1142, 1986.

Khorram O, Yeung M, Vu L, Yen SS. Effects of (norleucine27) growth hormone releasing hormone (GHRH) (1–29)-NH2 administration on the immune system of aging men and women. Journal of Clinical Endocrinology and Metabolism. 82: 3590–3596, 1997.

Kim D, Duran WR, Kobayashi I, Daniels AJ, Duran WN. Microcirculatory dynamics of neuropeptide Y. Microvascular Research. 48: 124–134, 1994.

Kimata H, Yoshida A. The effect of growth hormone and insulin-like growth factor-I on immunoglobulin production by and growth of human B cells. Journal of Clinical Endocrinology and Metabolism. 78: 635–641, 1994.

Kizaki T, Oh-ishi S, Ohno H. Acute cold stress induces suppressor macrophages in mice. Journal of Applied Physiology. 81: 393–399, 1996.

Kojima Y, Tsunoda Y, Owyang C. Adenosine 3′,5′-cyclic monophosphate-stimulated Ca^{++} efflux and acetylcholine release in ileal myenteric plexus are mediated by N-type Ca^{++} channels: Inhibition by the kappa opioid receptor agonist. Journal of Pharmacology and Experimental Therapeutics. 282: 403–409, 1997.

Koller M, Kotzmann H, Clodi M, Riedl M, Luger A. Effect of elevated serum prolactin concentrations on the immunophenotype of human lymphocytes, mitogen-induced proliferation and phagocytic activity of polymorphonuclear cells. European Journal of Clinical Investigation. 27: 662–666, 1997.

Komorowski J, Stepien H. Somatostatin (SRIF) stimulates the release of interleukin-6 from human peripheral blood monocytes (PBM) in vitro. Neuropeptides. 29: 77–81, 1995.

Kooijman R, Williams M, DeHaas CJ, Rijkers GT, Schuurmans AL, Van Buul-Offers SC, Heijnen CJ, Zegers BJ. Expression of type-I insulin-like growth factor receptors on human peripheral blood mononuclear cells. Endocrinology. 131: 2244–2250, 1992.

Kotzmann H, Koller M, Czernin S, Clodi M, Svoboda T, Riedl M, Boltz-Nitulescu G, Zielinski CC, Luger A. Effect of elevated growth hormone cncentrations on the phenotype and functions of human lymphocytes and natural killer cells. Neuroendocrinology. 60: 618–625, 1994.

Kronfol Z, Starkman M, Schteingart DE, Singh V, Zhang Q, Hill E. Immune regulation in Cushing's syndrome: Relationship to hypothalamic–pituitary–adrenal axis hormones. Psychoneuroendocrinology. 21: 599–608, 1996.

Kruger TE, Smith LR, Harbour DV, Blalock JE. Thyrotropin: An endogenous regulator of the in vitro immune response. Journal of Immunology. 142: 744–747, 1989.

Landmann RMA, Muller FB, Perini C, Wesp M, Erne P, Buhler FR. Changes of immunoregulatory cells induced by psychological and physical stress: Relationship to plasma catecholamines. Clinical and Experimental Immunology. 58: 127–135, 1984.

Larsen PJ, Mau SE. Effect of acute stress on the expression of hypothalamic messenger ribonucleic acids encoding the endogenous opioid precursors preproenkephalin a and proopiomelanocortin. Peptides. 15: 783–790, 1994.

Lattuada D, Casnici C, Gregori S, Berrini A, Secchi C, Franco P, Marelli O. Monoclonal antibodies against recombinant human growth hormone as probes to study immune function. Hybridoma. 15: 211–217, 1996.

Laudenslager ML, Rasmussen KLR, Berman CM, Suomi SJ, Berger CB. Specific antibody levels in free-ranging rhesus monkeys—Relationships to plasma hormones, cardiac parameters, and early behavior. Developmental Psychobiology. 26: 407–420, 1993.

Leceta J, Martinez C, Delgado M, Garrido E, Gomariz RP. Expression of vasoactive intestinal peptide in lymphocytes: A possible endogenous role in the regulation of the immune system. Advances in Neuroimmunology. 6: 29–36, 1996.

LeRoith D, Yanowski J, Kaldjian EP, Jaffe ES, LeRoith T, Purdue K, Cooper BD, Pyle R, Adler W. The effects of growth hormone and insulin-like growth factor I on the immune system of aged female monkeys. Endocrinology. 137: 1071–1079, 1996.

Lin J, Lojun S, Lei ZM, Wu WX, Peiner SC, Rao CV. Lymphocytes from pregnant women express human chorionic gonadotropin/luteinizing hormone receptor gene. Molecular and Cellular Endocrinology. 111: R13–R17, 1995.

Lotz M, Vaughan JH, Carson DA. Effect of neuropeptides on production of inflammatory cytokines by human monocytes. Science. 241: 1218–1221, 1988.

MacQueen G, Marshall J, Perdue M, Siegel S, Bienenstopck J. Pavlovian conditioning of rat mucosal mast cells to secrete rat mast cell protease II. Science. 243: 83–84, 1989.

Madden KS, Felten SY, Felten D, Hardy CA, Livnat S. Sympathetic nervous system modulation of the immune system. II. Induction of lymphocyte proliferation and migration in vivo by chemical sympathectomy. Journal of Neuroimmunology. 94: 67–75, 1994.

Maestroni GJM, Conti A, Pierpaoli W. Role of the pineal gland in immunity. Circadian synthesis and release of melatonin modulates the antibody response and antagonizes the immunosuppressive effect of corticosterone. Journal of Neuroimmunology. 13: 19–30, 1986.

Maestroni GJM, Conti A, Pierpaoli W. The pineal gland and the circadian, opiatergic, immunoregulatory role of melatonin. Annals of the New York Academy of Sciences. 496: 67–77, 1987.

Maestroni GJM, Conti A, Pierpaoli W. Pineal melatonin, its fundamental immunoregulatory role in aging and cancer. Annals of the New York Academy of Sciences. 521: 140–148, 1988.

Maisel AS, Fowler P, Rearden A, Motulsky HJ, Michel MC. A new method for isolation of human lymphocyte subsets reveals differential regulation of beta-adrenergic receptors by terbutaline treatment. Clinical Pharmacology and Therapapeutics. 46: 429–439, 1989.

Malarkey WB, Kiecolt-Glaser JK, Pearl D, Glaser R. Hostile behavior during marital conflict alters pituitary and adrenal hormones. Psychosomatic Medicine. 56: 41–51, 1994.

Manfredi R, Tumietto F, Azzaroli L, Zucchini A, Chiodo F, Manfredi G. Growth hormone (GH) and the immune system: Impaired phagocytic function in children with idiopathic GH deficiency is corrected by treatment with biosynthetic GH. Journal of Pediatric Endocrinology. 7: 245–251, 1994.

Manuck SB, Cohen S, Rabin BS, Muldoon MF, Bachen EA. Individual differences in cellular immune response to stress. Psychological Science. 2: 1–5, 1991.

Matera L, Cesano A, Bellone G, Oberholtzer E. Modulatory effect of prolactin on the resting and mitogen-induced activity of T, B, and NK lymphocytes. Brain, Behavior, and Immunity. 6: 409–417, 1992.

Mazumder S, Nath I, Dhar MM. Immunomodulation of human T cell responses with receptor selective enkephalins. Immunology Letters. 35: 33–38, 1993.

McGillis JP, Humphreys S, Rangnekar V, Ciallella J. Modulation of B lymphocyte differentiation by calcitonin gene-related peptide (CGRP). I. Characterization of high-affinity CGRP receptors on murine 70Z/3 cells. Cellular Immunology. 150: 391–404, 1993a.

McGillis JP, Humphreys S, Rangnekar V, Ciallella J. Modulation of B lymphocyte differentiation by calcitonin gene-related peptide (CGRP). II. Inhibition of LPS-induced kappa light chain expression by CGRP. Cellular Immunology. 150: 405–416, 1993b.

McGillis JP, Rangnekar V, Ciallella JR. A role for calcitonin gene related peptide (CGRP) in the regulation of early B lymphocyte differentiation. Canadian Journal of Physiology and Pharmacology. 73: 1057–1064, 1995.

Meltzer JC, Grimm PC, Greenberg AH, Nance DM. Enahnced immunohistochemical detection of autonomic nerve fibers, cytokines and inducible nitric oxide synthase by light and fluorescent microscopy n rat spleen. Journal of Histochemistry and Cytochemistry. 45: 599–610, 1997.

Merchav S, Tatarsky I, Hochberg Z. Enhancement of human granulopoiesis in vitro by biosynthetic insulin-like growth factor I/somatomedin C and human growth hormone. Journal of Clinical Investigation. 81: 791–797, 1988.

Merten MD, Tournier JM, Meckler Y, Figarella C. Epinephrine promotes growth and differentiation of human tracheal gland cells in culture. American Journal of Respiratory Cells and Molecular Biology. 9: 172–178, 1993.

Miller AH, Spencer RL, Trestman RL, Kim C, McEwen BS, Stein M. Adrenal steroid receptor activation in vivo and immune function. American Journal of Physiology. 261: E126–E131, 1991.

Miller AH, Spencer RL, Hasset J, Km C, Rhee R, Cira D, Dhabhar FS, McEwen BS, Stein M. Effects of selective Type I and Type II adrenal steroid receptor agonists on immune cell distribution. Endocrinology. 135: 1934–1944, 1994.

Mills PJ, Ziegler MG, Patterson T, Dimsdale JE, Hauger R, Irwin M, Grant I. Plasma catecholamine and lymphocyte beta 2-adrenergic receptor alterations in elderly Alzheimer caregivers under stress. Psychosomatic Medicine. 59: 251–256, 1997a.

Mills PJ, Karnik RS, Dillon E. L-selectin expression affects T-cell circulation following isoproterenol infusion in humans. Brain, Behavior, and Immunity. 11: 333–342, 1997b.

Miura S, Serizawa H, Tsuzuki Y, Kurose I, Suematsu M, Higuchi H, Shigematsu T, Hokari R, Hirokawa M, Kimura H, Ishii H. Vasoactive intestinal peptide modulates T lymphocyte migration in Peyer's patches of rat small intestine. American Journal of Physiology. 272: G92–99, 1997.

Moorhead JW, Claman HN. Thymus-derived lymphocytes and cortisol: Identification of subsets of theta-bearing cells and redistribution to bone marrow. Cellular Immunology. 5: 74–86, 1972.

Morgan EL. Regulation of human B lymphocyte activation by opioid peptide hormones. Inhibition of IgG production by opioid receptor class (mu-, kappa-, and delta-) selective agonists. Journal of Neuroimmunology. 65: 21–30, 1996.

Moyna NM, Acker GW, Weber KM, Fulton JR, Goss FL, Robertson RJ, Rabin BS. The effects of incremental submaximal exercise on circulating leukocytes in physically active and sedentary males and females. European Journal of Applied Physiology. 74: 211–218, 1996.

Nagy E, Berczi I, Wren G, Asa L, Kovacs K. Immunomodulation by bromocriptine. Immunopharmacology. 6: 231, 1983.

Nair MPN, Schwartz SA, Wu K, Kronfol Z. Effect of neuropeptide Y on natural killer activity of normal human lymphocytes. Brain, Behavior, and Immunity. 7: 70–78, 1993.

Naliboff BD, Benton D, Solomon GF, Morley JE, Fahey JL, Bloom ET, Makinodan T, Gilmore SL. Immunological changes in young and old adults during brief laboratory stress. Psychosomatic Medicine. 53: 121–132, 1991.

Nio DA, Moylan RN, Roche JK. Modulation of T lymphocyte function by neuropeptides. Evidence for their role as local immunoregulatory elements. Journal of Immunology. 150: 5281–5288, 1993.

O'Dorisio MS, Wood CL, Wenger GD, Vassalo LM. Cyclic AMP-dependent protein kinase in Molt 4b lymphoblasts: Identification by photoaffinity labeling and activation in intact cells by vasoactive intestinal polypeptide (VIP) and peptide histadine isoleucine (PHI). Journal of Immunology. 134: 4078–4086, 1985

Ottaway CA, Greenberg GR. Interaction of vasoactive intestinal peptide with mouse lymphocytes: Specific binding and the modulation of mitogen responses. Journal of Immunology. 132: 417–423, 1984.

Pahlavani MA, Harris MD. In vitro effects of melatonin on mitogen-induced lymphocyte proliferation and cytokine expression in young and old rats. Immunopharmacology and Immunotoxicology. 19: 327–337, 1997.

Pawlikowski M, Stepien H, Kunert J, Zelazowski P, Schally AV. Immunomodulatory activity of somatostatin. Annals of the New York Academy of Science. 496: 233–239, 1987.

Payan DG, Hess CA, Goetzl EJ. Inhibition by somatostatin of the proliferation of T lymphocytes and Molt-4 lymphoblasts. Cellular Immunology. 84: 433–438, 1984.

Payan DG, Neuropeptides and inflammation: The role of substance P. Annual Review of Medicine. 40: 341–352, 1989.

Peele ME, Carr FE, Baker JR, Wartofsky L, Burman KD. TSH beta subunit gene expression in human lymphocytes. American Journal of the Medical Sciences. 305: 1–7, 1993.

Pellegrini I, Lebrun JJ, Ali S, Kelly PA. Expression of prolactin and its receptor in human lymphoid cells. Molecular Endocrinology. 6 1023–1031, 1992.

Pepe S, Xiao RP, Hohl C, Altschuld R, Lakatta EG. "Cross talk" between opioid peptide and adrenergic receptor signaling in isolated rat heart. Circulation. 95: 2122–2129, 1997.

Petitto JM, Huang Z, McCarthy DB. Molecular cloning of NPY-Y1 receptor cDNA from rat splenic lymphocytes: Evidence of low levels of mRNA expression and NPY binding sites. Journal of Neuroimmunology. 54: 81–86, 1994.

Provinciali M, DiStefano G, Bulian D, Stronati S, Fabris N. Long-term melatonin supplementation does not recover the impairment of natural killer cell activity and lymphocyte proliferation in aging mice. Life Sciences. 61: 857–864, 1997.

Purcell ES, Wood GW, Gattone VH. Immune system of the spontaneously hypertensive rat. II. Morphology and function. Anatomical Record. 237: 236–242, 1993.

Raiden S, Polack E, Nahmod V, Labeur M, Holsboer F, Arzt E. TRH receptor on immune cells: In vitro and in vivo stimulation of human lymphocyte and rat splenocyte DNA synthesis by TRH. Journal of Clinical Immunology. 15: 242–249, 1995.

Rameshwar P, Gascon P, Ganea D. Stimulation of interleukin 2 production in murine lymphocytes by substance P and related tachykinins. Journal of Immunology. 151: 2482–2496, 1993.

Rapaport R, Oleske J, Ahdieh H, Skuza K, Holland BK, Passannante MR, Denny T. Effects of human growth hormone on immune functions: In vitro studies on cells of normal and growth deficient children. Life Sciences. 41: 2319–2324, 1987.

Rehman J, Mills PJ, Carter SM, Chou J, Thomas J, Maisel AS. Dynamic exercise leads to an increase in circulating ICAM-1: Further evidence for adrenergic modulation of cell adhesion. Brain, Behavior, and Immunity. 11: 343–351, 1997.

Rogers N, van den Heuvel C, Dawson D. Effect of melatonin and corticosteroid on in vitro cellular immune function in humans. Journal of Pineal Research. 22: 75–80, 1997.

Russell DH, Kibler R, Matrisian L, Larson DF, Poulos B, Magun BE. Prolactin receptors on human T and B lymphocytes: Antagonism of prolactin binding by cyclosporine. Journal of Immunology. 134: 3027–3031, 1985.

Saito T, Tazawa K, Yokoyama Y, Saito M. Surgical stress inhibits the growth of fibroblasts through elevation of plasma catecholamine and cortisol concentrations. Surgery Today. 27: 627–631, 1997.

Sauer J, Stalla GK, Muller OA, Arzt E. Inhibition of interleukin-2-mediated lymphocyte activation in patients with Cushing's syndrome: A comparison with hypocortisolemic patients. Neuroendocrinology. 59: 144–151, 1994.

Schedlowski M, Hosch W, Oberbeck R, Benschop RJ, Jacobs R, Raab HR, Schmidt RE. Catecholamines modulate human NK cell circulation and function via spleen-independent beta 2-adrenergic mechanisms. Journal of Immunology. 156: 93–99, 1996.

Schillaci R, Ribaudo CM, Rondinone CM, Roldan A. Role of insulin-like growth factor-I on the kinetics of human lymphocyte stimulation in serum free culture medium. Immunology and Cell Biology. 72: 300–305, 1994.

Schratzberger P, Reinisch N, Prodinger WM, Kahler CM, Sitte BA, Bellmann R, Fisher-Colbrie R, Winkler H, Wiedermann CJ. Differential chemotactic activities of sensory neuropeptides for human peripheral blood mononuclear cells. Journal of Immunology. 158: 3895–3901, 1997.

Schwarz H, Villiger PM, von Kempis J, Lotz M. Neuropeptide Y is an inducible gene in the human immune system. Journal of Neuroimmunology. 51: 53–61, 1994.

Sedqi M, Roy S, Mohanraj D, Ramakrishnan S, Loh HH. Activation of rat thymocytes selectively upregulates the expression of somatostatin receptor subtype-1. Biochemistry and Molecular Biology International. 38: 103–112, 1996.

Shahabi NA, Heagy W, Sharp BM. Beta-endorphin enhances Concanavalin-A stimulated calcium mobilization by murine splenic T cells. Endocrinology. 137: 3386–3393, 1996.

Shanahan F, Denburg JA, Fox J, Bienenstock J, Befus AD. Mast cell heterogeneity. Effects of neuroenteric peptides on histamine release. Journal of Immunology. 135: 1331–1337, 1985.

Shimozato T, Kincade PW. Indirect suppression of IL-7 responsive B cell precursors by vasoactive intestinal peptide. Journal of Immunology. 158: 5178–5184, 1997.

Singh A, Zelazowska EB, Petrides JS, Raybourne RB, Sternberg EM, Gold PW, Deuster PA. Lymphocyte subset responses to exercise and glucocorticoid suppression in healthy men. Medicine and Science in Sports and Exercise. 28: 822–828, 1996.

Smart BA, Rao KM, Cohen HJ. Substance P and adrenocorticotropin hormone do not affect T lymphocyte adhesion to vascular endothelium or surface expression of adhesion receptors. International Journal of Immunopharmacology. 16: 137–149, 1994.

Smith EM, Galin FS, LeBoeuf RD, Coppenhaver DH, Harbour DV, Blalock JE. Nucleotide and amino acid sequence of lymphocyte derived corticotropin: Endotoxin induction of a truncated peptide. Proceedings of the National Academy of Sciences USA. 87: 1057–1060, 1990.

Span JP, Pieters GF, Smals AG, Koopmans PW. Number and percentage of NK-cells are decreased in growth hormone deficient adults. Clinical Immunology and Immunopathology. 78: 90–92, 1996.

Spencer RL, Young EA, Choo PH, McEwen BS. Adrenal steroid type I and type II receptor binding: Estimates of in vivo receptor number, occupancy, and activation with varying level of steroid. Brain Research. 514: 37–48, 1990.

Spencer RL, Miller AH, Moday H, McEwen BS, Blanchard RJ, Blanchard DC, Sakai RR. Chronic social stress produces reductions in available splenic Type II corticosteroid receptor binding and plasma corticosteroid binding globulin levels. Psychoneuroendocrinology. 21: 95–109, 1996.

Sreedharan SP. Kodama KT, Peterson KE, Goetzl EJ. Distinct subsets of somatostatin receptors in cultures human lymphocytes. Journal of Biological Chemistry. 264: 949–952, 1989.

Staniek V, Misery L, Peguet-Navarro J, Abello J, Doutremepuich JD, Claudy A, Schmitt D. Binding and in vitro modulation of human epidermal Langerhans cell functions by substance P. Archives of Dermatological Research. 289: 285–291, 1997.

Stanisz AM, Befus D, Bienenstock J. Differential effects of vasoactive intestinal peptide, substance P, and somatostatin on immunoglobulin synthesis and proliferation by lymphocytes from Peyer's patches, mesenteric lymph nodes, and spleen. Journal of Immunology. 136: 152–156, 1986.

Stuart CA, Meehan RT, Neale LS, Cintron NM, Furlanetto RW. Insulin-like growth factor-I binds selectively to human peripheral blood monocytes and B lymphocytes. Journal of Clinical Endocrinology. 72: 1117–1122, 1991.

Takada Y, Ihara H, Urano T, Takada A. Changes in blood and plasma serotonergic measurements in rats—Effect of nicotine and/or exposure to different stresses. Thrombosis Research. 80: 307–316, 1995.

Tang SC, Fend F, Muller L, Braunsteiner H, Wiedermann CJ. High-affinity substance P binding sites of neurokinin-1 receptor type autoradiographically associated with vascular sinuses and high endothelial venules of human lymphoid tissues. Laboratory Investigation. 69: 86–93, 1993.

Teitelbaum DH, DelValle J, Reyas B, Post L, Gupta A, Mosely RL, Merion R. Intestinal intraepithelial lymphocytes influence the production of somatostatin. Surgery. 120: 227–232, 1996.

Terman GW, Shavit Y, Lewis JW, Cannon JT, Liebeskind JC. Intrinsic mechanisms of pain inhibition: Activation by stress. Science. 226: 1270–1277, 1984.

Toft P, Tonnesen E, Svendsen P, Rasmussen JW, Christensen NJ. The redistribution of lymphocytes during adrenaline infusion—An in vivo study with radiolabelled cells. Acta Pathologica, Microbiologica et Immunologica Scandinavica. 100: 593–597, 1992.

Torii H, Hosoi J, Beissert S, Xu S, Fox FE, Asahina A, Takashima A, Rook AH, Granstein RD. Regulation of cytokine expression in macrophages and the Langerhans cell-like line XS52 by calcitonin gene related peptide. Journal of Leukocyte Biology. 61: 216–223, 1997.

Tulen JHM, Moleman P, Blakenstein PJ, Manintveld AJ, Vansteenis HG, Boomsma F. Psychological cardiovascular, and endocrine changes during 6 hours of continuous infusion of epinephrine or norepinephrine in healthy volunteers. Psychosomatic Medicine. 55: 61–69, 1993.

Umeda Y, Takamiya M, Yoshizaka H, Arisawa M. Inhibition of mitogen stimulated T lymphocyte proliferation by calcitonin gene-related peptide. Biochemical and Biophysical Research Communication. 154: 227–235, 1988.

van Tits LJH, Michel MC, Grosse-Wilde H, Happel M, Eigler FW, Soliman A, Brodde OE. Catecholamines increase lymphocyte beta-2-adrenergic receptors via a beta-2-adrenergic, spleen dependent process. American Journal of Physiology. 258: E191–E202, 1990.

van Tits LJH, Graafsma SJ. Stress influences CD4$^+$ lymphocyte counts. Immunology Letters. 30: 141–142, 1991.

Vishwanath R, Mukherjee R. Substance P promotes lymphocyte endothelial cell adhesion preferentially via LFA-1/ICAM-1 interactions. Journal of Neuroimmunology. 71: 163–171, 1996.

Wagner F, Fink R, Hart R, Dancygier H. Substance P enhances interferon-γ production by human peripheral blood mononuclear cells. Regulatory Peptides. 19: 355–364, 1987.

Wang HY, Xin Z, Tang H. Ganea D. Vasoactive intestinal peptide inhibits IL-4 production in murine T cells by post-transcriptional mechanisms. Journal of Immunology. 156: 3243–3253, 1996.

Weigent DA, Blalock JE, LeBoeuf RD. An antisense oligonucleotide to growth hormone messenger ribonucleic acid inhibits lymphocyte proliferation. Endocrinology. 128: 2053–2057, 1991a.

Weigent DA, Riley JE, Galin FS, LeBoeuf RD, Blalock JE. Detection of growth hormone and growth hormone-releasing hormone-related messenger RNA in rat leukocytes by the polymerase chain reaction. Proceedings of the Society for Experimental Biology and Medicine. 198: 643–648, 1991b.

Wichmann MW, Zellweger R, DeMaso R, Ayala A, Chaudry IH. Melatonin administration attenuates depressed immune functions trauma-hemorrhage. Journal of Surgical Research. 63: 256–262, 1996.

Williamson SA, Knight RA, Lightman SL, Hobbs JR. Effects of β-endorphin specific immune response in man. Immunology. 65: 47–51, 1988.

Wilson TM, Yu-Lee LY, Kelley MR. Coordinate gene expression of lueinizing hormone-releasing hormone (LHRH) and the LHRH-receptor after prolactin stimulation in the rat Nb2 T cell line: Implications for a role in immunomodulation and cell cycle gene expression. Molecular Endocrinology. 9: 44–53, 1995.

Wood PG, Karol MH, Kusnecov AW, Rabin BS. Enhancement of antigen-specific humoral and cell-mediated immunity by electric footshock stress in rats. Brain, Behavior, and Immunity. 7: 121–134, 1993.

Wu CY, Sarfati M, Heusser C, Fournier S, Rubio-Trujillo M, Peleman R, Delespesse G. Glucocorticoids increase the synthesis of immunoglobulin E by interleukin-4 stimulated human lymphocytes. Journal of Clinical Investigation. 87: 870–877, 1991.

Wu JR, Chang HR, Huang TY, Chiang CH, Chen SS. Reduction in lymphocyte beta-adrenergic receptor density in infants and children with heart failure secondary to congenital heart disease. American Journal of Cardiology. 77: 170–174, 1996.

Wybran J, Appelboom T, Famaey JP, Govaerts A. Suggestive evidence for receptors for morphine and methionine-enkephalin on normal human blood T lymphocytes. Journal of Immunology. 123: 1068–1070, 1979.

Yun CH, Estrada A, Gajadhar AA, Redmond MJ, Laarveld B. Passive immunization against somatostatin increases resistance to Eimeria vermiformis infection in susceptible mice. Comparative Immunology, Microbiology, and Infectious Diseases. 19: 39–46, 1996.

Zurawski G, Benedik M, Kamb BJ, Abrams JS, Zurawski SM, Lee FD. Acyivation of mouse T-helper cells induces abundant preproenkephalin mRNA syntesis. Science. 232: 772–775, 1986.

Zwilling BS, Brown D, Pearl D. Induction of major histocompatibility complex class II glycoproteins by interferon-gamma: Attenuation of the effects of restraint stress. Journal of Neuroimmunology. 373: 115–122, 1991.

6

Stress Effects on Immune-Related Diseases

The immune system is involved in either causing or preventing several categories of disease.

Categories of disease caused by the immune system
   Autoimmune diseases
   Allergic diseases
Categories of disease prevented by the immune system
   Infectious diseases
   Malignant diseases

This chapter will discuss each of these categories of disease, how the immune system is involved in the disease pathogenesis or how the immune system prevents the disease, and how stress may modify the onset of disease or the course of the disease. This is the same question raised decades ago regarding whether stress can cause physiological changes that are responsible for the association of stress with altered health (Cannon, 1929; Selye, 1936). Although extensive research has been conducted and the association of stress with the onset and course of many immunologically mediated diseases is supported by published data, more work is needed to identify the specific mechanisms involved with the association, so that effective preventive strategies can be proposed, evaluated, and used.

GENERAL COMMENTS

The question asked in this chapter is relevant to the central theme of mind–body–health interaction: Is the quality of health susceptible to alteration by activities occurring within the brain? The following sections will present evidence for this association in the specific categories of disease listed above. However, as will be described, there is not yet enough convincing evidence to determine with absolute certainty that beneficial results on altering disease susceptibility or disease progression will be achieved with stress reduction interventions.

A summation of health and disease may be represented by measuring the duration of life. In a superficial manner, it may be considered that those who live longer have had healthier lives and were more resistant to succumbing to death from disease. It would be anticipated that factors which disrupt ones lifestyle by introducing a negative influence on mental affect would have a negative impact on health. Interestingly, a study of psychosocial factors associated with longevity has found parental divorce occurring before the subjects reached the age of 21 to be a factor in longevity (Friedman et al, 1995). Males whose parents divorced before the child was 21 had a median age of death of 76 years, in comparison with 80 years if parents remained married. For females, the ages were 82 and 86, respectively. There were no significant associations with a particular type of disease that was associated with earlier death. Children whose parents divorced early in their lives may have had behavioral alterations which contributed to their shortened duration of life (smoking, alcohol, lack of attention to medical care). The subjects in this long-term study were not representative of the general population as each had an IQ of >135. Therefore, the results may not be appropriate for application to the general population but they do suggest that similar investigations of additional populations may help clarify the importance of early negative life events on long-term physical health.

Other studies have related parental relationships with children to the long-term health of children (Russek and Schwartz, 1996). Healthy Harvard University students were asked to describe their parents. The health of those using positive words was compared with the health of those not using positive words. During 35 years of health assessment, those using fewer positive words had significantly more cardiovascular disease, hypertension, duodenal ulcers, and alcoholism. Disease onset occurred at a later age in those who used more positive words to describe their parents. Such studies present interesting questions regarding cause and effect. Did the subjects differ in regard to how they perceived their parents because they had different brain chemistries, which also had an influence on health parameters, including immune system function? Did subjects who had negative reactions to their parents engage in behaviors that affected their health because of a lack of self-respect? Did negative attitudes of the parents produce depression in the children and alter the function of their immune system and their health? Regardless of the cause, the study emphasizes the importance of the mind–body connection.

Five years after undergoing divorce, males were queried about the social and medical aspects of their lives. Although men living alone were similar to men who had reentered stable relationships on a number of factors, those living in a stable relationship with a new partner, or who had custody of their children, had fewer social and medical problems than men living alone (Hallberg, 1992). These findings are consistent with a variety of reports suggesting that social relationships are important for the maintenance of good health. There is also an indication that immune function differs between men who are separated or divorced and lonelier than married men (Kiecolt-Glaser et al, 1988). In addition to having decreased function of their immune system, the lonely men had more infectious disease illness than did the married men.

An association between immune function and longevity in elderly individuals has been reported. Evaluation of the responsiveness of lymphocytes to stimulation with nonspecific mitogens in older individuals found a broad range of responsiveness. Categorization of subjects, based on whether their lymphocytes responded more or less well to nonspecific stimulation, suggests that those individuals who have poor responsiveness, in comparison with other individuals of the same age with better lymphocyte responsiveness, will have a shortened life span (Murasko et al, 1988). It would have been interesting to know whether psychosocial factors contributed to the differences in immune function measured in these subjects. Of course, it must be remembered that those individuals who were more actively involved in social activities and who were involved in more physical activities may have slept better, ate better, sought medical care more readily, been more optimistic, and had a better sense of humor. After all, who can you laugh with if you don't have anyone to talk to?

However, not all studies support a generalized relationship between the mind and health. A recent long-term study of 113 males failed to find an association between negative life events occurring over 35 years (beginning at age 26) and physical health. There was an association between negative life events and psychological health, suggesting that, in some individuals, negative life events contribute to the onset of clinical depression (Cui and Vaillant, 1996).

The impact of negative life events on immune function, health, and longevity is, and will continue to be, an area of interest and concern. If negative life events have an impact on immune function and are indirectly found to have an impact on health and longevity, health practices that work to minimize negative life events and that promote immune function may become important as health management techniques. It is far less expensive to prevent disease than to treat chronic illness. Indeed, studies in humans and nonhuman primates have shown that affiliation and friendship can buffer the suppressive effects of stress on the immune system and enhance resistance to infection (Cohen et al, 1997a,b).

It is highly likely the mind does influence health, and health has an influence on longevity. The following discussion will review some diseases whose course and/or etiology are influenced by alterations of immune system function.

AUTOIMMUNE DISEASE

Autoimmune diseases occur when the immune system reacts to self-tissue as if the self-tissue were a foreign antigen. Elimination of the self-tissue would end the immune attack in the same way that elimination of an infectious agent ends the specific immune response. However, tissues such as the skin, liver, kidney, adrenal, central nervous system (CNS), eye, joint spaces, thyroid, muscles, intestine, and insulin-producing cells of the pancreas present large masses of antigen to the immune system, so that their removal presents a formidable task. Sometimes the immune system succeeds, and diseases such as insulin-dependent diabetes occur when the cells in the pancreas that produce insulin are destroyed. However, more often, the immune system produces continuous damage and inflammation to the tissue. The result is a long course of pain, discomfort, physiological abnormalities, and physical disability, along with the emotional effects mediated by chronic production of cytokines that induce feelings of tiredness and depression. Thus, not only does the immune process associated with autoimmune diseases produce tissue damage, but there are also behavioral changes that occur.

HOW CAN AN AUTOIMMUNE DISEASE BE INITIATED?

Failure to Eliminate Autoreactive B Lymphocytes

T and B lymphocytes can only recognize antigen that they can "see." The eyes of lymphocytes are the T-cell receptor and the immunoglobulin receptor. If all the lymphocytes that could recognize self-antigen were eliminated before they became functional cells, it would be impossible to develop an autoimmune disease. Therefore, because autoimmune diseases occur, elimination of autoreactive cells (the development of immune tolerance) is probably an inefficient process.

B lymphocytes mature in the bone marrow and binding of self-antigens to the immunoglobulin receptor of B lymphocytes during their maturation may eliminate the B lymphocyte by killing it or rendering it functionally inactive. For this to occur, the self-antigen must bind with a high affinity to the immunoglobulin receptor. The duration of time that the B cell is able to be tolerized to self-antigen is not known, nor is it known whether all self-antigens are present at all times in the marrow.

B lymphocytes are produced from the pluripotent lymphoid stem cells in the marrow. The immunoglobulin genes undergo rearrangement with the subsequent random generation of variable region combining sites. By chance, some of these will be reactive to self-antigens. This process continues throughout life, and removal of autoreactive B lymphocytes must also continue throughout life. However, nearly all normal individuals can be found to have antibodies (usually at low levels) directed to self-antigens, particularly as they age. This may indicate that the process of tolerization of newly developed B lymphocytes to self-antigens is less efficient as individuals age. Whether this is due to a decrease in the amount of circulating self-antigens, a decreased accessibility of self-antigens to the developing B lymphocytes in the marrow, or a decreased susceptibility to tolerization of the autoreactive B lymphocytes, or other reasons, is undetermined.

Another explanation for an increase of autoantibodies may relate to the process of affinity maturation of B lymphocytes that occurs in the germinal centers of lymphoid follicles (see Chapter 2). Once a B lymphocyte begins to synthesize antibody, the amino acid sequence of the variable region changes (the process of somatic hyper-mutation, which is unique to B lymphocytes). As part of this process, the B lympho-cyte may begin to release an antibody that binds to self-antigen. Theoretically, the B lymphocyte should die after 1–2 weeks because it would not be able to bind to anti-gen bound to the surface of a follicular dendritic cell. However, if an immune com-plex of autoantibody and self-antigen is formed and binds to the surface of follicular dendritic cells, autoantibody production will continue.

There is considerable information that still needs to be learned about the process of B-lymphocyte tolerization to self-antigens. With regard to tolerance of B lympho-cytes and hormones produced in response to stress, questions regarding whether stress hormones alter the process of the development of tolerance need to be ad-dressed. For example, do stress hormones:

Alter the kinetics of maturation of B lymphocytes so that there is a shorter win-dow of opportunity for B lymphocytes to become tolerant to self antigens

Alter blood flow to the bone marrow so that there is a decreased concentration of self antigens present

Alter the release of self antigens from tissue so that the concentration of these antigens is decreased in the blood

Interfere with the intracellular processes associated with apoptosis of autoreactive B lymphocytes or the B cell becoming unresponsive to its immunoglobulin molecule binding to self antigen

Lack of Elimination of Autoreactive T Lymphocytes

As described in Chapter 2, immature T lymphocytes migrate from the bone marrow to the thymus gland, where they undergo a maturation process to become T cells that can interact with antigen in the secondary lymphoid tissues and in the tissues and or-gans of the body. Assuming that the process eliminated all autoreactive T lympho-cytes whenever they were formed, there should be no autoimmune diseases involving antigens that must be presented by antigen-presenting cells (APC) to T lymphocytes, as there would be no T lymphocytes that could bind to the antigenic peptide in the major histocompatibility complex (MHC) molecule on the APC. That autoimmune diseases occur indicates that the process is not totally efficient.

Given that there must be some autoreactive T lymphocytes present that escape elimination in the thymus gland, the fate of these cells becomes important. One path-way that they could follow would be to be eliminated—either tolerized, so that they cannot be activated by antigen, or killed through a process such as apoptosis when they encounter antigen—in the tissues of the body. Alternatively, they could be acti-vated to produce tissue damage.

The mechanism of elimination of the autoreactive cells that do not become toler-ant in the thymus has been defined and is called "peripheral tolerization." Autoreac-tive lymphocytes that are not eliminated in the thymus enter the peripheral circulation as "naive lymphocytes." A percentage of the naive lymphocytes gain entrance to the extravascular tissue sites of the body, where they are exposed to the antigen that their T-cell receptor has specificity for. However, the antigen is not being presented by APC, such as dendritic cells, which have the costimulatory molecules required to activate a naive T lymphocyte. Rather, the antigen is being presented by tissue cells, or possibly by naive B lymphocytes, which lack costimulatory molecules. As a result, the T cell is inactivated or killed, resulting in the elimination of those autoreactive T cells that escaped tolerization in the thymus.

There are three possible types of cells that could present the autoantigen to the naive T lymphocyte:

1. Tissue cells within organs—As an example, if a cell of the proximal collecting duct of the kidney is synthesizing an antigen unique to the tissue cell, the antigen may be presented in MHC molecules on the surface of the kidney cell. If the naive T cell having a TCR that could bind to the antigen happened to roll over the kidney cell and the TCR bound to the MHC molecule, the activation of the T cell through the TCR without signals received from costimulatory molecules would eliminate the T cell.

2. Macrophages within the organ or that carry the antigen to lymph nodes, where the antigen is presented to naive T cells—Macrophages have a paucity of co-stimulation molecules in comparison to dendritic cells. Thus, a naive T lymphocyte interacting with autoantigen being presented in a MHC molecule on a macrophage may be eliminated as a functional cell that could contribute to autoimmune disease.

3. B lymphocytes—As indicated above, the elimination of autoreactive B lymphocytes is an inefficient process. Thus, there are B lymphocytes present in the secondary lymphatic tissues that have immunoglobulin molecules that can bind to self-antigen that passes through the lymphatic fluid filtering through the node. The autoreactive B lymphocytes will bind, internalize, and present the antigen on their surface in MHC II molecules. The usual situation is that the B lymphocyte would present the antigen to a CD4 T lymphocyte that had been activated by a dendritic cell. The interaction with the activated CD4 T cell would activate the B cell. However, if the B cell were to migrate out of the follicle, or a naive CD4 T cell were to pass through the follicle, the interaction of a naive antigen-presenting B cell to a naive CD4 T cell, would lead to inactivation of the T cell.

Infection may provide an environment that leads to activation of autoreactive T cells in the periphery rather than elimination of the autoreactive cells by a peripheral tolerance mechanism. If, for example a tissue is infected with a virus and an immune response is directed to the virus-infected tissue, cytokines will be released from CD4 Th1 cells and mononuclear phagocytic cells. If the cytokines induce the expression of costimulatory molecules on tissue cells, these cells may be converted from cells that induce peripheral tolerance to cells that activate autoreactive T cells that escaped tolerance in the thymus gland. This mechanism depends on the presence of naive T lymphocytes gaining entrance to organs of the body. As the pathway for trafficking of naive lymphocytes is primarily blood to lymph nodes, limited access of naive lymphocytes to parenchymal tissues should occur, limiting this pathway of development of autoimmune activation. However, if tissue inflammation changes the adhesion molecules on the local endothelial cells so that naive lymphocytes attach to them, the migration of naive lymphocytes into tissues where the tissue cells can become activated would become more likely. Indeed, this may actually occur, as cytokines are involved in converting flat endothelial cells to high endothelial cells to which naive lymphocytes adhere. An example is seen in the synovium of patients with rheumatoid arthritis.

Reaction to Cross-reactive Antigens

Another mechanism that results in activation of immune responses to self-antigens is that of overcoming the tolerance-inducing pathway. Three examples will be given, each depending on the presence of autoreactive B lymphocytes in the follicles of secondary lymphoid tissue.

Infection With a Bacteria That Has an Antigenic Determinant Identical to a Self-antigen. If a bacteria has an antigenic component on its surface that is identical to an antigen that is present on one's own tissues, tolerance can broken. The bacteria is ingested and digested by dendritic cells. Bacteria-specific antigens and the self-antigen are presented on the surface of the dendritic cell, which then moves to the parafollicular area of a secondary lymphoid tissue. A CD4 T lymphocyte is activated to one of the bacteria-specific antigens and the T cell then moves to a B-cell-rich follicle. Soluble antigens shed by the bacteria diffuse through the follicle. If the soluble molecule contains an epitope identical to a self-antigen, the epitope may bind to the immunoglobulin molecule on an autoreactive B lymphocyte. The antigen is internalized, digested, and presented on the surface of the B cell, along with many different peptides derived from the soluble molecule. Some of the peptides are specific for the bacteria.

However, even though the B cell is presenting many bacteria-specific peptides on its surface, the only antibody molecule that the B cell can produce is an antibody to the self-antigen. If the T cell that had been activated to bacterial antigen now binds to a MHC II molecule on the B cell that is presenting the same bacteria-specific peptide to which the T cell is activated, the T cell will begin to release cytokines that activate antibody production. As the B cell can only release antibody to the self peptide, the B cell will be releasing an autoantibody. That autoantibody has the potential of altering the function of tissue or damaging tissue.

An Immune Reaction to a Pathogen That Has Infected Tissue. Viruses infect tissue and immune reactions to the virus will kill the infected tissue cell. One of the mechanisms of cell killing is related to the release of enzymes from CD8 lymphocytes, neutrophils, and macrophages. The enzymes may degrade (denature) some of the molecules of self-antigen resulting in a self-molecule that retains a self-epitope and now has some epitopes that differ from self. This molecule may be taken up by dendritic cells where the denatured peptides are presented to CD4 T cells, causing them to become activated. The same molecule may also be taken in by an autoreactive B lymphocyte in the follicle, by binding to the self-reactive immunoglobulin molecule. Some of the denatured peptides would be presented on the surface of the B cell where the activated T cell could react with them. This would lead to activation of the B cell and autoantibody production. The infectious agent may also function to activate an autoimmune response by inducing macrophages to release IL-12. The IL-12 may stimulate autoreactive lymphocytes to become active. The autoreactive lymphocytes may only have to be near a macrophage that is releasing IL-12.

A Chemical That Gains Entry to the Body and Alters a Self-antigen. The environment that we live in contains numerous low-molecular-weight chemicals derived from air pollution, chemicals added to food, or the products of industrial processes. If a chemical gains entrance to the body, it may bind to a self-antigen (this is how the rash of poison ivy happens). The self-antigen may be bound to autoreactive B cells, which will present the chemical on the B cell surface bound to MHC II molecules. If the chemical had also been ingested by dendritic cells and CD4 T cells became sensitized to the chemical, the activated T cells could give help to the B cells to begin to release autoantibodies.

Alteration of Cell Regulation

An example of increased ability to produce autoantibody during aging has been reported in a strain of mice that are not susceptible to the development of autoimmune disease. B lymphocytes from 6-month-old and 21-month-old mice were stimulated, in vitro, with bacterial lipopolysaccharide, which induces all B cells to begin to release antibodies. The number of B cells releasing antibody that reacted with the erythrocytes of the strain of mouse being studied was approximately fourfold higher in the older mice. However, when young mice were treated with cyclophosphamide to reduce T-cell function, the younger mice had similar numbers of autoantibody producing B cells to those of the older mice (Meridith et al, 1979). This finding suggests that autoantibody production in older animals may be dependent on the loss of a regulatory T cell.

Other studies have shown that spleen or bone marrow cells from mice that are susceptible to the development of an autoimmune disease, but have not yet done so, will suppress the development of autoimmune disease in animals that would otherwise develop the disease (Hang et al, 1982). Regardless of the mechanism, it is important to consider that, in addition to producing antibodies to antigens on the surface of erythrocytes, autoantibodies may be produced to antigens involved in a variety of physiological processes.

Several categories of lymphoid cells may be considered regulatory in nature. These cells secrete soluble factors that alter the activity of other cells. Examples include:

1. Macrophages that produce transforming growth factor-β (TGF-β) and nitrous oxide—TGF-β inhibit proliferation of T and B lymphocytes and natural killer (NK) cell function, and nitric oxide is capable of killing a variety of intracellular

microbial pathogens and inhibits viral replication, and also has a regulatory role in immune function as it is capable of suppressing lymphocyte proliferation.

2. IL-4 and IL-10 production by CD4 Th2 lymphocytes, which suppresses CD4 Th1 lymphocyte function—This change in the balance between Th1 and Th2 function has been associated with activation of latent viral infections as Th1 activity suppresses viral replication.

3. Interferon-γ production by CD4 Th1 lymphocytes, which suppresses CD4 Th2 lymphocyte function—An increase of Th1 relative to Th2 activity has been associated with tissue damage in autoimmune disease.

Specific mechanisms of interaction and regulation are not well defined. Full understanding of the mechanisms whereby an alteration of regulatory lymphocyte function predisposes to the development of autoimmune disease will depend on the basic science investigations of how regulation works. However, as is obvious, the hormonal environment that is present at a given time may influence whether or not an autoimmune disease develops.

Another regulatory system involves Fas and Fas ligand (FasL). Fas is the designation of a molecule on the membrane of many different tissue cells, including activated B and T lymphocytes. Fas binds a molecule present on cell membranes that is called Fas ligand (FasL). When Fas and FasL bind together, the cell bearing Fas dies by apoptosis. Interestingly, during immune reactions and lymphocyte activation lymphocytes express both Fas and FasL. Thus, lymphocytes may actually kill each other. Tissues that contain high concentrations of FasL may be protected from immune attack by killing lymphocytes which have been activated to antigens on the tissue being presented in MHC molecules. On the other hand, expression of Fas and FasL on tissue cells may lead to the death of autologous tissues. If tissue cells, for example, the insulin-producing cells of the pancreas have Fas on their surface and are induced to express FasL, the tissue cells will kill each other (Chervonsky et al, 1997).

A mutation in the gene that codes for the FasL has been identified in a patient with systemic lupus erythematosus (Wu et al, 1996). The patient's lymphocytes had an increased in vitro proliferation to mitogenic stimulation, suggesting the importance of FasL in regulating cell growth.

AUTOIMMUNE DISEASE AND GENETIC FACTORS

There is a MHC association with the presence of autoimmune disease. For example, the HLA-B27 MHC I molecule is present in approximately 90% of individuals with the arthritic disease, ankylosing spondylitis.

The relative risk (the chance of individuals with a particular HLA allele developing a disease as compared with an individual without the allele) is significant for many autoimmune diseases. For example, an individual who has the HLA-DR 3 allele are approximately four times as likely to develop insulin-dependent diabetes than an individual who does not have HLA-DR3. Those who have both HLA-DR 3 and

HLA-DR4 have a relative risk of developing insulin-dependent diabetes of approximately 20. As the MHC molecules are involved in presenting antigen to T cells, part of the susceptibility for the development of autoimmunity may be associated with the ability of MHC molecules to bind self-antigens and with the ability of T cells to interact with autoantigen presenting cells.

However, studies of identical twins have suggested that there are factors, in addition to MHC molecules and antigen presentation, that are associated with susceptibility to the development of autoimmune disease. If all that were important were MHC molecules and T cells, it is unlikely that there would be sets of identical twins where one twin had an autoimmune disease and the other did not. Either both twins would have the disease or neither would. As concordance for autoimmune disease is approximately 30–50% in sets of identical twins, there must be factors other than those associated with MHC molecules and cell interactions that influence development of autoimmunity.

This suggests that the environment provides some of the susceptibility factors for the development of autoimmune diseases. Within the environment are infectious agents, chemical pollutants, dietary factors, and psychological and physical stressors. In addition, sex hormones influence autoimmune disease susceptibility, with most diseases being more common in females.

Does the Development of Autoimmune Disease Influence Life Span?

Certain strains of mice spontaneously develop autoimmune diseases. The autoimmune-prone strains of mice have a shorter duration of life than do mice that do not develop autoimmune disease. It is easy to hypothesize that the autoimmune response damages tissue and accelerates death. However, the properties of the immune system that predispose to, or that allow the development of, an autoimmune disease may also be immune parameters associated with an increased susceptibility to the development of infection. Infections and the immune response to an infection may produce damage to tissue, shortening life span. Thus, associations between an autoimmune process and whether the autoimmune process directly influences the duration of life must be interpreted with caution, as an abnormal immune system, rather than the autoimmune disease, may be the factor that is associated with a shortened life span.

There is an interesting observation regarding autoimmune responses in healthy humans who live to be greater than 100 years old (Mariotti et al, 1992). Subjects who were 70–85 years old had a significantly higher prevalence of thyroid antibodies than did the subjects who were less than 50 years old. However, the centenarians and the subjects aged less than 50 years had the same prevalence of thyroid antibodies. This observation may indicated that the development of autoimmune responses is associated with a shortened life span, which is related to the detrimental effect of the antibodies on physiological processes. It may also indicate that the immune system of the centenarians differs from the immune system of those who do not live to be centenarians, with the centenarians being more resistant to infections that could be detrimental to their health.

A full understanding of the association between longevity in animals and humans is complicated by the lack of therapeutic interventions in animals. Humans who develop autoimmune diseases are treated with specific medications (eg, insulin for diabetics or thyroid hormone for hypothyroid patients), or nonspecific medications (eg, anti-inflammatory and immune suppressant medications for multiple sclerosis or rheumatoid arthritis). Without these interventions the analogy between the development of autoimmune responses and longevity would likely be clearer in humans. However, it is likely that life-styles that encompass behaviors that promote immune system function that minimizes the susceptibility to the development of autoimmune responses, will enhance longevity.

If Stress Suppresses Immune Function, How Does Stress Predispose to the Development of Autoimmune Disease?

Stress is reported to increase susceptibility to infection because of a decrease of immune function, and to increase susceptibility to autoimmunity, which is associated with an increase of immune system function. These two results are not incompatible.

Increased susceptibility to infection may lead to tissue damage or infection with agents that contain antigens that cross-react with self-tissue. A decrease in the function of a regulatory component of the immune system may allow existing lymphocytes with an autoimmune potential, to become active. Obviously, there is not a simple relationship. Further complications are related to different patients, with the same disease having different etiologies to their disease. Eventually, clarification of the factors that contributed to the development of an autoimmune disease in a particular patient will depend on identifying the immune pathway responsible for the disease in that patient. That will allow a more precise characterization of the role of stress in the pathogenesis of autoimmune disease to be identified.

SPECIFIC AUTOIMMUNE DISEASES

The following section will discuss a variety of autoimmune diseases that have been shown to have an increased frequency of occurrence or that are exacerbated during stress, when the function of the immune system may be altered. Each disease will be presented with an explanation of how the stressor-induced immune alterations may affect the disease onset or course of disease.

There is a limit to the information that can be learned from the studies presented because:

The actual immune mechanisms involved in the onset or exacerbation of each disease are not precisely known.

Not every patient diagnosed as having a specific disease may have the same immune pathway causing the disease.

Not every exacerbation may be caused by the same immune mechanism.

Factors in a patient's environment may influence the course of their disease or have an influence on stress-reducing regimens experienced by the subject.

Some of these factors are the number and quality of friends the individual has, whether they are sedentary or physically active, or whether they are optimists or pessimists. These factors will be discussed in Chapter 7.

Thus, there are many unanswered questions with regard to the pathogenesis of autoimmune disease involving solid organs, their spontaneous remission, and their exacerbation. Indeed, in many diseases the contribution of immune factors is unclear and several immune pathways may be concurrently active. Research investigating an autoimmune disease focus on one or a few immune pathways. Associations may be found between the immune parameters being studied and the clinical course of the disease. However, without knowing all the immune pathways that may be contributing to the disease pathogenesis, and studying each of the pathways, associations may be made that are not biologically relevant. However, even though many of the data are epidemiological, and cause-and-effect relationships may not be clearly established, there is a wealth of data suggesting that there is a biologic relationship between stress and autoimmune disease.

Many of the studies in which stress in a person's life is associated with an autoimmune disease are flawed by the process itself. For example, if an individual diagnosed with an autoimmune disease is asked to recall negative events in their life, that individual may try harder to recall such events or add meaning to events that would seem less important if the individual did not have an autoimmune disease. A person experiencing negative life events may see a physician more frequently, just because they are not feeling well emotionally, and may be more likely to be diagnosed with a disease at an early stage. It is also possible that early stages of disease that produce metabolic alterations (eg, thyroid disease or diabetes) may have behavioral changes attributable to the altered concentration of endocrine hormones in their blood, increasing their likelihood of experiencing negative life events.

Psoriasis

Manifestation. Psoriasis is a skin disease that affects approximately 2% of the population. The involved areas of the skin are a pink color with white flaky scales. The skin lesions frequently undergo remissions and relapses. Blood vessels are dilated and often surrounded by lymphocytes and neutrophils.

Possible Pathogenesis. Psoriasis is likely to involve the production of cytokines by T lymphocytes in the skin. Considerable support for a T-cell-mediated pathogenesis is provided by the therapeutic efficiency of the immunosuppressive drug Cyclosporin A, which works by blocking production of IL-2. Reduction in the amount of adhesion molecules on blood vessels may also be caused by immunosuppressive treatment which would result in a decrease of the influx of lymphocytes into the skin (Danno et al, 1996).

The involved skin is infiltrated with T lymphocytes and streptococcal bacterial infections have been associated with psoriatic skin lesions. An immune response to the streptococci or superantigens released from streptococci may stimulate the cytokine release that is responsible for the skin lesions. The CD4 Th1 lymphocyte population may be responsible for the cytokines involved in psoriasis (Leung et al, 1995; Valdimarsson et al, 1997).

Skin keratinocytes in patients with psoriasis may have an enhanced propensity to proliferation when cytokines bind to them. In addition to decreasing cytokine production, Cyclosporin A may decrease the proliferation of the keratinocytes. This would suggest that both the appropriate cytokine environment and keratinocytes having a susceptibility to cytokine-induced proliferation are required for psoriasis to develop.

Influence of Stress on Disease. If psychological stress has an influence on the clinical course of patients with psoriasis, there may be evidence of stress altering the local skin environment where T lymphocytes will reside. A hypothetical scenario is partly based on the observation that the skin contains sensory nerve fibers that contain substance P (SP) (Wallengren et al, 1987).

SP can act on mast cells and induce the release of histamine (Foreman et al, 1983), and SP and histamine can increase vascular permeability. As T lymphocytes are involved in the pathogenesis of psoriasis (as supported by the therapeutic efficiency of Cyclosporin A), an enhanced migration of T cells into the skin through the blood vessels may be mediated by SP. In addition, T lymphocytes have a receptor for SP (Payan et al, 1984) and SP may stimulate T-cell proliferation (Payan et al, 1983).

Enhanced cytokine release by mononuclear phagocytic cells has been reported to be related to SP binding (Lotz et al, 1988), as has T-lymphocyte release of cytokine (Santoni et al, 1996). Thus, SP may be a neuropeptide that can contribute to T-cell infiltration and cytokine release in skin.

Stress has been associated with an increased release of SP in a rodent model. However, studies need to be performed to clarify whether there is also increased SP release from cutaneous nerves in patients with psoriasis (Chancellor-Freeland et al, 1995; Zhu et al, 1996). Of interest, individuals who have psoriasis and in whom innervation to the affected area of skin has been interrupted have a resultant amelioration of symptoms (Dewing, 1971; Farber et al, 1990). Thus, a hypothetical model can be constructed that supports the possibility that stress participates in the course of psoriasis by releasing neuropeptides that stimulate disease enhancing cytokine release from lymphocytes.

Clinical Studies. There are numerous published studies indicating that stress is associated with the exacerbation of symptoms in patients with psoriasis. As is the usual scenario with studies of stress effects on disease, many mitigating factors make interpretation of the studies difficult. Usually the number of subjects is low, the stage of disease and the actual pathogenesis of the disease in the subjects may vary, and coping skills (including psychosocial support, physical fitness, optimism, sense of humor, belief systems) that help buffer the effects of stress on the immune system may vary, whether the subject experienced high levels of stress as a youth or the subjects mother experienced high levels of stress during pregnancy (these topics will be discussed in Chapter 8). Given these contingencies, it would be highly unlikely, even if it is clearly established that stress influences the clinical course of a disease, that every patient would show the same susceptibility to having their disease clinically altered.

A summary of the literature evaluating stress effects on the course of psoriasis supports the role of stress as a modulator of disease activity and suggests that the severity of the stressor may be associated with more severe disease (Polenghi et al, 1989; Gaston et al, 1991; Al'Abadie et al, 1994; Gupta et al, 1996; Harvima et al, 1996). Additional studies have suggested that relaxation procedures that may produce a psychological relaxation (which would have an effect on the immune system if they decreased sympathetic nervous system activation) are capable of ameliorating the clinical appearance of disease in patients with psoriasis (Winchell and Watts, 1988; Zachariae et al, 1996).

Rheumatoid Arthritis

Manifestation. Rheumatoid arthritis (RA) is associated with a large accumulation of lymphocytes in the tissue covering the joints (the synovium). The amount of lymphocytes can be so large that the tissue looks like a lymph node. There is destruction of the joint spaces and considerable pain. Approximately 1% of the population has the disease and females are affected three times more than males. There is a genetic predisposition associated with the HLA-DR1 and DR4 genes, which have the same amino acid sequence in a portion of their groove that binds the antigenic peptide. Systemic manifestations include tendonitis, pericarditis, vasculitis, subcutaneous nodules, and pleuritis. The disease frequently has a relapsing and remitting course.

Possible Pathogenesis. As there is a large accumulation of lymphocytes in the synovium and numerous systemic manifestations (consumption of serum complement, circulating immune complexes, an HLA association, the presence of rheumatoid factor, responsiveness to immunosuppressive therapy) suggestive of an ongoing immune process, it is usually assumed that the disease is produced by activation of the immune system to an antigen. As identical twins are often discordant for RA, it is likely that an environmental (antigen) is involved in the disease pathogenesis. However, no specific antigen to which the immune response is directed has been identified.

Influence of Stress on Disease. An interesting animal model that indicates that stress can modify the development of experimentally induced arthritic disease was produced by immunization of rats with collagen and exposing them to a cat (Rogers et al, 1980). Not only did exposure of the rats to the cat ameliorate the disease, but just handling and transporting control rats ameliorated the disease. Although the investigators attempted to control for the presence of cat pheromones when the rats were handled, it is uncertain that all odors were eliminated, including pheromones from other frightened rats. As odor has been shown to affect the immune system (Moynihan et al, 1996), pheromones may have caused the disease amelioration in the control animals. This model suggests that stress may lessen the severity of immune system mediated arthritic disease. However, a direct comparison with human disease is difficult, as the animal model depends on specific immunization, and the time of immunization in relationship to exposure to the stressor is known. The human disease is a chronic disease and the severity, frequency, and strength of the stressors that modify the disease are difficult to characterize.

Another interesting experimental model produced arthritis in rats by injection of a material called Freund's adjuvant containing *Mycobactrium butyricum*. This material activates macrophages and monocytes. Arthritic changes develop approximately 21 days after injection. However, if the norepinephrine nerve terminals are depleted in the lymph nodes draining the site of injection, the disease develops within approximately 15 days, rather than 21 days. Depletion of SP by injection of capsaicin delayed the onset of disease and reduced disease severity (Felten et al, 1992). These studies, although investigating an arthritic disease with a different etiology, and possibly a different pathogenesis than that of RA, suggest that there may be a contribution of the central nervous system (CNS) to the clinical course of diseases such as RA, which involve lymphocyte accumulations in tissue.

Clinical Studies. There are several interesting aspects of the interrelationship between RA and the CNS:

1. If the disease is a response to an antigen (either an infectious agent or an autoantigen), the functional competency of the immune system and its modification by stress hormones could modify the disease course. Most studies of acute laboratory based or chronic life event psychological stress, report decreased antibody and cellular immune function. Thus, if stress does alter the course of RA, it may be through dysregulation of the normal relationship of the various lymphocyte subpopulations to each other. The effect of stress on the clinical course of RA has been variable and does not provide an unambiguous understanding regarding whether stress alters the onset or course of disease (Anderson et al, 1985; Rimon and Laakso, 1985).

   Another approach to evaluating whether stress influences the course of disease in patients with RA is to evaluate the effect of stress reduction interventions. Psychological interventions have suggested that slight clinical improvement can be achieved in patients with RA (Bradley et al, 1987; Parker et al, 1991). Thus, regardless of the difficulty in defining an immunologic etiology in RA, or a definitive understanding of the pathogenesis of the disease, there is suggestive evidence for an interaction between stress and the disease process.

2. As RA produces considerable pain and discomfort, the CNS hormonal response to pain and the subsequent effects on the immune system could influence the course of the disease. Patients with RA consider the associated pain as a major stressor. Thus, pain may activate stress pathways within the brain that lead to the production of hormones that modify immune system function.

   However, another pathway associated with pain may alter immune function. Pain elicits the release of opioid molecules from the brain and from cells of the immune system. The opioid molecules bind to specific receptors in the CNS and on sensory nerves that modify the sensation of pain. This may be a localized mechanism, within the joint space, to reduce the pain associated with bone destruction in patients with RA. However, there are opioid receptors on the cells of the immune system, and immune function is altered by opioids. The opioid-induced changes in immune function are variable, with both suppression and enhancement reported (Carr and Serou, 1995). Various effects of opioids on altering immune system function may be related to the concentration of the opioid, the specific type of opioid produced as well as the specific opioid receptors on the cells, the presence and concentration of other hormones or neuropeptides that bind to receptors on the immune cells, and the type of immune cells present.

Extensive studies indicate that psychological intervention programs can decrease the pain perceived by patients with RA (Young , 1993). Whether the pain reduction produces an alteration in the amount of opioid produced, both within the CNS and peripherally, and whether there is a subsequent change in immune system function that ameliorates the disease process, has not been determined.

3. The accumulation of lymphocytes, monocytes, and macrophages, in the synovium of the joints of RA patients may produce cytokines that alter CNS activity. The proinflammatory cytokines IL-1, TNF-α, and IL-6, are present in high concentration in synovial fluid. However, T-cell-derived cytokines are usually present in low concentration, if they are detectable at all. When T lymphocytes from the synovium of RA patients are studied in vitro, Th1-derived cytokines, but not Th2-derived cytokines, are produced. As the proinflammatory cytokines gain entrance to the systemic circulation of patients with RA (Houssiau et al, 1988), it is possible that they can then enter the CNS and affect the behavior and immune function of the subject. Indeed, a correlation between sIL-2R levels in serum and fluctuations in the daily mood of patients with RA (assayed by the Daily Profile of Mood States-B) has been reported (Harrington et al, 1993).

Recently diagnosed subjects with RA have a lower activation of the sympathetic nervous system following a mental challenge stress task than do control subjects without RA. Those subjects with the greatest amount of pain had the lowest sympathetic activation (Geenen et al, 1996). The lack of an intact stress response in RA subjects may indicate that the immune pathogenesis of RA differs from the immune pathogenesis of other autoimmune diseases or that RA is more likely to occur in subjects who have an impaired hormonal response to stress.

An impaired hormonal response to stress may cause the immune system to become overactivated, promoting an autoimmune process. Indeed, experimental animals that have an increased susceptibility to the induction of arthritis have been found to have functional differences of their HPA axis (susceptible animals have a decreased production of corticosterone) in comparison to experimental animals which are resistant to the induction of arthritis (Sternberg, 1995; Bernardini et al, 1996). An abnormal HPA response to immune and inflammatory stimuli has been reported in patients with RA (Chikanza et al, 1992).

Whether humans with RA have an altered response to stress because of modification of CNS function by cytokines, or whether there is an innate difference within the CNS that modifies their response to stress, has not been defined. However, subjects with another autoimmune disease, multiple sclerosis, have an intact response to the same psychological stressor that produced a diminished response in subjects with RA (Ackerman et al, 1996).

Clinical depression is also noted in patients with RA. The relative contributions of increased concentrations of peripheral cytokines, chronic pain, and decreased mobility to depression are unclear. Most likely, each contributes. However, clinical depression is known to be associated with immune alteration, and the effect on the course of RA is undefined.

As suggested above, RA is a complex disease whose course may be influenced by pain, systemic cytokines, and possibly impaired HPA axis or autonomic nervous system activity. Further complication occurs because an antigen-related pathogenesis is not obvious, different patients may have different systemic manifestations, the extent of disease may vary, psychological coping skills may vary, and different patients may engage in different amounts of physical activity. There has even been the suggestion that the presence or absence of rheumatoid factor may be related to a stress-associated disease onset (Stewart et al, 1994). Given such disease-related variability, the question of stress-induced alteration of the clinical course of disease in patients with RA will require better identification of homogeneous groups of patients for future studies.

The two autoimmune diseases described above (psoriasis and RA) involve T-cell-mediated immune reactions. Stress can also have an impact on an antibody-mediated autoimmune disease.

Graves' Thyroid Disease

Manifestation. Patients with Graves' disease have symptoms of hyperthyroidism. These include weakness, nervousness, weight loss, fatigue, warm and sweaty skin, menstrual irregularities, heat sensitivity (feeling hot when it is cool), and protrusion of the eyes, along with an enlarged thyroid gland. The disease is more common among females than among males.

Possible Pathogenesis. The pathogenesis of Graves' disease involves an antibody that binds to a receptor on thyroid epithelial cells that binds thyroid-stimulating hormone (TSH). When TSH binds to its receptor, the thyroid releases the thyroid hormones T3 or T4. The thyroid-stimulating antibody mimics the binding of TSH and stimulates the release of thyroid hormone. However, unlike TSH, which decreases in concentration as the concentration of thyroid hormone increases (reducing the releases of thyroid hormone), there is no inhibition of the physiological effects of the thyroid-stimulating antibody. Therefore, patients who have this antibody develop symptoms of hyperthyroidism.

Influence of Stress on Disease. If stress is a factor in the pathogenesis of Graves' disease, hypotheses that account for the production of thyroid-stimulating antibodies need to be proposed. Two can be considered:

1. *Loss of regulatory cells*—An extensive series of studies has been conducted evaluating whether patients with autoimmune thyroid disease have altered regulation of the immune system. It has been proposed that loss of the function of a "suppressor" lymphocyte allows autoreactive lymphocytes that will mediate both T-cell-mediated and autoantibody-mediated pathology of the thyroid gland to become activated (Yoshikawa et al, 1993; Volpe, 1993). Whether the proposed alterations of regulatory lymphocyte activity precede or result from the disease process is unclear.

   Another autoimmune disease that is also caused by an antibody directed to a cell surface receptor is myasthenia gravis (MG). An antibody directed to the acetylcholine receptor at the neuromuscular junction of striated muscle induces a decrease in the number of receptor molecules. Release of acetylcholine from the motor nerve is then unable to stimulate muscle contraction. Thus, there is a similarity in the pathogenesis of Graves' and MG in that both diseases are antibody mediated. However, a literature review failed to find support for a stress-related onset of MG. In one small study, 16 of 46 patients perceived a connection between the onset of MG and stress (Knieling et al, 1995). However, the nature of the study with few subjects and requiring self-reports makes interpretations difficult. Another study, of four patients, reported that the symptoms would disappear during psychotherapy (Kutemeyer, 1979). Anecdotally, some physicians caring for patients with MG, and patients with MG, believe that stress does influence the severity of the disease symptoms.

   However, why stress has been found to participate prominentally as a factor in the development of one antibody-mediated autoimmune disease (Graves' disease) and is not linked to another (MG) is unclear. There may be more interest in studying patients with Graves' disease, the patients may be more vocal, the association may be more clearly identifiable, or there may be no true association with MG, and the anecdotal nature of the reported association may not be valid.

2. *Alteration of the target organ*—Stress has been reported to produce physiological alteration of thyroid gland function. An acute stressor in rats has been found to produce an increase in the release of thyroid hormone (Turakulov et al, 1993), while chronic stress decreases thyroid hormone production (Servatius et al, 1994). However, acute stress may only increase thyroid hormone secretion when the experimental subject cannot control (terminate) the stressor (Josko, 1996). In association with decreased thyroid hormone production in chronic stress, there is a decreased production of TSH (Reist et al,, 1995; Marti et al, 1996). Chronic stress is associated with an increase in the weight of the thyroid gland, which is interesting as the concentration of TSH is decreased in chronic stress (Sardessai et al, 1993). Thus, even though there is a decrease of thyroid function, there is a stimulus for increased thyroid mass.

The data suggest that stress may participate in stimulating an antibody response to the TSH receptor. If chronic stress decreases TSH production (either directly by stress hormones acting on the pituitary or indirectly through a decreased production of thyrotropin stimulating hormone by the hypothalamus) an increase in production of the TSH receptor may occur. If the receptor is shed into the circulation, and if immune tolerance had not been established to it because it normally is bound to the membrane of thyroid epithelial cells and does not circulate, an immune response to the receptor may ensue. Both antibody and cell-mediated immunity would be expected to occur.

The mechanism for antibody production to initiate Graves' disease is unknown. Future research will require the testing of hypotheses to determine the role of stress hormones in the pathogenesis of the disease.

Clinical Studies. Patients who have Graves' disease have been queried in regard to whether they have experienced more stress in their lives than control individuals who do not develop Graves' disease. Such studies are often difficult to interpret, as the presence of a disease may increase an individual's awareness of negative life events. A significant problem with this approach is the definition of the control group. Matching for age, sex, and socioeconomic status, although important may not include all the factors that need to be considered. Approximately 56% of patients with Graves' disease are HLA-DR3 positive, but only 26% of healthy controls are HLA-DR3 positive. Selection of controls without matching for MHC markers will bias the control group in the direction of decreased likelihood for developing Graves' disease. A properly matched group may be found to develop Graves' regardless of stressors in their lives.

Noting the concerns expressed above, several studies found that high levels of stress are more likely to occur in an individual who develops Graves' disease than in individuals who do not develop Graves' disease (Winsa et al, 1991; Harris et al, 1992; Sonono et al, 1993; Kung, 1995). These studies suggest that patients had more negative life events during the months preceding the clinical diagnosis of disease. There is also a suggestion that stress may be more of a predisposing factor in women than in men (Yoshiuchi et al, 1998). However, not all studies support an association between prior stress and the onset of Graves' disease (Rosch, 1974).

If thyroid hormones are increased in concentration before the clinical diagnosis of disease, it is possible that behavioral alterations will be induced that either contribute to negative life events or to the subject's awareness of negative life events. As thyroid hormone measurements are not made during the months preceding the appearance of clinical manifestation of Graves' disease, a possible influence of thyroid hormones on life events cannot be ruled out.

A literature review failed to identify an association between stress and the diagnosis of Hashimoto's disease (autoimmune thyroiditis). Hashimoto's disease is caused by an immune attack on the thyroid gland involving both cell-mediated immunity and antibodies to thyroglobulin and an enzyme (thyroid peroxidase) located within the thyroid epithelial cells. Patients with Hashimoto's disease are initially euthyroid and frequently become hypothyroid as the disease progresses. Whether the lack of reports of an association between disease onset and stress is due to the slow development of Hashimoto's disease so that stressful life events may have been forgotten, the lack of rigorous investigations, or the lack of an association, cannot be determined at this time.

Multiple Sclerosis

Manifestation. Multiple sclerosis (MS) produces weakness, visual dysfunction, and paralysis due to destruction of nerve function. MS lesions develop in the brain and the spinal cord where myelin surrounding nerve fibers are destroyed by lymphocytes and macrophages. There is an infiltrate of CD4 and CD8 lymphocytes, macrophages, and plasma cells. Nerve conduction is impaired. Identical twins have an approximately 50% concordance for MS, indicating that both genetic and environmental factors are involved with the pathogenesis of the disease.

Possible Pathogenesis. The precise pathogenesis of MS is uncertain, but there is considerable evidence suggesting participation of the immune system. This includes characteristic changes in the immunoglobulins of cerebrospinal fluid (CSF), which suggest an immune reaction within the CNS, the mitogenic responsive of lymphocytes from patients with MS to antigens derived from the CNS, the clinical response to immunosuppressive therapy, and the existence of an experimental model induced by immunization with myelin basic protein (MBP), an antigen found in myelin.

Influence of Stress on Disease. As is common with regard to determining the influence of stress on the clinical course of patients with autoimmune disease, studies of MS are not definitive. Such studies suffer from the faults of small sample size, heterogeneity of the extent and pathogenesis of disease, influence of standard therapies, various stress-buffering capabilities of subjects, and concomitant clinical depression, having an effect on immune system function. Definition of the precise immune mechanism(s) that produce demyelination is also a hindrance, as without knowing which immune mechanisms are responsible for the tissue damage, it is impossible to know whether that pathway is being altered by stress. Even if an immune pathway is altered by stress, it must be altered in a direction that will lead to disease onset or exacerbation. An increase of Th1 lymphocyte function would be compatible with such an immune change. Interestingly, the CSF of patients with MS contains cytokines that promote CD4 Th1 lymphocyte activity (Drulovic et al, 1997).

An indirect indication of predominant Th1 activity in MS patients is the paucity of IgE-mediated disease in MS patients (Oro et al, 1996), as Th1-derived cytokines suppress the Th2 cells that promote B lymphocytes to synthesize IgE. As reviewed in Chapter 2, stress has been found to increase the production of cytokines from Th1 lymphocytes, while sparing alteration of cytokine production by Th2 lymphocytes.

To help clarify the relationship between stress and MS clinical activity, we exposed patients with MS to a psychological stressor and monitored the resultant changes in components of the immune system. MS patients responded to the stressor in the same manner as did healthy control individuals (Ackerman et al, 1996). The quantitative changes in the lymphocyte populations were compatible with what would be predicated to produce damage within the CNS (an increase in the numbers of cytotoxic CD8 lymphocytes and NK lymphocytes). In the same subjects, cytokine production by peripheral blood lymphocytes was determined. There was a stressor-induced increase in Th1-derived cytokines, with no change in Th2-derived cytokines.

Therefore, if stress is a factor in the clinical course of MS, the immune alterations induced by stress are compatible with those that would be expected to exacerbate the disease.

Another interesting observation is that a respiratory viral infection frequently precedes the exacerbation of MS (Panitch et al, 1987). There are at least three interpretations to this observation. First, stress suppressed immune system function, increasing susceptibility to viral infection (possibly the virus causing the respiratory infection, but also infection with another virus that infects cells in the CNS). Restoration of immune function to normal after termination of the stressor activates an immune response to the virus in the infected cells producing CNS damage. Second, stress suppresses immune system function, which becomes clinically apparent by the development of a respiratory infection. Unrelated to the respiratory infection, but occurring because of immune system suppression, a latent viral infection becomes activated in the CNS. An immune response to the activated virus produces tissue damage. Third, stress alters the immune system predisposing to a viral respiratory infection. Unrelated to the viral infection, the stress-induced changes in the immune system (increased CD8 and NK cells and increased Th1 cytokine production) promote destruction of myelin in the CNS by reactions to autologous antigens.

Clearly, the mechanisms cannot be defined at this time, but if stress is found to be a factor in the course of disease, stress interventions will become increasingly important as a clinical therapeutic modality.

Clinical Studies. Many studies have looked at the association of stress with the clinical course of patients with MS. The data are variable and are subject to criticism for the reasons stated above. However, they are suggestive that stress and the clinical course of MS are related (Warren et al, 1982; Grant et al, 1989; Stip and Truelle, 1994). These studies found that MS patients had significantly more life stress before the onset of disease or disease exacerbation than did controls. The most common life events related to exacerbation were those involving financial or interpersonal concerns.

An interesting observation regarding stress and disease activity in MS was made during the Persian Gulf War (Nisipeanu and Korczyn, 1993). This study reported a decreased rate of exacerbations of MS during the war. This observation indicates that an intense psychological stressor can have a profound effect on suppressing immune system function and can actually decrease disease activity. However, this is a unique situation that does not argue against less intense life-event stressors having an influence on the exacerbation of the clinical course of MS.

Studies that question the relationship between stress and the course of MS have also been published (Pratt, 1951; Antonovsky et al, 1968). Experimental animal studies in which immunization to MBP is used are difficult to relate to the clinical observations of MS patients, where the onset of the immune process is unknown. Stressing an animal in proximity to the time of immunization with MBP may alter the primary development of the immune response to the antigen and attenuate the disease process (Griffin et al, 1993).

Overall, the clinical observations and the possible stressor-induced immune changes suggest that stress can alter the course of MS. Studies of stress intervention are needed to confirm or refute this hypothesis. Care will have to be directed toward the clinical homogeneity of the patient population, including HLA characteristics, social support and other buffering systems available to the patient, use of medications by the patient, and how strongly the patient believes in the potential effectiveness of the intervention therapy.

Insulin-Dependent Diabetes Mellitus

Manifestation. Insulin-dependent diabetes mellitus (IDDM) occurs when the pancreas produces abnormally low concentrations of insulin, resulting in inadequate glucose uptake and utilization. Insulin is produced by cells located in distinct clusters, or "islets," within the pancreas. The insulin-producing cells are termed "beta islet" cells. Other cells in the islets produce different hormones. Patients with IDDM have reduced numbers of insulin-producing beta islet cells, but cells in the islets producing other hormones (glucagon produced by alpha islet cells and somatostatin produced by delta islet cells) are unaltered. This suggests that a specific reaction damages the insulin-producing cells. Once damaged, the insulin-producing cells do not regrow. Treatment consists of insulin replacement, on a daily basis, or possibly, the transplantation of insulin-producing cells.

Possible Pathogenesis. The usual pathogenesis of IDDM is probably related to immune destruction of the beta islet cells. Antibodies to insulin and islet cell antigens are present before the clinical onset of disease and may indicate a destructive inflammatory process is occurring. Sensitized T lymphocytes that have a cytotoxic effect on islet cells are also present. Studies designed to characterize the lymphocytes present in the islet during the process of islet cell destruction have identified CD4, CD8, B, plasma cells, NK, and macrophages.

The disease is frequently preceded by a viral infection and may be initiated by an immune response to a virus that specifically infects beta islet cells. Indeed, virus has been isolated from the islets of newly diagnosed diabetic subjects and, when the virus is injected into mice, IDDM has occurred with an associated immune-mediated destruction of the beta islet cells. Active viral infection is suggested because of a rising antibody titer in the patients serum to the isolated virus.

There is a strong HLA association with IDDM. Approximately 95% of Caucasian patients have the HLA-DR3 and/or HLA-DR4, which are linked to the HLA-DQ3.2 allele. Interestingly, in IDDM patients, position 57 of the HLA-DQ molecule, which contributes to the antigenic peptide binding cleft, frequently contains either valine, alanine, or serine, but not aspartic acid. Aspartic acid may contribute to a conformation of the peptide binding groove that interferes with binding of the relevant islet cell antigen. However, there are numerous exceptions to this general rule, suggesting that different peptides may be associated with the immune response that causes beta islet cell destruction.

The actual destruction of the islet cells may be due to cytotoxic CD8 lymphocytes reacting to a viral antigen in the groove of a MHC I molecule, an inflammatory reaction brought about by a CD4 lymphocyte reacting to a viral antigen in a MHC II molecule, cytokines (IL-1, tumor necrosis factor [TNF], interferon-γ [IFN-γ]) released from infiltrating cells that have a direct cytotoxic effect on the islet cells or the production of Fas and Fas ligand on the islet cells, resulting in their destruction of each other. Regardless of the cause, the only treatment is insulin replacement.

There have been several reports of giving patients immunosuppressive therapy (usually cyclosporin) at the time of diagnosis of IDDM. The objective is to prevent the immune system from destroying all the islets and allowing the pancreas to contribute some insulin, thereby lowering the amount required to be injected and also to maintain a more normal physiological rhythm to insulin levels. When this is done, insulin requirements are lowered during the time that the immunosuppressive therapy is given, indicating that the immune system is involved in the pathogenesis of IDDM. However, patients are eventually removed from the immunosuppressive drug because of potential serious side effects, which include infection, malignancy, and kidney or liver toxicity, at which time they become fully insulin dependent.

Influence of Stress on Disease. There are several reports associating life event stressors with the onset of IDDM. Unlike diseases such as RA or MS, which have a relapsing and remitting course, IDDM does not remit. Therefore, studies showing an association of stress with alteration of clinical activity are nonexistent, but studies showing an association of stress with disease onset are numerous.

Similar to stressor-induced increased susceptibility to MS, studies of IDDM suffer from the lack of a definitive etiology in a given patient. However, stressor-induced alterations of immune function may contribute to disease onset by:

1. Suppressing immune function and increasing susceptibility to viral infection
2. Altering the balance of regulatory lymphocyte populations which then allows an autoimmune response to occur

Early reports linking stressors in an individual's life with an increased susceptibility to the development of IDDM were not rigorously controlled and presented small sample sizes (Hinkle et al, 1951; Treuting, 1962; Stein and Charles, 1971). However, there are studies that suggest a possible association between stress and susceptibility to the onset of IDDM. These studies should be considered preliminary, as they have not addressed important questions. Specifically, does stress increase the risk of IDDM onset in all individuals, or only in those who are HLA-DR3 and/or HLA-DR4? If this association only occurs in HLA-susceptible individuals, should the control group of individuals who do not have high levels of stress be restricted to HLA-DR 3 and/or HLA-DR-4-positive individuals?

Does the stress-associated increased risk only occur in individuals who have antibodies to antigens associated with the beta islet cells of the pancreas? If it does, should the control group only consist of individuals who have these antibodies but who do not experience high levels of stress in their lives?

The only way to control for genetic differences between subjects is to study identical twins. The concordance for IDDM in identical twins is approximately 50%. Environmental factors are usually designated as explaining the lack of 100% concordance. Environmental factors may include viruses, but they may also include stress and the ability of a subject to cope with the stressor. A study conducted in identical twins (both concordant and discordant for IDDM) in which such factors as stress, psychosocial support, physical fitness, belief systems, sense of humor, and being an optimist or a pessimist, are considered would make a significant contribution to our understanding of the relationship between stress and susceptibility to autoimmune disease. If identical twins discordant for IDDM experience the same stressors, does the twin who doesn't develop IDDM have better coping skills?

Studies that have contributed to the suggestion of an association between stress and the onset of IDDM in children have found that severe emotional stress, usually associated with parental loss, especially occurring early in life, increased the risk of the subsequent development of IDDM (Leaverton et al, 1980; Hagglof et al, 1991; Thernlund et al, 1995).

The list of autoimmune disease that has been presented is not comprehensive but is representative of cell-mediated and antibody-mediated diseases. For example, inflammatory bowel diseases (ulcerative colitis and Crohn's disease) and uveitis have a relapsing and remitting course, have evidence of an immunological pathogenesis, and have been reported to exacerbate with stress.

Autoimmune diseases in which stress is not noted as a factor include:

Autoimmune adrenal disease (caused by antibody- and cell-mediated immunity to antigens of the adrenal)

Pemphigus vulgaris (caused by antibodies to an antigen in the skin)

Goodpasture's disease (caused by antibodies to the basement membrane of the renal glomerulus and the alveoli of the lung)

Primary biliary cirrhosis (caused by antibody- and cell-mediated immunity to an antigen of the biliary system of the liver)

Diseases involving circulating blood elements, such as autoimmune hemolytic anemia, autoimmune thrombocytopenia, or autoimmune agranulocytosis, are not included among the diseases in which stress is believed to contribute to the clinical activity. There is little, if any evidence to associate stress with the onset or exacerbation of these antibody mediated diseases. That does not mean that these diseases do not have a stress-associated component. This association may not have been noted and reported. Alternatively, the association with stress may not exist, even though it is likely that some antibody-mediated autoimmune diseases are likely to be associated with stress (eg, Graves' disease).

If there is no stressor-related component to the diseases of circulating blood elements, it will be interesting to determine why. This may be related to the need for a contribution of the target tissue to the process (eg, an alteration of the antigenic structure of the tissue by a viral infection or other process that modifies antigens on the tissue) or the difficulty in breaking tolerance to antigens that are in the circulation.

If there is a relationship between life events, hormonal alterations, altered immune system function, and the course of an autoimmune disease, the use of intervention strategies to lower the impact of stressors on the onset or exacerbation of autoimmune disease would be beneficial. Strategies that do not require immune suppression and that are able to maintain normal hormonal rhythms may lessen the risks of side effects associated with current therapies. Although there are many anecdotal indications that stress reduction may be beneficial in this regard, rigorous appropriately controlled studies are needed.

It is likely that cell-mediated immune reactions, including CD 4 Th1-mediated, CD 8, and NK-mediated reactions, are involved in autoimmune damage to solid tissue. Antibodies are involved in autoimmune diseases of the circulating blood elements. Antibodies may also be produced that react with surface molecules on cells that have physiological relevancy (eg, in Graves' disease and myasthenia gravis). Whether other antibodies to physiologically important molecules on cell surfaces exist, and whether they contribute to the decline of function associated with aging, has not been determined. However, if autoantibodies are associated with a "wearing out" of tissue, understanding of factors that predispose to their development, or that may impede their development, will be of great importance.

Diseases commonly classified as having an allergic component to them, but that are not autoimmune, such as asthma, have been reported to be associated with becoming activated at times of stress and with responding to behavioral intervention (Agle and Baum, 1977; Erskine-Milliss and Schonell 1981; Lehrer et al, 1996). The mechanism may involve a stressor induced release of chemical mediators from mast cells which produce constriction of bronchial smooth muscle. A possible scenario involves the stressor-induced release of substance P from nerve terminals with the subsequent degranulation and release of chemical mediators from mast cells (MacQueen et al, 1989; Bienenstock et al,, 1991; Heiman and Newton, 1995). Thus, a pathway of brain activation, release of substance P from nerve terminals, the binding of substance P to a receptor on mast cells with the subsequent release of mediators of smooth muscle contraction, and alterations of vascular permeability may be operative and associated with the symptoms of asthma and other allergic diseases.

INFECTIOUS DISEASES

As the primary purpose of the immune system is to provide protection from infectious diseases, stressor-induced alteration of susceptibility to infectious diseases induced through alteration of immune system function would be anticipated and is supported by epidemiological and experimental studies. Most reported studies are of upper respiratory viral infection or activation of latent viral infection. Deliberate infection of human subjects with viruses that infect the upper respiratory tract clearly indicates that high levels of stress in ones life increases the susceptibility to infection and that social support can modify susceptibility to experimentally induced infection (Cohen et al, 1991, 1997a).

Gram-positive and gram-negative bacterial infections, fungal infections, and protozoan and parasitic infections related to stress are not frequently reported. However, this does not mean that stress does not predispose to such infections, but rather that appropriate studies have not been done to evaluate this relationship.

I believe it less likely that stress alters immune function in a manner that increases the susceptibility to bacterial infection than to viral infection. The reason lies in the mechanism of immune resistance to the different types of infection. Antibody has a significant role in preventing susceptibility to bacterial infection, and serum antibody levels (with a half-life of IgG of approximately 21 days) are not likely to be altered by short-term stress.

Gram-Positive Bacterial Infection

Resistance to infection requires opsonization (by complement activated through the alternate pathway or the classic pathway), followed by ingestion and killing by phagocytic cells. The components of the host defense system that are involved with this protective mechanism are antibody, complement, and phagocytic cells. These will be individually addressed:

Antibody. Existing antibody levels would not be affected by stress unless stress increased the rate of protein catabolism. Primary antibody responses are attenuated when the response to antigen is elicited at a time of stress.

The question that needs to be addressed is: How much antibody is enough? That is not an easy question to answer. As a general rule, if the total amount of IgG is greater than 150 mg/dl (and the subclasses of IgG are present in normal ratios), bacterial infections do not occur. However, the total amount of IgG does not provide information regarding the amount of antibody that is present for a specific bacteria. Even though stress reduces the antibody titer during a primary immune response, there are no studies indicating that the reduced amount of antibody will result in an increased risk of bacterial infection.

If chronic stress were coupled with a severely decreased appetite, and malnutrition were to develop, antibody levels might decrease and predispose to bacterial infection (Gross and Newberne, 1980). However, chronic stress, by itself, has not been studied with regard to its ability to reduce antibody levels, so that there would be insufficient protection against gram-positive bacterial infections.

Complement. Antibody without complement can provide opsonization of bacteria. However, the process is much less efficient than when complement is present. The question of stressor-induced alteration of complement component levels and function has not been adequately addressed. However, studies that have looked at total complement activity or components find modest alterations by stress, with both increased and decreased levels reported (Ayensu et al, 1995; Cannon et al, 1994). It is possible that chronic stress along with malnutrition will lower complement component levels to a point where they are no longer able to provide protection, but that is an unknown, as there are no studies to support it.

Phagocytic Cells. Once a gram-positive bacteria has been opsonized by antibody and/or complement, the bacteria is ingested and killed by neutrophil phagocytes. The ability of these cells to carry out this process is influenced by stress (discussed in Chapter 2).

Gram-Negative Bacterial Infection

The innate defense to gram-negative bacteria is through the killing of bacteria by activation of the alternate complement pathway. Immune-mediated resistance is due to antibody binding to the outer membrane and activating the classic complement cascade. Activated complement kills the bacteria by damaging the membrane of the bacterium. Antibody directed to antigens of the bacteria membrane will cause complement binding and killing of the bacteria. The same concerns regarding antibody as addressed in the response to gram-positive bacterial infections apply to gram-negative infections.

Intracellular Bacteria Infection

There are bacteria that escape the antibody and complement host defenses by infecting and multiplying within macrophages. Bacteria included in this group are *Listeria, Legionella, Brucella,* and *Mycobacterium tuberculosis.* Some of the intracellular bacterial antigens will be presented on the surface of the macrophage in MHC molecules. Lymphocytes that have become sensitized to the bacterial antigens presented by dendritic cells in secondary lymphoid tissue may interact with the infected macrophages. Release of IFN-γ by Th1 lymphocytes will activate the macrophages to kill the intracellular bacteria (see Chapter 2, Figure 17). As stress can decrease the production of IFN-γ and decrease MHC expression, stress may be associated with an increased susceptibility to intracellular bacterial infection. Indeed, the association between mycobacterial infection and stress has been noted for a considerable time (Lerner, 1996).

Viral Infection

Resistance to viral infection depends on a variety of functional immune factors that are known to become modified by stress.

Antibody. Antibody that is specific for antigens present on a virus that are important for the pathogenesis of the virus is an important defense factor (Barclay et al, 1989). A virus is located extracellularly when it first enters the body and when it is released from the cells in which it is multiplying. During its extracellular phase, virus can be neutralized by antibody.

If there has been no prior exposure to a virus, either occurring naturally or through vaccination, there will be no antibody-mediated resistance; this mechanism will only become important in reexposure to a virus. Although stress may not be a factor in modifying the level of existing antibody unless coupled with other behaviors which will result in a reduced antibody level (eg, malnutrition), stress may modify the amount of antibody produced in a primary response.

A decreased ability to produce antibody to viral immunization when individuals are immunized at times of high levels of stress has been documented (Glaser et al, 1992; Kiecolt-Glaser et al, 1996). Thus, immunization at times of stress may result in lower antibody levels as compared with levels that may have resulted from immunization at times of no stress. However, whether there is a biological effect of the lower amount of antibody (ie, an increased susceptibility to infection) upon reexposure to the virus in one's environment has not been determined.

Once a virus has entered the tissue spaces, IgG antibody (which is equally distributed between the intra- and extravascular fluid) can bind to the virus. If the antibody binds to a site on the virus that is essential for viral binding to receptors on cells required for viral penetration, the ability of the virus to infect cells may be impaired (see Chapter 2, Fig. 2.29). Whether stressor-induced alteration of a primary antibody response or the inability to produce an adequate secondary response increases susceptibility to infection has not been determined. However, I believe it unlikely that short-term acute stressors or moderate levels of chronic stress are likely to be associated with an altered susceptibility to viral infection because of their effects on antibody production. However, high levels of chronic stress associated with nutritional deficiencies and engaging in behaviors that impair immune function (eg, alcohol consumption, smoking, inadequate sleep, poor personal hygiene) may contribute to an increased susceptibility to infection through a deficiency of protective antibody levels. Indeed, although the mechanism of increased susceptibility to becoming infected with an upper respiratory virus was not determined, severe life events of less than 1 month's duration were not found to be associated with an increased susceptibility to infection, but chronic stress of longer than 1 month's duration was associated with such susceptibility (Cohen et al, 1998).

The mucosal surfaces of the body are bathed in secretory IgA and IgA binding to the virus will prevent the virus from penetrating the tissue. This defense mechanism is the basis of the Sabin attenuated polio vaccine. The effect of stress on secretory IgA concentrations in saliva has been discussed in Chapter 4.

Cytokines. Interferons are a group of proteins that interfere with the ability of viruses to bind to and replicate in tissue cells and that also increase the reactivity of immune cells to tissue cells infected with a virus. There are three classes of interferon: α, β, and γ. IFN-α and IFN-β inhibit viral replication and increase the expression of MHC I molecules on tissue cells that may function to increase the ability of CD8 lymphocytes to kill virus-infected cells. The function of NK lymphocytes is increased by IFN-γ.

IFN-γ increases the expression of MHC I and II molecules on cells and increases the activity of NK lymphocytes. As described in Chapter 2, NK lymphocytes are potent killers of cells that have been infected with a virus that is likely due to conformational changes in the MHC I molecule that contains a viral peptide in its antigen binding groove. It is also possible that a viral infection will interfere with the synthesis of MHC I molecules in an infected cell. This would decrease the ability of activated CD8 cells to kill the infected cell but would increase the ability of NK cells to kill the tissue cells.

Thus, decreased cytokine production induced by stress may alter susceptibility or resistance to viral infection. Stress has been shown to inhibit the production of IFN-γ (Sonnenfeld et al, 1992; Bonneau, 1996).

IFN-α and IFN-β are capable of stimulating the HPA axis and of elevating plasma glucocorticoid concentrations (Menzies et al, 1996). Decreased interferon-induced activation of the HPA axis would be expected to increase the function of the immune system due to the removal of the inhibiting effects of glucocorticoid. How this would affect the balance of the protective effect of the immune system on susceptibility to infection needs to be explored.

Lymphocyte Populations. Lymphocytes are involved in resistance to viral infections by mediating an inflammatory response (CD4 cells) at the site of the infected cells or by direct killing of the virus-infected cells (CD8 and NK cells). Alterations of their function may alter susceptibility to, or the course of, a viral infectious disease. However, the net effect of alterations of the function of these cell populations on biologic processes, such as resistance to viral infections, is not well defined.

Infection with the hepatitis B virus with destruction of liver hepatocytes, jaundice, and lethargy is likely to be a stressful situation for many individuals. Yet most infected individuals fully recover after the immune system kills all the infected hepatocytes and interferons, and antibody prevents the released viral particles from infecting new cells. There are individuals who become infected with hepatitis B and who then are incapable of completely eliminating the infected cells. The result is a continuous infection, with hepatocytes being destroyed as new hepatocytes are formed (the liver has the unique capability of being able to regenerate itself after it is damaged). The condition is called "chronic active hepatitis" and is associated with an impaired ability of the immune system to kill all the infected hepatocytes. Whether stress hormones contribute to the deficient immune response has not been determined. However, most infected individuals completely recover, even though they are experiencing stress during the time that they have an active hepatitis infection. Thus, it is probably unrealistic to suspect that stress prevents recovery from viral infections, even though stress may increase susceptibility to infection.

Association of Natural Infection With Stress. Studies have been conducted that show a relationship between upper respiratory infections and stressors in an individual's life. Obvious problems with this approach relate to the following factors:

1. The accurate identification of a viral infection (as distinct from an allergic response, upper respiratory irritation due to environmental pollution, bacterial infections)
2. The coping capabilities of the subject
3. Whether the reported stressor was upsetting to the individual (divorce may be perceived in either a positive or a negative way)
4. How an individual perceives that physical symptoms may differ, when experiencing negative events in their lives (more attention may be paid to physical symptoms) or experiencing events which make them feel happy

Even with these concerns, the available studies suggest that there is an association between stressors in an individual's life and an increased susceptibility to viral infectious disease. For example:

1. Families with children between the ages of 1 and 18 were studied for the presence of naturally occurring infection with the influenza virus and a relationship with stress. A lack of family cohesion and adaptability was found to be associated with an increased risk of the development of infection (Clover et al, 1989). The effect of family function on immune function and the presence of an elevation of hormones that are increased in concentration in the blood by stress was not investigated. Thus, it cannot be determined why the association exists as a lack of harmony in a family may produce poor hygiene, poor nutrition, inadequate sleep, and stress.

2. A correlation between stress and the subsequent onset of symptoms associated with upper respiratory viral infection has been reported (Roghmann and Haggerty, 1973). Following life events that were perceived as being stressful, there was an approximate doubling of individuals who had symptoms of upper respiratory illness in comparison with individuals who did not experience stressors.

3. Data have been reported indicating that "undesirable" events occur in an individual's life 3–5 days preceding the onset of an upper respiratory illness, while 3–5 days preceding good health it is less likely that undesirable events occur (Stone et al, 1987). However, a replication of this study failed to find the association of undesirable events preceding an illness (Stone et al, 1993). Whether there was a lack of standardization of the analytical procedures used to assess clinical illness and the psychological variables between the two studies, or whether there was an actual difference in the association, has not been determined. However, the discrepancy emphasizes the difficulties of obtaining reproducible data from this type of experimental approach.

4. Whether everyday stressors in an individuals life are perceived by the individual as being stressful, and the social support available to the subject as a mediator of susceptibility to naturally occurring infection, has been assessed (Turner Cobb and Steptoe, 1996). Of 107 study subjects, 29 developed an upper respiratory infection (URI) during the study. There was a significant association of increased stress during the year preceding the study and during the 15 weeks of the study in those who developed URI in comparison with those who did not. Interestingly, during the 3 weeks preceding the onset of URI there was a decrease in the actual number of everyday stressors, but an increase in how those stressors that were present were perceived.

   There were no differences between those who did or did not develop URI with regard to sleeping patterns, smoking, alcohol consumption, or exercise. Interestingly, individuals who had a coping style that kept them away from the stressors that produced anxiety (an avoidant psychological coping style) were less likely to develop colds. High levels of stress and a coping style that did not employ avoidance of the stressor were associated with susceptibility to colds.

   Social support was determined to be a factor in protection from illness, but only when the level of stress was low. Low stress and high social support levels were associated with a low level of infectious disease. Thus, both psychological variables and buffering effects are identified by this study. However, mechanistic information regarding why and how stress and social support interact to modify disease susceptibility was not determined.

5. A study of children and susceptibility to URI suggests that not all children who are exposed to high levels of stress have an increased susceptibility to infection (Boyce et al, 1995). Those children who reacted to a stressor with greater elevations of heart rate and blood pressure than other children, were those most likely to develop infectious disease, even though the stressors in their lives were the same.

   This study suggests that individual differences in physiological reactivity to a stressor are associated with whether an altered susceptibility to an infectious disease will occur. It is likely that increased sympathetic nervous system reactivity to a stressor is associated with greater immune alteration than that which occurs in individuals who have less sympathetic nervous system activation to a stressor. Indeed, our studies have found that association (Manuck et al, 1991).

The above studies suggest that high levels of stress can increase an individual's susceptibility to infection, usually with an upper respiratory viral infection. However, buffering factors that influence whether there is sympathetic nervous system activation to the stressor will contribute to the eventual clinical outcome regarding the possible development of an infectious disease.

Association of Experimental Infection With Stress. an approach that can overcome some of the concerns regarding whether a viral infection was actually occurring in a subject who reports clinical symptoms suggestive of an upper respiratory infection would be to deliberately infect a subject after having determined the extent of stressors that the subject had been experiencing in their life. Studies of this design can address the question of the status of the psychological and immunological aspects of the subjects at the time of being infected. The studies are analogous to test tube approaches where a virus is incubated with tissue cells incubated in different types of tissue culture medium. In in vivo studies, the psychological aspects of the subject contribute to defining the composition of the tissue culture fluid (actually the hormonal content of plasma).

   Although psychoneuroimmunologists and health psychologists study stress as a factor that contributes to immune alteration and an increased susceptibility to infection, there are factors in addition to stress that may determine whether infection will occur. The virus must attach to a specific viral receptor in order to infect a cell. Whether stress hormones alter cell metabolism to increase or decrease receptor expression has not been determined. Accessibility to receptors may be altered if stress hormones alter the production of mucus in the respiratory tract with a subsequent altered accessibility of the virus to receptors on the cell membrane. It is also possible that stress hormones alter metabolism within infected cells, with a resultant increase or decrease of viral replication. Thus, although experimental studies related susceptibility to infection to psychological factors, the mechanisms accounting for increased susceptibility to infection in subjects experiencing higher levels of life stress are not well defined. Indeed, as has been emphasized, the extent of immune alteration induced by stress does not produce large quantitative changes in immune system function.

Regardless of the mechanism, higher levels of stress are associated with an increased susceptibility to becoming infected when a subject is deliberately exposed to a virus that can produce URI:

1. Exposing healthy volunteer subjects to one of five different viruses that cause URI revealed a correlation between susceptibility to infection and the development of the symptoms of colds and stress. Stressful life events, perceived stress, and negative affect (for the week before the study) each predicted the probability of becoming infected or developing a cold 7–10 days after infection (Cohen et al, 1991, 1993). Age, sex, smoking, or alcohol consumption were not related to the differences in susceptibility to infection.

   Infection was determined by isolating the virus in nasal washes and by an increase in the amount of antibody produced to the virus. Colds were determined by clinical symptoms. Even those subjects who reported low levels of stress in their lives became infected (approximately 75% of subjects). However, 90% of subjects reporting the highest levels of stress became infected. Clinical colds developed in 30% of subjects with low stress levels and in 45% of subjects with high stress levels.

   A subsequent study, using a similar experimental approach, determined that the extent of an individual's social ties could be related to whether an individual developed a cold subsequent to deliberate infection with a rhinovirus that produces URI (Cohen et al, 1997a). The actual number of social contacts that an individual had was not related to susceptibility to becoming infected. Rather, those individuals with more diversity (spouse, parents, inlaws, children, other close family members, close neighbors, friends, workmates, schoolmates, members of groups with or without religious affiliations, and volunteering with others in charitable activities) of their social groups were less susceptible to infection. In addition to an increased resistance to developing a cold, those subjects with more social diversity shed less virus (although this did not appear to be related to the differences in the development of colds between those with more or less social diversity), produced less mucus, and had greater ciliary activity in their nasal passages (which may produce a more rapid clearance of the virus and decrease the time that the virus is in contact with nasal cells, with a resultant decrease in infectivity). Interestingly, urine catecholamine levels were higher in those subjects who developed colds. This may reflect an increased activity of the sympathetic nervous system, which has been associated with decreased immune function. NK cell function was measured in this study and did not differ between subjects with more or less social diversity. Thus, this study suggests that social diversity modulates an individuals mental state which subsequently influences the hormonal milieu of the body which then alters, through an undefined mechanism, susceptibility to becoming infected when an upper respiratory infective virus is placed into the nose.

2. Another group of investigators performed a similar study of deliberate infection with a rhinovirus and obtained similar results (Stone et al, 1992). Those subjects who did not develop a cold after deliberate infection had fewer negative and more positive life events than did those who developed colds. What the actual effects of the different mental states are on altering the hormonal milieu of the body remains to be determined.

Activation of Latent Viral Infection. Suppression of the immune system, which occurs when transplant patients are treated with immunosuppressive drugs, or when patients with malignancy are treated with chemotherapeutic drugs, is often associated with activation of a latent viral infection. Thus, it is likely that either a particular pattern of cytokine production, a certain amount of immune system function, or particular concentrations of hormones, are associated with maintaining the virus in a latent state. If stress alters the concentration and the relationship of different hormones in plasma, or alters the function of the immune system and cytokine production, activation of virus production may occur.

Examples of virus that are associated with the development of latent viral infections are herpes simplex (causes cold sores), herpes zoster (causes shingles), Epstein-Barr virus (causes infectious mononucleosis), and possibly, and the human immunodeficiency virus (HIV) (causes acquired immunodeficiency syndrome [AIDS]).

Herpes Simplex Virus. Subjects who have recurrent herpes simplex virus (HSV) activation, either oral or genital infections, frequently report stress as a factor in disease activation. However, when subjected to careful study, the association of stress with either oral or genital herpes cannot be conclusively established. Some studies find an association (Schmidt et al, 1985; VanderPlate et al, 1988; Dalkvist et al, 1995), while others do not (Katcher et al, 1973; Silver et al, 1986; Goldmeier et al, 1986; Kemeny et al, 1989; Green and Kocsis, 1997). It has been suggested that an individual's ability to cope with stress, rather than the actual amount of stress experienced, is associated with recurrence of genital herpes (Cassidy et al, 1997).

The reasons for the differences in the study outcomes are not readily evident. Differences in experimental design, varying interpretations of infectious and psychological criteria, failure to evaluate the subjects' reactivity to stress, and coping mechanisms available to the subjects, may have contributed to the different outcomes. Obviously, from an immunological perspective, the function of the immune system and the concentration of stress hormones in blood are important parameters that need to be evaluated during times of stress in subjects when HSV becomes activated and in subjects with latent HSV who experience and perceive the same stress, but who do not reactivate HSV. If the same hormonal and immunological changes occur in both groups of subjects, it would be unlikely that the viral activation was related to these parameters. However, if there were differences between the hormonal and immune parameters in those who reactivated versus those who did not reactivate the virus, an explanation for the reactivation could be proposed. If a particular hormonal and immunologic profile were found to be associated with HSV reactivation, it may then be suggested that it is not a specific mental state associated with HSV reactivation, but rather a combination of stress and coping skills that produces the particular hormonal and immunological profile. Again, it is not the experience of stress that is the final determinant of whether or not viral reactivation will occur, but an interaction between how the stress is perceived and an individuals coping capabilities, that determine an outcome.

Herpes Zoster. Zoster (shingles) is caused by activation of the virus that causes chickenpox. The virus may remain latent in neurons in ganglia of the spinal cord. When activated, the virus moves down the nerve to the skin, and a rash appears in the skin innervated by the nerves that were infected. Although there has been an indication that perceived stress is greater in subjects who develop shingles in comparison with those who do not, limited data are available for careful analysis (Schmader et al, 1990). It would be important to know whether all subjects who carried zoster in a latent state reactivated the virus when events in their life resulted in a hormonal and immune milieu that supported viral reactivation. If this were found to occur, the combination of external environmental factors and internal regulatory processes (coping skills and perception of a stressor) that resulted in the immune and hormonal milieu would become critical to understand.

Epstein-Barr Virus. Epstein-Barr virus (EBV) infects B lymphocytes by binding to a receptor on the cell surface. Infection causes the B cells to proliferate leading to an increase of large lymphocytes in the blood (mononucleosis). Many of the infected B cells are killed by CD8 lymphocytes, which become activated to EBV antigen and react to the antigen as it is presented on the membrane of B cells in MHC I molecules. However, some of the infected B cells are not removed and remain with a latent EBV infection.

A series of studies have been performed that have shown that stress in combination with loneliness may result in reactivation of EBV (Glaser et al, 1985a,b, 1991). The proposed mechanism is a stressor-induced suppression of the cellular immune system. When fully functional, the cellular immune system contributes to maintaining the virus in a latent state. However, the interaction of elevated concentrations of stress hormones with an altered immune system as contributors to viral activation has not been fully explored. In vitro studies indicate that glucocorticoids, CRH, and ACTH, are capable of enhancing replication of EBV (Glaser et al, 1995), while in vivo studies suggest that hormones other than glucocorticoids are associated with activation of latent EBV infection (Glaser et al, 1994).

It is also unclear whether a specific level of immune function is required to maintain the virus in a latent state or whether each individual has their own baseline level of immune function and a suppression of their baseline function allows viral reactivation. As the stressor-induced depression of cellular immune function is not profound, certainly much less than is found in individuals with immune deficiency diseases, the mechanism associated with viral activation may involve physiologic parameters in addition to altered immune function. However, precise studies cannot be done until the biochemical pathways that maintain viral latency are established and the contribution of the immune system and stress-related hormones to maintaining the biochemical pathways are clarified.

Human Immunodeficiency Virus. Following infection with HIV, there is a variable time period for the development of AIDS, and not every HIV-positive individual will develop AIDS. Some of the variability may be related to different strains of HIV, whether the subject has a deficiency of the CC-CKR-5 chemokine receptor on macrophages and T cells that is required for entry of the HIV virus into cells, the presence of concurrent infections, and how well immune competency is maintained in the subject. It is logical to suspect that if maintenance of immune function is associated with delayed conversion from being HIV positive to developing AIDS, and if stress hormones can increase viral expression (Markham et al, 1986), stress may participate as a factor in the development of AIDS in HIV-positive subjects.

The basic premise of an interaction between the development of AIDS in subjects who are HIV positive and stress is the same as for other viral diseases associated with activation of a latent viral infection, although it is unclear whether HIV is actually latent. Rather, in HIV infection, there may be continual replication of the HIV virus and destruction of CD4 lymphocytes, but a continued production of new CD4 lymphocytes from the bone marrow. As long as the balance between production and destruction is able to maintain adequate numbers of CD4 lymphocytes, the subject does well clinically and is able to maintain effective immune function. This scenario is analogous to that of chronic active hepatitis, in which there is a balance between destruction of hepatocytes in the liver and the generation of new hepatocytes. However, once destruction of cells predominates and the production of new cells is unable to maintain adequate cell numbers, illness results. Stress may contribute to upsetting the balance in HIV- positive subjects.

Stress may exert its effect on the balance by decreasing immune function, which may increase HIV viral replication, by increasing glucocorticoid production, which may increase HIV production, or by promoting detrimental behaviors in the subject. For example, individuals who have difficulty accepting that they are HIV positive and who deny being HIV positive may not seek proper medical care or follow the medical advice they are given. They may even practice unsafe sex. If they experience emotional anxiety about their state and do not use buffers (friends, exercise, optimism) to help alleviate the anxiety, their stress levels may increase, further suppressing their immune system function.

Studies of the effect of stress on the progression of HIV infection have produced a variety of inconsistent results for which an explanation can be provided. How an individual perceives stressful events in their life is likely to be more important than the existence of stress. When an individual is stressed, they may engage in behaviors that are not beneficial to their health (eg, not obtaining proper health care advise, not taking proper medications, not avoiding nonprescription drugs that could be detrimental to health, not reducing or eliminating smoking and excessive alcohol consumption, not eating nutritious foods, not getting adequate amounts of sleep). How these behaviors interact with the neural–endocrine–immune systems to maintain viral latency needs to be determined.

Studies of stress and the course of disease in HIV-positive individuals do not evaluate the hormones that influence immune function. Therefore, attempting to relate different psychological parameters to disease progression, without characterizing the hormonal content of plasma and without being able to identify the immune functions that are important for regulating viral production, it is not surprising that there is variation in the reported literature. In addition, much of the literature does not take into consideration newer ways to assess the extent of disease. Although the numbers of CD4 lymphocytes have provided a useful way to assess disease progression, the amount of virus in a patients plasma provides a more reliable means of assessing the extent of disease and fluctuation in disease activity. Thus, studies that have evaluated the interaction between stress and disease progression are compromised not only by failing to identify and evaluate the relevant hormonal and immune profiles in study subjects, but also by not knowing whether all study subjects had the same viral load and how the viral load was influenced by the psychological and environmental parameters being evaluated.

Given the above concerns regarding the lack of consistency of the reported data and the concerns regarding current methodologies for assessing disease extent and progression, there are several reports indicating an association between disease state and stress (Goodkin et al, 1992a,b; Reed et al, 1994; Ironson et al, 1994; Kemeny et al, 1994, 1995; Evans et al, 1997; Leserman et al, 1997). There are also reports that fail to find an association between stress and disease progression (Kessler et al, 1991; Rabkin et al, 1991; Perry et al, 1992; EichHochli et al, 1997).

Differences in progression of HIV infection have also been reported between individuals who either do or do not conceal their homosexuality with more rapid progression occurring in those who conceal their homosexuality (Cole et al, 1996). The differences were not found to be related to health practices, sexual behavior, antiretroviral therapy, clinical depression, anxiety, social support, or a repressive coping style.

Studies in monkeys also support the influence of social interactions on the course of simian imunodeficiency virus infection. The concentration of simian imunodeficiency virus RNA (an indication of the amount of virus present in blood) was measured in the plasma of infected rhesus monkeys maintained in stable or unstable housing conditions. The unstable condition involves adjustment to being periodically rehoused with new monkeys. The monkeys housed in unstable conditions displayed less affiliation and more antagonism to other monkeys and had a shorter duration of life after being infected. Those monkeys who showed higher levels of affiliation had lower concentrations of viral RNA in their plasma while those being the object of social threats had higher levels (Capitanio et al, 1998).

Diseases which have their etiology or pathogenesis related to an infection may be more prevalent than our current awareness. For example, atherosclerotic lesions of blood vessels in the heart have been linked to infection with *Chlamydia pneumoniae,* an organism which causes pneumonia (Davidson et al., 1998). As anti-inflammatory agents have been shown to ameliorate the progress of Alzheimer's disease, it could be hypothesized that in some individuals with Alzheimer's disease an immune response to an infectious agent participates in the pathogenesis of disease. As the immune alterations induced by stress have been associated with an increased susceptibility to infection or to activation of latent infection, the influence of stressor induced immune alteration on each disease that is shown to have an infectious component to its pathogenesis, will have to be assessed.

MALIGNANT DISEASE

The hypothesized association between the mind and the development and course of malignant disease continually receives attention. The association is a double-edged sword. If subjects with malignancy are told that they can improve their chances of survival by learning to reduce the level of stress in their lives, it is possible for the subject to believe that their response to stressors in their life had contributed to the development of malignancy. This belief may serve to increase the amount of stress that they experience.

The underlying theme of the interrelationship between the mind and the development of malignancy is that malignancy is more likely to develop in individuals who have an immune system that is incapable of eliminating spontaneously occurring malignant cells. For example, lymphoproliferative malignancies occur in some individuals who receive immunosuppression for the maintenance of tissue transplants and reduction of the immunosuppression results in a reversal of tumor growth (Nalesnik and Starzl, 1994). Immunosuppression for the treatment of autoimmune disease has also been associated with the development of malignancy (Radis, 1995).

However, not all patients who receive immunosuppression develop malignancies, and the types of malignancies that occur are limited. For example, breast cancer rarely occurs in transplant recipients with a suppressed immune system. Even in patients with congenital immune deficiency diseases involving either the humoral or cellular components of the immune system, there is an increased likelihood for the development of malignant disease, but not all patients with congenital immune deficiency diseases develop malignancies. This finding suggests that the association between immune deficiency and the predisposition to the development of a malignancy is multifactorial.

Could stress contribute in ways other than alteration of immune function to the development of malignancy? As stress alters the hormonal milieu of the body, it is possible that changes in the concentration of various hormones could, for example, lead to virus activation or production of growth factors that promote the growth of malignant cells. Oxidation-induced breaks in cellular DNA have also been reported to be induced by psychological stress (Adachi et al, 1993). Thus, an association between stress or the reduction of stress and the growth of malignant tissues may exist, but the mechanism responsible for the association has not been defined.

Another consideration is whether any malignancy will have an increased likelihood of developing when an individual is experiencing a high degree of stress or whether the course of any existing malignancy will be altered by stress. Therapeutic modalities employing the concept of "biologic response modification" designed to increase the activity of the immune system against the growth of malignant tissues are mostly effective against a limited number of types of malignancy, primarily malignant melanoma and renal cell carcinoma. This would suggest that behavioral alterations which enhance immune system function would not be effective modifiers of the growth and/or development of all malignant tissues.

It is also likely that augmentation of immune function as a therapeutic modality against malignant tissue will be most effective when the mass of tumor tissue is small. Thus, if immune augmentation is capable of having an ameliorative effect on the course of malignancy, immune enhancement should be used at the early stages of growth. However, it is also more likely that chemotherapy will be more effective when the tumor is small. Yet, chemotherapy will decrease the ability of the immune stem to function. Therefore, the clinical effectiveness of combining immune-enhancing modalities at the same time as that immune suppressing drugs are used will be difficult to determine. However, if stress reduction and enhancement of immune function through behavioral modification is found to provide a means of limiting tumor development or growth, it would have the advantage of minimal, if any, deleterious side effects. Certainly, it may contribute to the maintenance of health when used as a preventative modality by healthy individuals without tumors.

How does the immune system prevent malignancy? The likely scenario is that an antigen is present on the tumor and that immunologic tolerance has not developed to the antigen. The unique antigen, which would be referred to as a "tumor-specific antigen" may be derived from a chemical toxin or an infectious agent, or may be produced as the result of a mutation in an expressed gene. The formation and growth of a malignant tissue may therefore, indicate that the tumor specific antigen was not recognized and responded to by the immune system.

There are dramatic reports of an association between the ability of a patient with malignancy to learn to relax and cope with stress and an improved clinical course, often including a prolonged life span. However, these associations require careful evaluation, as an individual who has survived beyond the time that they expected to live may make the assumption that their behavior influenced their survival, when there is no actual relationship. It is even possible that having a malignancy will influence an individual to have increased recollections of prior stress in their life. Even when an individual with malignancy deliberately modifies their behavior and has a prolonged life span, the association is difficult to establish as cause-and-effect.

One study found increased work-related problems during the preceding 10 years among individuals who had colorectal cancer in comparison with individuals who did not have colorectal cancer (Courtney et al, 1993). Death of a spouse or change of residence was also associated with increased risk of colorectal cancer, but the increased risk was not as great as that of work-related stress. On the basis of the data from this study one can consider that the stress one experiences in their life may induce physiologic changes (possibly of the immune system) that increases the risk of developing a malignancy. One also could wonder what would have been the results if the investigators had selected another malignancy for consideration. Fortunately, another group of investigators performed that study.

A group of patients with breast cancer (258 subjects) and matched controls (614 subjects) were queried regarding stressors that occurred in their lives during the preceding 5 years (Roberts et al, 1996). There were no differences in the stressors experienced between the two groups. Thus, this would suggest that the stressors in one's life do not predispose to the development of breast cancer, although colon cancer (found to be increased by work-related stress in the study reported above) was not evaluated in this group of subjects. Other similar studies of subjects with breast cancer find an association with increased stress before the diagnosis (Forsen, 1991) or fail to find an association (Hilakivi-Clarke et al, 1994).

The effect of severe stress was studied in 11,231 parents who had a child who developed a malignancy (Johansen and Olsen, 1997). Even though experiencing a severe stressor in their lives, there was no increase of malignancies, allergic, or autoimmune diseases in the parents. Coping skills and resources were not evaluated. Therefore, it was not determined whether parents who had good social support, who were physically active, and who experienced less bereavement differed in the development of malignancy as compared with parents who lacked coping skills and social support.

As was previously emphasized in the discussion of stress and infectious diseases, the perception of stress is important to be aware of. If an event in one's life that can induce stress does so for one individual and not for another, the physiological importance of the stressor will differ between the two individuals. This has been considered in a study of stress and breast cancer (Ginsberg et al, 1996). The study measured the stress of events in the subjects' lives and the psychological impact of changes in their lives that were caused by the stressor. Information for the preceding 10 years was obtained from 99 subjects with, and from 99 without, breast cancer. The subjects who were in the highest 25% of life event change and distress had 4.67 times the risk of breast cancer in comparison with the women in the lowest 25%. Thus, it is suggested that it is important to be aware of the psychological impact of a stressor in addition to the frequency of stressor occurrence. It is also unclear whether the physiological effects of stress are cumulative. Of course, it would be better to be able to identify the hormonal and immune measures that might be associated with an increased risk of developing a malignancy. The impact of events in one's life could then be measured by means of laboratory assays.

It remains unknown whether the differences are due to better recall on the part of some patients, to the particular stressors surveyed for, to changes induced in other behaviors by the stress such as a change in diet or smoking habits, or to differences in the type of breast cancer. For example, do different histological types of breast cancer have different associations with stressor-induced immune alteration, or do malignancies that have estrogen receptors differ in their association with stress from malignancies that do not have estrogen receptors.

Programs designed to provide relaxation and improved coping skills may be capable of increasing some aspects of immune function. NK cell function increases in patients with malignancy who have undergone psychologic intervention programs designed to produce relaxation and greater ability to cope with the diagnosis of malignancy (Gruber et al, 1988; Fawzy et al, 1990). Such studies are important as they indicate that the immune system in patients with malignancy can be susceptible to alteration when an individual experiences different emotions.

Although there are many studies that can be looked at in which emotional distress and survival or disease course in patients with malignancy were evaluated, few have been comprehensive in regard to the evaluation of altered emotional states, immune function, and clinical course. One study, of patients with malignant melanoma, does provide interesting information (Fawzy et al, 1990a,b, 1993). Subjects of the study had been treated surgically for the removal of malignant melanoma tissue and were considered to have a good prognosis for survival. Subjects underwent six weekly group sessions that provided social interaction, health education, stress management, and an improved ability to cope with stress. Subjects experiencing the intervention program, as opposed to controls who did not receive the intervention, had pronounced differences in several psychological parameters. They experienced less depression and more vigor and had developed better coping skills. The number and function of NK lymphocytes in the blood were increased in those undergoing the intervention. The increase of NK function correlated with a lower level of depression and anxiety. The higher level of NK function correlated with a lower likelihood of disease recurrence. There were significantly fewer deaths in the treatment group than in the control group at 5 years after the intervention therapy. Thus, this study suggests that psychological intervention in patients who have been surgically treated for malignant melanoma and who have a good prognosis will experience positive psychologic effects of a program designed to increase coping skills and reduce anxiety, will have an increase of NK cell function, and will have a prolonged mean life span—certainly encouraging data.

Another study of psychological intervention that provided enhanced coping skills and social support and interaction was conducted in patients with breast cancer (Spiegel et al, 1989). The intervention lasted 1 year, and the rate of death was the same in the intervention and control groups for the next 8 months. There was then a divergence of the survival of subjects in the intervention group and the control group with those in the intervention group surviving longer (the mean survival for the intervention group was 36.6 months and 18.9 months for the control group). However, a recent abstract suggested that social support groups for women with breast cancer have a better outcome among women who lack social support. Women with strong social support were not found to benefit from peer counseling; in fact, they may actually become more depressed. Thus, as with most studies, there are going to be subpopulations of the total subject pool who receive benefit from the intervention.

The interrelationship between the development of a malignancy and the clinical course of malignancy with stress and anxiety in an individual's life has been suggested by several studies. However, there is considerable evidence contradicting the association. Stress may influence susceptibility or the course of a malignant disease by contributing to the deleterious behavior of an individual (reduced sleep, unhealthy diet, lack of physical activity, smoking, alcohol consumption, use of nonprescription drugs). Stress may also produce hormonal changes that alter the function of the immune system with an associated increased susceptibility to infection or activation of latent infections, or stress may produce hormonal changes which contribute to chromosomal damage. Once specific mechanisms for the induction of malignancy can be defined in a particular patient, appropriate studies that evaluate how stress affects the mechanism leading to the development of cancer can be initiated. Until then, data concerning associations will be accumulated without an understanding of the relevant biochemical and physiological pathways.

Stress alone does not determine how well or poorly the immune system will function and how that will affect an individual's resistance to infectious disease, autoimmune disease, or malignancy. Rather, it is the balance between the amount of stress in an individual life (both acute and chronic) and the ability of an individual to cope with the stress. Thus, a high stress level with excellent coping skills may result in minimal effects on immune system function. A low level of stress in an individual who has poor coping skills may produce alterations of immune function with a resultant altered susceptibility to disease. The actual amount of stress is only part of the information needed in evaluating the effect of stress on immune function. Determination of the coping skills that will optimize immune system function, because of their effect on the hormonal response to stress, is needed.

REFERENCES

Ackerman KD, Martino M, Heyman R, Moyna NM, Rabin BS. Immunologic response to acute psychological stress in MS patients and controls. Journal of Neuroimmunology. 68: 85–94, 1996.

Adachi S, Kawamura K, Takemoto K. Oxidative damage of nuclear DNA in liver of rats exposed to psychological stress. Cancer Research. 53: 4153–4155, 1993.

Agle DP, Baum GL. Psychological aspects of chronic obstructive pulmonary disease. Medical Clinics of North America. 61: 749–758, 1977.

Al'Abadie MS, Kent GG, Gawkrodger DJ. The relationship between stress and the onset and exacerbation of psoriasis and other skin conditions. British Journal of Dermatology. 130: 199–203, 1994.

Anderson KO, Bradley LA, Young LD, McDaniel LK, Wise CM. Rheumatoid arthritis: Review of the psychological factors relating to etiology, effects and treatment. Psychological Bulletin. 98: 358–387, 1985.

Antonovsky A, Leibowitz U, Medalie JM, Smith HA, Halpern L, Alter M. Reappraisal of possible etiologic factors in multiple sclerosis. American Journal of Public Health. 58: 836–848, 1968.

Ayensu WK, Pucilowski O, Mason GA, Overstreet DH, Rezvani AH, Janowsky DS. Effects of chronic mild stress on serum complement activity, saccharine preference, and corticosterone levels in Flinders lines of rats. Physiology and Behavior. 57: 165–169, 1995.

Barclay W, al-Nakib W, Higgins P, Tyrrell D. The time course of the humoral immune responses to rhinovirus infection. Epidemiology and Infection. 103: 659–663, 1989.

Bernardini R, Iurato MP, Chiarenza A, Lempereur L, Calogero AE, Sternberg EM. Adenylate-cyclase-dependent pituitary adrenocorticotropin secretion is defective in the inflammatory-disease-susceptible Lewis rat. Neuroendocrinology. 63: 468–474, 1996.

Bienenstock J, MacQueen G, Sestini P, Marshall JS, Stead RH, Perdue MH. Mast cell/nerve interactions in vitro and in vivo. American Review of Respiratory Diseases. 143: S55–S58, 1991.

Bonneau RH. Stress induced effects on integral immune components in herpes simplex virus (HSV)–specific memory cytotoxic T lymphocyte activation. Brain, Behavior, and Immunity. 10: 139–163, 1996.

Boyce WT, Chesney M, Alkon A, Tschann JM, Adams S, Chesterman B, Cohen F, Kaiser P,

Folkman S, Wara D. Psychobiologic reactivity to stress and childhood respiratory illness: Results of two prospective studies. Psychosomatic Medicine. 57: 411–422, 1995.

Bradley LA, Young LD, Anderson KO, Turner RA, Agudelo CA, McDaniel LK, Pisko EJ, Semble EL, Morgan TM. Effects of psychological therapy on pain behavior of rheumatoid arthritis patients: Treatment outcome and six-month follow-up. Arthritis and Rheumatism. 30: 1105–1114, 1987.

Cannon JG, Fiatarone MA, Fielding RA, Evans WJ. Aging and stress induced changes in complement activation and neutrophil mobilization. Journal of Applied Physiology. 76: 2616–2620, 1994.

Cannon WB. Bodily Changes in Pain, Hunger, Fear, Rage. Appleton, New York, 1929.

Capitanio JP, Mendoza SP, Lerche NW, Mason WA. Social stress results in altered glucocorticoid regulation and shorter survival in simian acquired immune deficiency syndrome. Proceedings USA. 95: 4714–4719, 1998.

Carr DJJ, Serou M. Exogenous and endogenous opioids as biological response modifiers. Immunopharmacology. 31: 59–71, 1995.

Cassidy L, Meadows J, Catalan J, Barton S. Are reported stress and coping style associated with frequent recurrence of genital herpes? Genitourinary Medicine. 73: 263–266, 1997.

Chancellor-Freeland C, Zhu GF, Kage R, Beller DI, Leeman SE, Black PH. Substance P and stress-induced changes in macrophages. Annals of the New York Academy of Sciences. 771: 472–84, 1995.

Chervonsky AV, Wang Y, Wong FS, Visintin I, Flavell RA, Janeway CA, Matis LA. The role of Fas in autoimmune diabetes. Cell. 89: 17–24, 1997.

Chikanza IC, Petrou P, Kingsley G, Chrousos G, Panayi GS. Defective hypothalamic response to immune and inflammatory stimuli in patients with rheumatoid arthritis. Arthritis and Rheumatism. 35: 1281–1288, 1992.

Clover RD, Abell T, Becker LA, Crawford S, Ramsey CN Jr. Family functioning and stress as predictors of influenza B infection. Journal of Family Practice. 28: 535–539, 1989.

Cohen S, Tyrrell DAJ, Smith AP. Psychological stress and susceptibility to the common cold. New England Journal of Medicine. 325: 606–612, 1991.

Cohen S, Tyrrell DAJ, Smith AP. Negative life events, perceived stress, negative affect, and susceptibility to the common cold. Journal of Personality and Social Psychology. 64: 131–40, 1993.

Cohen S, Doyle WJ, Skoner DP, Rabin BS, Gwaltney JM. Social ties and susceptibility to the common cold. Journal of the American Medical Association. 277: 1940–1944, 1997a.

Cohen S, Line S, Manuck SB, Rabin BS, Heise ER, Kaplan JR. Chronic social stress, social status, and susceptibility to upper respiratory infections in nonhuman primates. Psychosomatic Medicine. 59: 213–221, 1997b.

Cohen S, Frank E, Doyle WJ, Skoner DP, Rabin BS, Gwaltney JM. Types of stressor that increase susceptibility to the common cold in healthy adults. Health Psychology. 17: 214–223, 1998.

Cole SW, Kemeny ME, Taylor SE, Visscher BR, Fahey JL. Accelerated course of human immunodeficiency virus infection in gay men who conceal their homosexual identity. Psychosomatic Medicine. 58: 219–231, 1996.

Courtney JG, Longnecker MP, Theorell T, Gerhardsson de Verdier M. Stressful life events and the risk of colorectal cancer. Epidemiology. 4: 407–414, 1993.

Cui XC, Vaillant GE. Antecedents and consequences of negative life events in adulthood: A longitudinal study. American Journal of Psychiatry. 153: 21–26, 1996.

Dalkvist J, Wahlin TB, Bartsch E, Forsbeck M. Herpes simplex and mood: A prospective study. Psychosomatic Medicine. 57: 127–37, 1995.

Danno K, Kaji A, Mochizuki T. Alterations in ICAM-1 and ELAM-1 expression in psoriatic lesions following various treatments. Journal of Dermatological Science. 13: 49–55, 1996.

Davidson M, Cho-Chou K, Middaugh JP, Campbell LA, Wang AP, Newmann WP, Finley JC, Grayston JT. Confirmed previous infection with *Chlamydia pneumoniae* (TWAR) and its presence in early coronary atherosclerosis. Circulation. 98: 628–633, 1998.

Dewing SB, Remission of psoriasis associated with cutaneous nerve section. Archives of Dermatology. 104: 220–221, 1971.

Drulovic J, MostaricaStojkovic M, Levic Z, Stojsavljevic N, Pravica V, Mesaros S. Interleukin-12 and tumor necrosis factor-alpha levels in cerebrospinal fluid of multiple sclerosis patients. Journal of Neurological Sciences. 147: 145–150, 1997.

EichHochli D, Niklowitz MW, Luthy R, Opravil M. Are immunological markers, social and personal respurces, or a complaint-free state predictors of progression among HIV-infected patients? Acta Psychiatria Scandinavica. 95: 476–484, 1997.

Erskine-Milliss J, Schonell M. Relaxation therapy in asthma: A critical review. Psychosomatic Medicine. 43: 363–593, 1981.

Evans DL, Leserman J, Perkins DO, Stern RA, Murphy C, Zheng B, Gettes D, Longmate JA, Silva SG, van der Horst CM, Hall CD, Folds JD, Golden RN, Petitto JM. Severe life stress as a predictor of early disease progression in HIV infection. American Journal of Psychiatry. 154: 630–634, 1997.

Farber EM, Lanigan SW, Boer J. The role of cutaneous sensory nerves in the maintenance of psoriasis. International Journal of Dermatology. 29: 418–420, 1990.

Fawzy FI, Cousins N, Fawzy NW, Kemeny ME, Elashoff R, Morton D. A structured psychiatric intervention for cancer patients. I. Changes over time in methods of coping and affective disturbance. Archives of General Psychiatry. 47: 720–725, 1990a.

Fawzy FI, Kemeny ME, Fawzy NW, Elashoff R, Morton D, Cousins N, Fahey JL. A structured psychiatric intervention for cancer patients. II. Changes over time in immunological measures. Archives of General Psychiatry. 47: 729–735, 1990b.

Fawzy FI, Fawzy NW, Hyun CS, Elashoff R, Guthrie D, Fahey JL, Morton D. Effects of an early structured psychiatric intervention, coping and affective state on recurrence and survival 6 years later. Archives of General Psychiatry. 50: 681–690, 1993.

Felten DL, Felten SY, Bellinger DL, Lorton D. Noradrenergic and peptidergic innervation of secondary lymphoid organs: Role in experimental rheumatoid arthritis. European Journal of Clinical Investigation. 22(suppl 1): 37–41, 1992.

Foreman JC, Jordan CC, Oehme P, Renner H. Structure–activity relationships for some substance P-related peptides that cause wheal and flare reactions in human skin. Journal of Physiology. 335: 449–465,1983

Forsen A. Psychosocial stress as a risk for breast cancer. Psychotherapy and Psychosomatics. 55: 176–185, 1991.

Friedman HS, Tucker JS, Schwartz JE, Tomlinson-Keasey C, Martin LR, Wingard DL, Criqui MH. Psychological and behavioral predictors of longevity. The aging and death of the "Termites." American Psychologist. 50: 69–78, 1995.

Gaston L, Crombez JC, Lassonde M, Bernier-Buzzanga J, Hodgins S. Psychological stress and psoriasis: Experimental and prospective correlational studies. Acta Dermato-Venereologica (Stockholm). 156: 37–43, 1991.

Geenen R, Godaert GLR, Jacobs JWG, Peters ML, Bijlsma JWJ. Diminished autonomic nervous system responsiveness in rheumatoid arthritis of recent onset. Journal of Rheumatology. 23: 258–264, 1996.

Ginsberg A, Price S, Ingram D, Nottage E. Life events and the risk of breast cancer: A case-control study. European Journal of Cancer. 32A: 2049–2052, 1996.

Glaser R, Kiecolt-Glaser JK, Stout JC, Tarr KL, Speicher CE, Holliday JE. Stress-related impairments in cellular immunity. Psychiatry Research. 16: 233–239, 1985a.

Glaser R, Kiecolt-Glaser JK, Speicher CE, Holliday JE. Stress, loneliness, and changes in herpesvirus latency. Journal of Behavioral Medicine. 8: 249–260, 1985b.

Glaser R, Pearson GR, Jones JF, Hillhouse J, Kennedy S, Mao HY, Kiecolt-Glaser JK. Stress-related activation of Epstein-Barr virus. Brain, Behavior, and Immunity. 5: 219–232, 1991.

Glaser R, Kiecolt-Glaser JK, Bonneau R, Malarkey W, Hughes J. Stress-induced modulation of the immune response to recombinant hepatitis B vaccine. Psychosomatic Medicine. 54: 22–29, 1992.

Glaser R, Pearl DK, Kiecolt-Glaser JK, Malarkey WB. Plasma cortisol levels and reactivation of latent Epstein-Barr virus in response to examination stress. Psychoneuroendocrinology. 19: 765–772, 1994.

Glaser R, Kutz LA, MacCallum RC, Malarkey WB. Hormonal modulation of Epstein-Barr virus replication. Neuroendocrinology. 62: 356–361, 1995.

Goldmeier D, Johnson A, Jeffries D, Walker GD, Underhill G, Robinson G, Ribbans H. Psychological aspects of recurrences of genital herpes. Journal of Psychosomatic Research. 30: 601–608, 1986.

Goodkin K, Blaney NT, Feaster D, Fletcher MA, Baum MK, Mantero-Atienza E, Klimas NG, Millon C, Szapocznik J, Eisdorfer C. Active coping style is associated with natural killer cell cytotoxicity in asymptomatic HIV-1 seropositive homosexual men. Journal of Psychosomatic Research. 36: 635–650, 1992a.

Goodkin K, Fuchs I, Feaster D, Leeka J, Rishel DD. Life stressors and coping style are associated with immune measures in HIV-1 infection—A preliminary report. International Journal of Psychiatry in Medicine. 22: 155–172, 1992b.

Grant I, Brown GW, Harris T, McDonald WI, Patterson T, Trimble MR. Severely threatening events and marked life difficulties preceding onset or exacerbation of multiple sclerosis. Journal of Neurology, Neurosurgery, and Psychiatry. 52: 8–13, 1989.

Green J, Kocsis A. Psychological factors in recurrent genital herpes. Genitourinary Medicine. 73: 253–258, 1997.

Griffin AC, Lo WD, Wolny AC, Whitacre CC. Suppression of experimental autoimmune encephalomyelitis by restraint stress: Sex differences. Journal of Neuroimmunology. 44: 103–116, 1993.

Gross RL, Newberne PM. Role of nutrition in immunologic function. Physiological Reviews. 60: 188–302, 1980.

Gruber B, Hall N, Hersh S, Dubois P. Immune system and psychologic changes in metastatic cancer patients while using ritualized relaxation and guided imagery. Scandinavian Journal of Behavioral Therapy. 17: 25–46, 1988.

Gupta MA, Gupta AK, Watteel GN. Early onset (<40 years age) psoriasis is comorbid with greater psychopathology than late onset psoriasis: A study of 137 patients. Acta Dermato-Venereologica. 76: 464–466, 1996.

Hagglof B, Blom L, Dahlquist G, Lonnberg G, Sahlin B. The swedish childhood diabetes study: Indications of severe psychological stress as a risk factor for Type I (insulin-dependent) diabetes mellitus in childhood. Diabetologia. 34: 579–583, 1991.

Hallberg H. Life after divorce—A five-year follow-up study of divorced middle-aged men in Sweden. Family Practice. 9: 49–56, 1992.

Hang L, Izui S, Theofilopoulos AN, Dixon FJ. Suppression of transferred BXSB male SLE disease by female spleen cells. Journal of Immunology. 128: 1805–1808, 1982.

Harrington L, Affleck G, Urrows S, Tennen H, Higgins P, Zautra A, Hoffman S. Temporal co-variation of soluble interleukin-2 receptor levels, daily stress, and disease activity in rheumatoid arthritis. Arthritis and Rheumatism. 36: 199–203, 1993.

Harris T, Creed F, Brugha TS. Stressful life events and Graves' disease. British Journal of Psychiatry. 161: 535–541, 1992.

Harvima RJ, Viinamaki H, Harvima IT, Naukkarinen A, Savolainen L, Aalto ML, Horsman-heimo M. Association of psychic stress with clinical severity and symptoms of psoriatic patients. Acta Dermato-Venereologica. 76: 467–471, 1996.

Heiman AS, Newton L. Effect of hydrocortisone and disodium cromogloycate on mast cell mediator release induced by substance P. Pharmacology. 50: 218–228, 1995.

Hilakivi-Clarke L, Rowland J, Clarke R, Lippman ME. Psychosocial factors in the development and progression of breast cancer. Breast Cancer Research and Treatment. 29: 141–160, 1994.

Hinkle LE, Evans FM, Wolf S. Studies in diabetes mellitus. III. Life history of 3 persons with labile diabetes and relationship of significant experiences in their lives to the onset of disease. Psychosomatic Medicine. 13: 160–183, 1951.

Houssiau FA, Devogelaer JP, Van Damme J, de Deuxchaisnes CN, Van Snick J. Interleukin-6 in synovial fluid and serum of patients with rheumatoid arthritis and other inflammatory arthritides. Arthritis and Rheumatism. 31: 784–788, 1988.

Ironson G, Friedman A, Klimas N, Antoni, M, Fletcher MA, LaPerriere A, Simoneau J, Schneiderman N. Distress, denial, and low adherence to behavioral interventions in gay men infected with human imunodeficiency virus. International Journal of Behavioral Medicine. 1: 90–105, 1994.

Johansen C, Olsen JH. Psychological stress, cancer incidence and mortality from non-malignant disease. British Journal of Cancer. 75: 144–148, 1997.

Josko J. Liberation of thyreotropin, thyroxine and triiodothyronine in the controllable and uncontrollable stress and after administration of naloxone in rats. Journal of Physiology and Pharmacology. 47: 303–310, 1996.

Katcher AH, Brightman V, Luborsky L, Ship I. Prediction of the incidence of recurrent herpes labialis and systemic illness from psychological measurements. Journal of Dental Research. 52: 49–58, 1973.

Kemeny ME, Cohen F, Zegans LS, Conant MA. Psychological and immunological predictors of genital herpes recurrence. Psychosomatic Medicine. 51: 195–208, 1989.

Kemeny ME, Weiner H, Taylor SE, Schneider S, Visscher B, Fahey JL. Repeated bereavement, depressed mood, and immune parameters in HIV seropositive and seronegative gay men. Health Psychology. 13: 14–24, 1994.

Kemeny ME, Weiner H, Duran R, Taylor SE, Visscher B, Fahey JL. Immune system changes after the death of a partner in HIV-positive gay men. Psychosomatic Medicine. 57: 547–554, 1995.

Kessler RC, Foster C, Joseph J, Ostrow D, Wortman C, Phair J, Chmiel J. Stressful life events and symptom onset in HIV infection. American Journal of Psychiatry. 148: 733–738, 1991.

Kiecolt-Glaser JK, Kennedy S, Malkoff S, Fisher L, Speicher CE, Glaser R. Marital discord and immunity in males. Psychosomatic Medicine. 50: 213–229, 1988.

Kiecolt-Glaser JK, Glaser R, Gravenstein S, Malarkey W, Sheridan J. Chronic stress alters the immune response to influenza virus vaccine in older adults. Proceedings of the National Academy of Sciences USA. 93: 3043–3047, 1996.

Knieling J, Weiss H, Faller H, Lang H. Psychosocial causal attributions by Myasthenia Gravis patients. A longitudinal study of the significance of subjective illness theories after diagnosis and in follow-up. Psychotherapie, Psychosomatik, Medizinische Psychologie. 45: 373–380, 1995.

Kung AWC. Life events, daily stresses and coping in patients with Graves' disease. Clinical Endocrinology. 42: 303–308, 1995.

Kutemeyer M. Symptom changes during the psychotherapy of patients with myasthenia gravis. Psychotherapy and Psychosomatics. 32: 279–286, 1979.

Leaverton DR, White CA, McCormick CR, Smith P, Sheikholislmm B. Parental loss antecedent to childhood diabetes. Journal of the American Academy of Child Psychiatry. 19: 678–689, 1980.

Lehrer PM, Hochron S, Carr R, Edelberg R, Hamer R, Jackson A, Porges S. Behavioral task-induced bronchodilation in asthma during active and passive tasks: A possible cholinergic link to psychologically induced airway changes. Psychosomatic Medicine. 58: 413–422, 1996.

Lerner BH. Can stress cause disease—Revisiting the tuberculosis research of Holmes, Thomas, 1949–1961. Annals of Internal Medicine. 124: 673–680, 1996.

Leserman J, Petitto JM, Perkins DO, Folds JD, Golden RN, Evans DL. Severe stress, depressive symptoms, and changes in lymphocyte subsets in human imunodeficiency virus infected men—A 2 year follow-up study. Archives of General Psychiatry. 54: 279–285, 1997.

Leung DY, Travers JB, Norris DA, The role of superantigens in skin disease. Journal of Investigative Dermatology. 105(suppl 1): 37S–42S, 1995.

Lotz M, Vaughan JH, Carson DA. Effects of neuropeptides on production of inflammatory cytokines by human monocytes. Science. 241: 1218–1221, 1988.

MacQueen G, Marshall J, Perdue M, Siegel S, Bienenstock J. Pavlovian conditioning of rat mucosal mast cells to secrete rat mast cell protease II. Science. 243: 83–85, 1989.

Manuck SB, Cohen S, Rabin BS, Muldoon MF, Bachen EA. Individual differences in cellular immune response to stress. Psychological Science. 2: 1–5, 1991.

Mariotti S, Sansoni P, Barbesino G, Caturegli P, Monti D, Cossarizza A, Giacomelli T, Passeri G, Fagiolo U, Pinchera A, Franceshi C. Thyroid and other organ-specific autoantibodies in healthy centenarians. Lancet. 339: 1506–1508, 1992.

Markham PD, Salahuddin SZ, Veren K, Orndorff S, Gallo RC. Hydrocortisone and some other hormones enhance the expression of HTLV-III. International Journal of Cancer. 37: 67–72, 1986.

Marti O, Gavalda A, Jolin T, Armario A. Acute stress attenuates but does not abolish circadian rhythmicity of serum thyrotropin and growth hormone in the rat. European Journal of Endocrinology. 135: 703–708, 1996.

Menzies R, Phelps C, Wiranowska M, Oliver J, Chen L, Horvath E, Hall N. The effect of interferon-alpha on the pituitary–adrenal axis. Journal of Interferon and Cytokine Research. 16: 619–629, 1996.

Meridith PJ, Kristie JA, Walford RL. Aging increases expression of LPS-induced autoantibody secreting B cells. Journal of Immunology. 123: 87–91, 1979.

Moynihan JA, Karp JD, Cohen N, Cocke R. Alterations in interleukin-4 and antibody production following pheromone exposure: Role of glucocorticoids. Journal of Neuroimmunology. 54: 51–58, 1996.

Murasko DM, Weiner P, Kaye D. Association of lack of mitogen-induced lymphocyte proliferation with increased mortality in the elderly. Aging: Immunology and Infectious Disease. 1: 1–6, 1988.

Nalesnik MA, Starzl TE. Epstein-Barr virus, infectious mononucleosis, and posttransplant lymphoproliferative disorders. Transplantation Science. 4: 61–79, 1994.

Nisipeanu P, Korczyn AD. Psychological stress as a risk factor for exacerbations in multiple sclerosis. Neurology. 43: 1311–1312, 1993.

Oro AS, Guarino TJ, Driver R, Steinman L, Umetsu DT. Regulation of disease susceptibility: Decreased prevalence of IgE mediated allergic disease in patients with multiple sclerosis. Journal of Allergy and Clinical Immunology. 97: 1402–1408, 1996.

Panitch HS, Hirsch RL, Schindler J, Johnson JP. Treatment of multiple sclerosis with gamma-interferon: Exacerbations with activation of the immune system. Neurology. 37: 97–102, 1987.

Parker JC, Smarr KL, Walker SE, Hagglund KJ, Anderson SK, Hewett JE, Bridges AJ, Caldwell CW. Biopsychosocial parameters of disease activity in rheumatoid arthritis. Arthritis Care and Research. 4: 73–80, 1991.

Payan DG, Brewster DR, Goetzl EJ. Specific stimulation of human T lymphocytes by substance P. Journal of Immunology. 13: 1613–1615, 1983.

Payan DG, Brewster DR, Missirian-Bastian A, Goetzl EJ. Substance P recognition by a subset of human T lymphocytes. Journal of Clinical Investigation. 74: 1532–1539, 1984.

Perry S, Fishman B, Jacobsberg L, Frances A. Relationships over 1 year between lymphocyte subsets and psychosocial variables among adults with infection by human immunodeficiency virus. Archives of General Psychiatry. 49: 396–401, 1992.

Polenghi M, Gals C, Citeri A, Manca G, Guzzi R, Barcella M, Finzi A. Psychoneurophysiological implications in the pathogenesis and treatment of psoriasis. Acta Dermato-Venereologica (Stockholm). 146: 84–86, 1989.

Pratt RTC. An investigation of the psychiatric aspects of disseminated sclerosis. Journal of Neurology, Neurosurgery, and Psychiatry. 14: 326–336, 1951.

Rabkin JG, Williams JB, Remien RH, Goetz R, Kertzner R, Gorman JM. Depression, distress, lymphocyte subsets, and human immunodeficiency virus symptoms on two occasions in HIV-positive homosexual men. Archives of General Psychiatry. 48: 111–119, 1991.

Radis CD. Effects of cyclophosphamide on the development of malignancy and on long-term survival of patients with rheumatoid arthritis—A 20 year followup study. Arthritis and Rheumatism. 38: 11–20, 1995.

Reed GM, Kemeny ME, Taylor SE, Wang HY, Visscher BR. Realistic acceptance as a predictor of decreased survival time in gay men with AIDS. Health Psychology. 13: 299–307, 1994.

Reist C, Kauffmann CD, Chicz-Demet A, Chen CC, Demet EM. REM latency, dexamethasone suppression test, and thyroid releasing hormone stimulation test in posttraumatic stress disorder. Progress in Neuro-Psychopharmacology and Biological Psychiatry. 19: 433–443, 1995.

Rimon R, Laakso R. Life stress with rheumatoid arthritis: A 15 year follow-up study. Psychotherapy and Psychosomatics. 43: 38–43, 1985.

Roberts FD, Newcomb PA, Trentham-Dietz A, Storer BE. Self-reported stress and risk of breast cancer. Cancer. 77: 1089–1093, 1996.

Rogers MP, Trentham DE, McCune WJ, Ginsberg BI, Rennke HG, Reich P, David JR. Effect of psychological stress on the induction of arthritis in rats. Arthritis and Rheumatism. 23: 1337–1342, 1980.

Roghmann KJ, Haggerty RJ. Daily stress, illness, and use of health services in young families. Pediatric Research. 7: 520–526, 1973.

Rosch PJ. Stress and Graves' disease. Lancet. 339: 577–578, 1974.

Russek LG, Schwartz G. Narative descriptions of parental love and caring predict health status in midlife: A 35-year follow-up of the Harvard Mastery of Stress Study. Alternative Therapies in Health and Medicine. 2: 55–62, 1996.

Santoni G, Perfumi M, Bressan AM, Piccoli M. Capsaicin-induced inhibition of mitogen and interleukin-2-stimulated T cell proliferation: Its reversal by in vivo substance P administration. Journal of Neuroimmunology. 68: 131–138, 1996.

Sardessai SR, Abraham ME, Mascarenhas JF. Effect of stress on organ weights in rats. Indian Journal of Physiology and Pharmacology. 37: 104–108, 1993.

Schmader K, Studenski S, MacMillan J, Grufferman S, Cohen HJ. Are stressful life events risk factors for Herpes zoster. Journal of the American Geriatric Society. 38: 1188–1194, 1990.

Schmidt DD, Zyzanski S, Ellner J, Kumar ML, Arno J. Stress as a precipitating factor in subjects with recurrent herpes labialis. Journal of Family Practice. 20: 359–66, 1985.

Selye H. A syndrome produced by diverse nocuous agents. Nature. 138: 32, 1936.

Servatius RJ, Ottenweller JE, Natelson BH. A comparison of the effects of repeated stressor exposures and corticosterone injections on plasma cholesterol, thyroid hormones and corticosterone levels in rats. Life Sciences. 55: 1611–1617, 1994.

Silver PS, Auerbach SM, Vishniavsky N, Kaplowitz LG. Psychological factors in recurrent genital herpes infection: Stress, coping style, social support, emotional dysfunction, and symptom recurrence. Journal of Psychosomatic Research. 30: 163–171, 1986.

Sonnenfeld G, Cunnick JE, Armfield AV, Wood PG, Rabin BS. Stress induced alterations in interferon production and class II MHC histocompatibility antigen expression. Brain, Behavior, and Immunity. 6: 170–178, 1992.

Sonono N, Girelli ME, Boscaro M, Fallo F, Busnardo B, Fava GA. Life events in the pathogenesis of Graves' disease. A controlled study. Acta Endocrinologica. 128: 293–296, 1993.

Spiegel D, Bloom JR, Kraemer HC, Gottheil E. Effect of psychosocial treatment on survival of patients with metastatic breast cancer. Lancet 2: 888–891, 1989.

Stein SP, Charles ES. Emotional factors in juvenile diabetes mellitus: A study of early life experience of adolescent diabetes. American Journal of Psychology. 128: 700–704, 1971.

Sternberg EM. Neuroendocrine factors in susceptibility to inflammatory disease: Focus on the hypothalamic–pituitary–adrenal axis. Hormone Research. 43: 159–161, 1995.

Stewart MW, Knight RG, Palmer DG, Highton J. Differential relationships between stress and disease activity for immunologically distinct subgroups of people with rheumatoid arthritis. Journal of Abnormal Psychology. 103: 251–258, 1994.

Stip E, Truelle JL. Organic personality syndrome in multiple sclerosis and effect of stress on recurrent attacks. Canadian Journal of Psychiatry. 39: 27–33, 1994.

Stone A, Reed B, Neale J. Changes in daily events frequency precede episodes of physical symptoms. Journal of Human Stress. 13: 70–74, 1987.

Stone AA, Bovbjerg DH, Neale JM, Napoli A, Valdimarsdottir H, Cox D, Hayden F, Gwlatney

J. Development of common cold symptoms following experimental rhinovirus infection is related to prior stressful life events. Behavioral Medicine. 18: 115–120, 1992.

Stone A, Porter L, Neale J. Daily events and mood prior to the onset of respiratory illness episodes: A non-replication of the 3–5 day 'desirability dip'. British Journal of Medical Psychology. 66: 383–393, 1993.

Thernlund GM, Dahlquist G, Hansson K, Ivarsson SA, Ludvigsson J, Sjoblad S, Hagglof B. Psychological stress and the onset of IDDM in children—A case control study. Diabetes Care. 18: 1323–1329, 1995.

Treuting TF. The role of emotional factors in the aetiology and course of diabetes mellitus: A review of the recent literature. American Journal of Medical Science. 244: 131–147, 1962.

Turakulov I, Burikhanov RB, Patkhitdinov PP, Myslitskaia AI. Effect of immobilization stress on the level of thyroid hormone secretion. Problemy Endokrinologii. 39: 47–48, 1993.

Turner Cobb JM, Steptoe A. Psychosocial stress and susceptibility to upper respiratory tract illness in an adult population sample. Psychosomatic Medicine. 58: 404–412, 1996.

Valdimarsson H, Sigmundsdottir H, Jonsdottir I. Is psoriasis induced by streptococcal super-antigens and maintained by M-protein-specific T cells that cross-react with keratin? Clinical and Experimental Immunology. 107(suppl 1): 21–24, 1997.

VanderPlate C, Aral SO, Magder L. The relationship among genital herpes simplex virus, stress, and social support. Health Psychology. 7: 159–68, 1988.

Volpe R. Suppressor T lymphocyte dysfunction is important in the pathogenesis of autoimmune thyroid disease—A perspective. Thyroid. 3: 345–352, 1993.

Wallengren J, Ekman R, Sundler F. Occurrence and distribution of neuropeptides in the human skin. Acta Dermato-Venereologica. 67: 185–92, 1987.

Warren S, Greenhill S, Warren KG. Emotional stress and the development of multiple sclerosis: Case control evidence of a relationship. Journal of Chronic Diseases. 35: 821–831, 1982.

Winchell SA, Watts RA. Relaxation therapies in the treatment of psoriasis and possible psychologic mechanisms. Journal of the American Academy of Dermatology. 18: 101–104, 1988.

Winsa B, Adami HO, Bergstrom R, Gamstedt A, Dahlberg PA, Adamson U, Jansson R, Karlsson A. Stressful life events and Graves' disease. Lancet. 338: 1475–1479, 1991.

Wu JG, Wilson J, He J, Xiang LB, Schur PH, Mountz JD. Fas ligand mutation in a patient with systemic lupus erythematosus and lymphoproliferative disease. Journal of Clinical Investigation. 98: 1107–1113, 1996.

Yoshikawa N, Morita T, Resetkova E, Arreanza G, Carayon P, Volpe R. Reduced activation of suppressor T lymphocytes by specific antigens in autoimmune thyroid disease. Journal of Edocrinological Investigation. 16: 609–617, 1993.

Yoshiuchi K, Kumano H, Nomura S, Yoshimura H, Ito K, Kanaji Y, Ohashi Y, Kuboki T, Suematsu H. Stressful life events and smoking were associated with Graves' disease in women, but not in men. Psychosomatic Medicine. 60: 182–185, 1998.

Young LD. Rheumatoid arthritis. In Psychophysiological Disorders. Gatchel RJ, Blanchard EB (eds). American Psychological Association, Washington, DC, 1993, p 269.

Zachariae R, Oster H, Bjerring P, Kragballe K. Effects of psychologic intervention on psoriasis: A preliminary report. Journal of the American Academy of Dermatology. 34: 1008–1015, 1996.

Zhu GF, Chancellor-Freeland C, Berman AS, Kage R, Leeman SE, Beller DI, Black PH. Endogenous substance P mediates cold water stress-induced increase in interleukin-6 secretion from peritoneal macrophages. Journal of Neuroscience. 16: 3745–3752, 1996.

7

Behaviors That Can Be Used to Buffer the Detrimental Effects of Stress on the Immune System and Health

Can a Stress-Resistant Brain Be Engineered?

Is the stressor-induced increase in the plasma and tissue concentrations of hormones that modify immune function an all-or-none phenomenon, or are buffers used by the brain to ameliorate stress-induced hormonal elevations?

It is likely that the negative effects of stress on the quality of health can be ameliorated by adopting stress-buffering behaviors. This would be easier than trying to eliminate the sources of stress in ones life. The ability to develop coping skills to buffer the effect of stress on health is important, as demonstrated by the lack of control of ones work environment in association with increased morbidity (Marmot et al, 1991).

The concept developed in this chapter is that stressor-induced alteration of the hormonal milieu of plasma can be modulated by the behavioral characteristics of an individual. It is not exclusively the characteristics of the stressor that are of importance in determining the hormonal alterations, but rather it is how the stressor is perceived by the brain and the availability of coping skills that will influence how the stress will alter the hormonal milieu in which the immune system resides.

Physiologic alterations that influence the quality of health may be influenced by numerous circumstances in an individual's life. An area that has received attention is satisfaction with one's job and how high up on the hierarchy one is at work (Marmot et al, 1997). As individuals with low job grades, but with stable employment, are at increased risk of cardiovascular disease, it is suggested that their physiological response to frustrating circumstances in the conditions of their employment elicit either behaviors (smoking, alcohol use) or a hormonal response that effects health. In fact, increased mortality was found to be associated with a lower grade of employment (Marmot et al, 1984).

Studies of health and employment status suggest that low control of the work environment may be more of a risk factor to inducing psychological changes that affect health than is working hard. Not having control of the workplace may be the same as being highly controlled. If you don't have control, someone else does. Being highly controlled may be stressful for many individuals, especially talented individuals who are not given the opportunity to make a contribution to their work environment. A relationship suggesting ties between psychology and physiology is found in increased susceptibility to diseases such as asthma, allergies, and autoimmune diseases in subjects with depression (Vogt et al, 1994).

The baseline physiology in an individual while experiencing a stressor will influence the physiological alterations that are induced. For example, an acute stressor may not produce the same changes in an individual who is experiencing chronic stress as compared with an individual who is not experiencing chronic stress (Pike et al, 1997). Early life experiences may modify an individual's later life hormonal response to stress (see Chapter 8). Clearly, it is not just experiencing an acute stressor that influences the central nervous system (CNS) and hormonal response as the background on which the acute stressor is applied contributes to the characteristics of the response.

If the effect of stress on the production of hormones that modify physiological processes differs in the brains of different individuals, consideration should be directed toward creating a brain with qualities that will be the least stimulated by a stressor. This may involve the development of skills that provide coping capabilities to minimize the effect of stress on altering physiological parameters.

Whether the functional alterations of the immune system produced by stress-induced hormonal alterations are minimal or extensive is not well defined. However, as previously indicated, the immune alterations are not so extensive that the in vitro or in vivo measurement of immune function produces abnormal results.

In this chapter, we will consider behaviors that may attenuate a stressor from altering the immune system in a manner that is detrimental to health. There are individuals who easily participate in behaviors that help minimize stress effects on health. Examples include social interactions and regular exercise. Other individuals do not comfortably engage in stress-buffering behaviors. Do individuals who engage in behaviors that minimize stressor-induced immune alterations have such behaviors because of a specific brain chemistry? Is that particular brain chemistry associated with stress being unable to produce high concentrations of immune altering hormones? Is there a linkage between the brain chemistry associated with increased skills at socialization with a brain chemistry that ameliorates stress from producing immune changes?

Will better health be achieved if behaviors can be adopted that ameliorate the effects of stress on activating hormonal changes that alter immune changes? A tough question. There are two answers—one relating to a specific individual, and one to a population:

1. No! It is unrealistic to tell a specific individual that if they were to adopt stress-buffering behaviors they will healthier because of better immune function. At this time, there is no way to predict how a specific individual will be affected.

2. Yes! It is realistic to predict that the adoption of stress-buffering behaviors will have a beneficial effect on the health of a large population of individuals. However, within that population, it cannot be predicted which individuals will benefit.

If the assumption can be made that the characteristics of an individual's work environment (especially the amount of stress present), the amount of control one has over the characteristics of their work environment, and the coping resources that are available can have an effect on health, a relationship between the environment outside of an individual's body and within their body is evident. The brain connects the outside world with the inside world. One has to wonder whether a chaotic, unsatisfactory, depressing, work environment outside the body creates a chaotic state in the hormonal milieu within the body.

The brain may mirror the outside world and may bring an exact image to the inside. Chaos outside may be mirrored as chaos inside. However, the brain may act as a filter that alters the impact of the characteristics of the outside environment so that the alteration of the internal hormonal milieu is less or greater than the alteration that would be induced if there were no intervention of the brain. The brain is the buffer between the outside world and the inside hormonal milieu. Whether environmental factors such as social support, physical fitness, a sense of humor, and (Sergerstrom et al, 1998) optimism can contribute to the ability of the brain to filter the outside world from hormonal milieu in the body is certainly speculative. However, there does appear to be a basis for making the assumption that there are behaviors that can add to the buffering capacities of the brain.

An example of being able to have an influence on the quality of one's own life has been demonstrated in older individuals. Older individuals with lower capabilities of caring for themselves show a more rapid functional decline than do individuals with higher self-care capabilities (Mendes et al, 1996). It was also found that in older individuals, social interactions and participating in an active regimen of exercise were associated with better physical capabilities of gait, lower body strength, coordination, and manual dexterity (Seeman et al, 1995).

Interestingly, simply believing that one is in good health, regardless of the actual state of health, may be capable of positively influencing longevity (Schoenfeld et al, 1994). Individuals who self-rate their health as poor are more likely to live a shorter period of time than are individuals who do not have a self-perception of poor health.

It may be possible that individuals with medically defined diseases would live longer if they believed that they had a chance to live a long life rather than a short life in poor health (Mossey and Shapiro, 1982). The belief in self-rated good health may affect the hormonal milieu of plasma in a beneficial way or promote other health-enhancing behaviors. If a person does not believe that they will be healthy, they may promote a hormonal milieu and behaviors that do not promote optimal physiologic function (Idler and Kasl, 1991). It is also possible that knowledge of a family history of short life duration and chronic illness will motivate self-ratings of poor health. If that belief contributes to a hormonal milieu that is associated with suboptimal immune function, a self-fulfilling prophecy may ensue.

SOCIAL INTERACTIONS

There have been consistent indications that social interactions have a positive effect on reducing morbidity and mortality (Cassel, 1976; Cobb, 1976; Berkman and Syme; Smith et al, 1994; Seeman et al, 1993; Berkman, 1995). Even the perception of receiving emotional support through social interactions may be an important contributing factor to the reduction of mortality (Penninx et al, 1997). Although a loss of social ties contributes to an increased rate of mortality, sustained low levels of social ties have a stronger association with mortality (Cerhan and Wallace, 1997) than does the loss of social ties.

Individuals who engage in social interactions through marriage, close friends, religious beliefs, and group associations have lower mortality rates than those of individuals without such interactions (Berkman and Syme, 1979; Schoenbach et al, 1986). The perception of social support may actually be more important than actual social support (Blazer, 1982). The importance of perception may indicate that a positive perception of the environment can influence the mind to influence the hormonal milieu of the body.

Health-promoting effects of social interaction are reported for divorced men who reentered a stable relationship or who had custody of their children. They had fewer health problems than did divorced men who lived alone (House et al, 1988; Hallberg, 1992).

Aspects of social support that promote better health by activating pathways in the brain that provide a hormonal milieu in plasma that optimizes physiological function may be those that provide feelings of self-respect, desirability, or competency. The effect of these emotional states on suppressing the stress hormone-producing areas of the brain may contribute to immunological functions that enhance good health.

A relationship between aspects of the social network and the mortality of women aged 65–74 and greater than 75 years was investigated. Women in the older group who had no contact with children, friends, or group activities had greater mortality than that of those who used these resources. No influence of social contact was noted for women in the younger group. Thus, there may be an age associated influence on social interactions and mortality (Yasuda et al, 1997) with the loneliness that may occur with advanced age being more significant in producing detrimental physiological responses.

A relationship between negative life events (events perceived by the subject as being undesirable), health, and social support has been found. The association of negative life events with illness is strongest in individuals with lower levels of social support (Sarason et al, 1985).

Negative life events may:

Activate pathways in the brain that alter the hormonal milieu in which the immune systems resides and suppress immune function

Prevent buffering skills from ameliorating stress effects on hormonal alterations

Alter nutrition or sleep habits

Increase the use of alcohol, tobacco, or nonprescription drugs.

Obviously, the effect of negative life events on increasing susceptibility to illness is important to health.

The perception one has of being loved and cared about by one's parents (one of our earliest social relationships) has been found to have an influence on disease susceptibility (Russek and Schwartz, 1997). It was found that 87% of adult subjects who rated both parents as being low in parental caring had diagnosed medical problems, including cardiovascular disease, hypertension, ulcers, and alcoholism, while only 25% of the subjects who perceived their parents as having high levels of caring, had these diseases. Low caring was associated with infrequent use of descriptions such as loving, friendly, warm, open, understanding, sympathetic, and just.

Why the perception of parental caring is capable of modifying health remains an unanswered question. Whether individuals who grow up feeling loved and cared about follow better health practices, including those related to exercise, diet, and routine medical care, is undetermined. A mental state created by early perceptions of being cared about may induce the development of happier emotions with more optimism and humor and may promote a desire for social interactions with others. Certainly, experiencing positive emotional interactions with one's parent(s) could serve as a role model for similar interactions during adolescence and adult life. Relationships between parents and children may have a significant impact on physical health, and the joke related to blaming the mother for one's emotional problems needs to be extended to health problems.

Children whose parents divorced before their 21st birthday have a decreased life span, as compared with those of parents who did not divorce. For males the predicted age of death was 76 vs 80 years, and for females 82 vs 86 years (Schwartz et al, 1995; Friedman et al, 1995). It is possible that in some individuals early life emotional impact of parental divorce can influence health, possibly by long-term modification of the production of stress-related hormones or promoting behaviors that are detrimental to health. Thus, the social environment that one experiences during adolescence can influence one's longevity.

A number of interesting studies reflect on the beneficial influence of social interactions in individuals who have experienced a stroke or a myocardial infarction. Although it has not been established that these diseases have an immunological component to them, the data contribute to the important influence of social interactions on health. After an initial stroke more rapid recovery and better post-stroke function is present in subjects with more social support (Glass et al, 1993; Reifman, 1995). Having interactions with family members, friends, religious organizations, and community activities reduced the extent of functional impairment after a stroke (Colantonio et al, 1993).

A consideration that may influence the relationship between social interactions and morbidity and mortality is that individuals with medical illness may have less social interactions because of their illness (Welin et al, 1985). Thus, there may be a bias in the data indicating that less social interaction predisposes to illness, if illness, or even the perception of illness, decreases an individual's involvement in social interactions.

A possible difference in males and females in regard to an effect of social interactions has also been suggested, with men receiving greater benefit with regard to mortality (House et al, 1982). However, not all studies have found a gender effect and clarification is needed (Seeman et al, 1993).

Obviously, some individuals are more comfortable than others in social situations. Your own experience with others supports the existence of different levels of ease and comfort interactions with different social contacts. This may be a reflection of the attribute called "personality." Factors that contribute to this aspect of behavior likely include how external events and people are perceived by the brain and how comfortable or uncomfortable the brain makes an individual feel in social interactions. As the brain must be the primary organ that determines personality, and the brain modulates immune function, it would not be surprising to find correlations between personality characteristics and disease.

Indeed, characteristics of personality have been associated with predisposition to different types of disease (Scheier et al, 1995). Personality characteristics were grouped into four clusters, and the effect of each on disease was evaluated:

1. Expression of anger and hostility—individuals who have high levels of hostility have an increased risk of developing cardiovascular heart disease
2. Emotional suppression—associated with increased risk of cancer
3. Depression and depressed affect—there is an increased risk of death after a myocardial infarction in depressed patients, in comparison with nondepressed patients
4. Pessimistic (the tendency to expect negative outcomes in the future) or fatalistic attitude (the belief that outcomes are predetermined)—such individuals have an influence on survival in patients with AIDS, cancer, and cardiovascular disease

An association between personality characteristics and the hormonal response to stress has been reported (Kirschbaum et al, 1995). Healthy male subjects were exposed to the same psychological stressor on each of 5 days. Two different response patterns were detected. One pattern was a lower cortisol response on day 2, in comparison with day 1, with no further decline of cortisol on subsequent days. The other pattern was a stressor induced elevation of cortisol on each of the 5 days. Interestingly, the two groups had different personality characteristics. The group that had daily cortisol elevations to the same stressor had the personality characteristics of low self-esteem, negative self-concept, depressed mood, and more health problems. The categories of health problems in each group would be of interest.

Why may different personality characteristics be associated with different categories of disease? Do hormonal patterns in plasma differ with personality and predispose to different diseases? Do behaviors associated with different personalities predispose to different diseases? Do different personalities have different stress-buffering capabilities? Obviously, this is a fascinating area of research. If biochemical, hormonal, immune, and physiological responses are related to the characteristics of an individual's personality (Kirschbaum et al, 1995), it is not surprising that different personalities have different responses to stress and different health consequences of their response. Whether a change of socialization skills and frequency of time spent in personally meaningful social activities interact with personality characteristics to inhibit disease and mortality would be of significant interest to public health and preventive medicine.

How Can Social Support Improve Health?

In regard to the effect of social support on immune function, the important point is probably that social support is capable of producing a hormonal milieu that promotes the effective function (resistance to infectious disease) of the immune system. Whether social support achieves its benefit by providing a feeling of happiness, being cared about and respected, not feeling lonely, or merely allowing an individual to cite a list of acquaintances is irrelevant. What is essential is that the individual perceive the unique characteristics of their social support system as meaningful to them. Thus, it is likely that different types of social support will be beneficial for different subjects.

It is not the actual characteristics of the support that is available; rather, it is how the subject perceives the support. Can the perception of social support and activities that are considered meaningful to an individual influence the hormonal composition of plasma and immune function? Is it as trivial as a happy perception produces happy hormones that produce a happy immune system that produces good health?

Social support may work because it promotes an alteration of hormones that enhance beneficial physiologic processes. However, social support may also promote other beneficial health practices, such as:

Earlier seeking out of appropriate medical treatment

Involvement in a program of exercise

Less use of alcohol and cigarettes

A better diet

A better sleep pattern

Studies in nonhuman primates have indicated the possibility that there are aspects of social relationships (eg, stable or unstable) that can influence physiologic processes. Lower resting plasma cortisol levels are characteristic of dominant male baboons who are in a stable social environment (Sapolsky, 1989). This, of course, indicates that there are higher resting cortisol levels in subordinate baboons. However, nonhuman male primates who are dominant and in an unstable social environment have higher adrenocorticotropic hormone (ACTH) and cortisol and increased sympathetic nervous system activity (Sapolsky, 1983; Kaplan et al, 1991a). A relevant question is whether those animals with low resting cortisol levels in stable social environments are dominant because the physiologic processes within the brain that regulate cortisol production also influence personality.

Can an individual's social environment influence physiological processes in the brain? A study performed on fish tries to answer this question and suggests that neuroanatomical changes can be induced by the local environment of a fish. However, the implications of this study should be interpreted with caution until similar studies are performed in mammals.

Fish were studied that were either dominant males in a territory of nondominant males (Francis et al, 1993). Gonadotropin-releasing hormone (GnRH) neurons in the preoptic area (POA) of the ventral hypothalamus were significantly larger in the territorial males that dominate the nonterritorial males. When conditions were modified so that the nonterritorial males became territorial, the size of the GnRH neurons in the POA increased to the same size as the territorial males. This finding suggests that the experimentally induced change in the social status of the fish is reflected in a change in the size of a population of neurons in the brain. Although a mechanism for the change in neuronal size is not defined, the data indicate that the environment is capable of inducing physiological and neuroanatomical alterations. It would be of immense interest to know whether, in selected areas of the human brain, individuals with social support have different-size neuron and numbers of neurons as compared with the size of neurons among subjects who lack social support.

Plasma hormonal differences in subjects with different levels of social support have been found in humans. Males with more frequent high levels of social support had lower levels of urinary cortisol, epinephrine, and norepinephrine than did individuals who had less frequent social support. Note that lower concentrations of hormones are associated with enhanced immune function. The effect was not found in females (Kemp and Hatmaker, 1989; Seeman et al, 1994). The interaction of the social environment that one is a part of and the effect of the social environment on physiological characteristics is therefore suggested (Seeman and McEwen, 1996).

Subjects who were given a stress-eliciting task to perform had less heart rate elevation and blood pressure elevation when a friend was present, as compared with subjects who performed the task without the presence of a friend (Kamarck et al, 1990). It is unknown how the benefit of a friend's presence is able to buffer the effects of a stressor on cardiovascular reactivity. However, the presence of a stranger is not as effective as having a friend present in buffering cardiovascular reactivity to a stressor (Christenfeld et al, 1997). This suggests that there must be an element of familiarity or comfort associated with the presence of the other person. It is not merely the presence of a warm body. This is not surprising. We select other individuals for friendship based on some aspect of CNS activity that promotes pleasure with the sharing of events and activities with the other person. It is possible that pheromones contribute to how we perceive someone. We generally do not become friends with someone whom we find annoying. The study conducted by Kamarck et al (1990) suggests that those elements within the brain that are activated and that motivate the desire for friendship are capable of buffering stress effects on physiological reactivity. These apparently are not activated by someone with whom there is no emotional or comfort feelings.

As discussed in Chapter 2, the lack of an immune response to antigens of an individuals own body is called "tolerance." However, the absence of an immune response is not a passive process. It is an active process that requires complex immunological interactions. By analogy, it is possible that the lack of a physiological response to a stressor is a very active process, requiring significant activity within the CNS. If this is a valid assumption, the critical question becomes whether an individual can develop the CNS functions that will prevent stressor-induced immune alteration.

The concept is comparable to a train track extending from point A to point B. The train can go directly along the track. However, over time, spurs may be built along the track, allowing the train to take a more meandering course, possibly never getting to its original destination. More to the point of this analogy, the development of spurs may allow other trains to get onto the main track, preventing the original train from reaching its destination. Can the brain develop the means of preventing stress signals from reaching an area of the brain where they will induce detrimental physiological change? As an example of activities that can affect CNS function and susceptibility to disease, having at least six social ties is associated with a decreased risk of becoming infected upon deliberate exposure to an influenza virus (Cohen et al, 1997).

What are some possible pathways that may be involved in social support decreasing susceptibility to infection?

1. The presence of friends or the knowledge that one has a social support system may activate areas of brain (let's call them friendship perception areas [FPA]) that inhibit stressor-induced activation of the HPA axis or the sympathetic nervous system (SNS). The inhibitory pathways may be complex, going through several synapses, or possibly directly connected to stress hormone-eliciting areas such as the locus coeruleus or hypothalamus.
2. The FPAs of the brain are the same as some of the areas of the brain that are involved in activation of the HPA axis or the SNS, or both. Repeated activation of these areas by the perception of social support contributes to habituating them to activation, leading to the need for increased intensity of input for their activation.

Social Support and Immune Function

The effect of companionship on immune function has been studied in nonhuman primates. In one study, 10 juvenile monkeys were separated from groups of monkeys they were living with and combined into a new group of 10 (Gust et al, 1996). Some of the monkeys were separated from other monkeys of the original group, while others were brought into the new group of 10 along with another monkey from their original group. Control monkeys were left with their original group. In comparison with the monkeys left undisturbed, the monkeys transferred to the new group of 10 exhibited significant suppression of circulating CD4 lymphocyte numbers. Those monkeys transferred alone, without another monkey from their group, had significantly greater CD4 suppression than did the monkeys transferred along with another monkey. One week after formation of the group of 10, the monkeys transferred alone had significantly higher concentrations of cortisol than did the monkeys transferred with another monkey. Thus, this study provides information that companions may modulate stressor-induced hormonal and immune alterations.

In another study, juvenile monkeys were separated from their mothers but remained with peers or were separated and remained alone (Boccia et al, 1997). The monkeys that were separated without friends showed more depression and suppression of in vitro lymphocyte function as compared with those that were separated but that retained the presence of a peer.

Our research group found that when monkeys were stressed by living in an unstable housing condition, the lymphocytes of monkeys that had the characteristic of affiliating with other monkeys had greater responsiveness to nonspecific mitogenic stimulation than did lymphocytes from monkeys that did not affiliate with other monkeys (Kaplan et al, 1991b). However, affiliation was only important as a modifier of lymphocyte function in monkeys that were low in aggressive characteristics. Interestingly, natural killer (NK) cell activity was highest in affiliative monkeys, regardless of whether they were aggressive. Hormone measurements were not performed. However, the data raise the question of whether the personality characteristics of affiliation and aggression can influence the effect of stress on immune function. Similar findings have been reported by others (Laudenslager and Boccia, 1996). Studies of stressor-induced immune alteration often do not take these behavioral characteristics into consideration as modulators of the impact of components of the environment on activities of the brain.

Studies in humans have found that social support can modulate immune function. Current and former caregivers to a spouse with Alzheimer's disease were studied for the function of their NK cells (Esterling et al, 1996). Although NK function was decreased in the caregivers in comparison to non caregiving controls, not all caregivers had equally suppressed NK function. Those subjects with more social support had greater NK function than did subjects without social support.

Differences in immune function and health were studied in separated or divorced men and matched married controls (Kiecolt-Glaser et al, 1988). The married controls had fewer reported episodes of illness and produced significantly more antibody in response to immunization with antigen. A similar beneficial effect of social support was found in individuals who cared for a spouse with Alzheimer's disease (Kiecolt-Glaser et al, 1987) and in medical students at a time of stress (Glaser et al, 1985).

Thus, it is possible that socialization skills are a useful stress-buffering tool. However, this may not be totally correct. Socialization may only be effective in those individuals who want to have increased social contacts but do not have them. These may be the individuals who, when they do have social interactions, will benefit by a reduction of the magnitude of stressor-induced immune alteration. Individuals who do not want to have social interactions may, in fact, not benefit if told that they should have these interactions. Indeed, this may actually be harmful to them, as it may increase the activation of the stress-responsive areas of the brain.

The one study done in fish would suggest that a change in the environment can induce changes within the brain. Supporting data need to be obtained from human studies. No study reported in humans or nonhuman primates indicates that environment can change neuroanatomy. Rather, the data can be interpreted to suggest that there are fixed CNS differences in different humans and that these differences are associated with the development of socialization skills or the lack of socialization skills, and less immune alteration is induced by stress in those subjects with the CNS capacity for more socialization.

BELIEF SYSTEMS

Although social support has not been found to have a mechanism associated with it that can be determined to be responsible for less stressor-induced alteration of (1) HPA axis and SNS activation, and (2) immune function, it is well established that social support does have a beneficial role in the maintenance of better-quality health. Another activity (if being involved in social support can be called an activity) that has been found to have a beneficial effect on health and may function as a buffer that prevents stress from altering the immune system is religious beliefs.

Certainly, when faced with a catastrophic illness that may be associated with a high risk of mortality or that may leave an individual in a chronic debilitated state, it is not unusual for individuals to turn to prayer. There is little question that the practice of religious principles and belief in the teachings of a religion can have a beneficial health influence, although many of the beneficial effects may be due to an influence on life style.

Not all studies have found an increase of longevity and health with increased religious participation (Blaser and Palmore, 1976; Simons and West, 1985). However, an increased feeling of happiness and a feeling of usefulness was associated with religious beliefs.

Positive examples include the following:

1. There is decreased atherosclerotic heart disease, emphysema, and cirrhosis of the liver in individuals who regularly attend church services (Comstock and Partridge, 1972). These beneficial health effects may have been due to church goers having a better diet, better sleep patterns, and more concern about seeking medical care. Regardless of the reason, church attendance had a beneficial health effect. Blood pressure can also be modified by religious beliefs (Levin and Vanderpool, 1989).

2. Mortality has been found to be significantly lower for those who regularly attend religious services in comparison with those who do not (Levin, 1994;

Strawbridge et al, 1997). There was a stronger association in females than in males. Interestingly, those who were more active in their attendance at religious services followed better health-promoting behaviors and had more social interactions and stable marriages. These are obvious behaviors that are capable of contributing to good health. However, not all studies have found a relationship between the frequency of church attendance and social support, even when there was a relationship between church attendance and health (Koenig et al, 1997a). Possibly, church attendance fulfilled all the health-promoting CNS functions that are provided through social support.

A study of the the health of Mormon men was based on how closely they followed church teachings regarding not using alcohol and tobacco (Gradner and Lyon, 1982). Not all Mormons abstain from using alcohol and tobacco. Those men who were adherent to the church policy had significantly less risk of developing cancer of the lung, stomach, lip, oral cavity, pharynx, esophagus , larynx, bladder, leukemia, and lymphoma. There were no differences for cancer of the prostate, pancreas, colon and rectum. Similar data was obtained from a study of Dutch Seventh Day Adventists (Berkel and DeWaard, 1983). Seventh Day Adventists do not smoke and have excellent dietary habits. They were found to have less cancer and cardiovascular disease and a longer life expectancy in comparison with the Dutch population. Thus, health-promoting benefits of religious teachings may partially relate to health-promoting activities.

There are both religious and secular kibbutzes in Israel. There are some interesting health-related differences between the two types of kibbutz. For example, between 1970 and 1985, mortality was approximately double in the secular kibbutz. The members of the religious kibbutz reported a higher sense of coherence and lower levels of hostility (Kark et al, 1996). There were no differences between the two types of kibbutz with regard to social support or social contact. It is possible that the sharing of religious activities produced a sense of coherence in the religious kibbutz that was reflected in the reduced mortality due to stress-buffering activities within the brain that ameliorated stress-induced hormonal alterations. It is also possible—even likely—that individuals who affiliate with a religious kibbutz have different personality characteristics than those of individuals who affiliate with a secular kibbutz. The different personality characteristics may relate to less stressor-induced activation of the CNS in individuals who affiliate with a religious kibbutz.

Interleukin-6 (IL-6) is produced by several different cell types, one of which is the macrophage. Synthesis of IL-6 is induced when macrophages ingest a bacteria. Thus, an increased plasma concentration of IL-6 may indicate the presence of an infection and an inflammatory response to limit the spread of the infection. IL-6 was measured in the plasma of older individuals who either regularly attended church services or did not regularly attend church services (Koenig et al, 1997b). An elevated plasma concentration of IL-6 was present in the plasma of significantly fewer church going individuals than individuals who did not attend church regularly. This may be interpreted to indicate that there was less infectious disease or inflammatory processes present in the church going subjects. Alternatively, as IL-6 has been reported to increase in plasma during stress (Zhou et al, 1993), the church attending subjects may have had less of a response to stress than did the non-church-attending subjects.

Indeed, church attendance may provide a mental state that is associated with a hormonal environment which facilitates greater resistance to the development of infectious disease. Alternatively, church attendance may promote better dietary, sleep, and exercise habits and discourage the use of alcohol and cigarettes. Either psychological or physical stress can increase the concentration of IL-6 in plasma (Zhou et al, 1993; Hisano et al, 1997; Gannon et al, 1997). Thus, it is unclear whether the church attendance was associated with lower IL-6 in plasma because of fewer episodes of infection or because of a reduced stress response.

Is involvement in religious activities capable of contributing to a better state of health and increased longevity if practiced throughout life? Possibly! If this is a valid association, the mechanism is unclear and may relate to the maintenance of better health practices, more social interactions, more stable marriages, and an enhanced ability to cope with stress. The emotional feeling provided through religion of greater satisfaction with life, personal happiness, and fewer negative psychosocial consequences associated with traumatic life events are all likely to be important factors in the health-promoting influence of religion (Ellison, 1991).

Can turning to religion at a time of medical illness contribute to ameliorating the course of the illness? This is an area that needs to be carefully addressed. Different diseases, different extents of disease, different ages of the subjects, and the availability of other support behaviors such as social support must be considered in the evaluation of the association of the effect of turning to religion at a time of crisis.

The mechanism as to how participation in religious activities achieves a beneficial health effect is unknown. One possible consideration is that there is a reduction of SNS activation associated with participation in activities centered around a religious structure. Such activities may be considered relaxing if they reduce SNS activity and enhance immune function. Does involvement in religious activities have the same effect on the CNS as does the positive and personally meaningful perception of social support?

An association between techniques that are believed to induce mental relaxation and reduced SNS activity is not readily evident. A physical stressor produced the same alteration in blood pressure and heart rate in subjects who were trained to relax or untrained controls (Hoffman et al, 1982). However, in the relaxation trained subjects, there was a greater increase in physical stressor-induced plasma norepinephrine than in the control subjects. This finding was interpreted to indicate that more catecholamine stimulation was required to produce the increase in heart rate and blood pressure, suggesting that there was less responsiveness to catecholamines in the relaxation trained group. The hormonal response to a psychological stressor was not evaluated.

A similar finding of higher plasma catecholamine concentrations in subjects trained in transcendental meditation than in nontrained subjects has been reported (Cooper et al, 1985). The effect of a response to a psychological stressor on altering catecholamine concentrations was not determined. Another report suggested that transcendental meditation can produce lower systolic blood pressure than was associated with population means (Wallace et al, 1983). It is unfortunate that the practitioners of transcendental meditation were not compared with a group of controls that were carefully matched for age and medical conditions and evaluated in the experimenter's laboratory, rather than population means.

Health care utilization by subjects who practice transcendental meditation is lower in all age groups (Orme-Johnson, 1983). Both inpatient days and outpatient visits were lower as compared with the norms of large health care providers. Thus, regardless of whether physiologic or hormonal differences were detectable between the transcendental meditators and controls, there were differences in use of health care facilities, possibly suggesting differences in health. However, it is also possible that the meditators were more stoic, were healthier to begin with and were thus a selected population, or that health benefits were achieved through mechanisms not related to hormonal systems (eg, healthier diets, more exercise, better sleep patterns, more social support).

Another possible explanation for a positive effect of belief systems on health is a placebo response. There is considerable evidence that if an individual believes in the effectiveness of a treatment that many individuals will have a meaningful therapeutic response (Lupoarello et al, 1970; Roberts, 1995). I certainly do not want to suggest any aspect of disrespect for the importance of religion and religious beliefs in an individuals life. However, if individuals receive health benefits through belief systems associated with religious beliefs, regardless of the mechanism, a significant benefit of religion will have been provided to those who are or may become involved in religious activities.

SENSE OF HUMOR

It is possible that there is a specific site within the brain that, when activated, induces laughter (Fried et al, 1998). It is possible that when this area, which may be located in the supplementary motor area of the cortex, is activated, inhibitory signals are received at the areas of the brain that induce the activation of the SNS and HPA axis. Indeed, hearty laughter has been found to decrease plasma levels of cortisol and epinephrine (Berk et al, 1989), and humor tends to reduce the stressor-induced elevation of heart rate (Newman and Stone, 1996). Salivary concentrations of IgA are also reported to increase when subjects are experiencing a humorous episode (Dillon et al, 1985).

Laughter produces an emotional state that is quite different than that associated with bereavement, an emotion that is associated with decreased immune function (Bartrop et al, 1977). A lower plasma concentration of glucocorticoids and catecholamines suggests that laughter may produce a hormonal milieu similar to the beneficial hormonal milieu that may be produced by social support with its associated beneficial health effects. Certainly, the best example that one can cite to indicate a beneficial health effect of laughter has been provided by Norman Cousins (1991).

EXERCISE

Numerous studies in humans show that exercise produces alteration of the function of the immune system. There are also studies showing that exercise is capable of minimizing the effect of stress on altering the function of the immune system, primarily conducted in experimental animal systems, and that exercise has a beneficial effect on health by reducing cardiovascular disease, cerebrovascular accidents, and malignancy.

The stress-buffering behaviors discussed in this chapter involve influences on the mind (social support or the perception of social support, a belief system, and a sense of humor), but exercise is a physical activity. To produce alteration of the function of the immune system probably requires activation of areas of the brain that activate the SNS and HPA axis. Finding less alteration of the immune system in subjects who are physically fit suggests that chronic exercise may attenuate activation of the areas of the brain that modify immune function, and this has an influence on the response of the brain to psychological stress.

An important question is whether exercise can have a beneficial effect on the health (both mental and physical) of every individual who participates in an exercise program. It is possible that those who are physically active comprise a population of subjects quite different from subjects who do not exercise. The question revolves around the consideration of whether the brain of an individual who exercises differs from the brain of an individual who does not exercise and whether the differences within the CNS are associated with different states of health. For example, individuals who participate in physical activities rather than maintaining a sedentary life style may:

Be more comfortable in social interactions and have more social support

Eat a better diet

Seek out medical care more readily when appropriate

Have less activation of the SNS and HPA axis when experiencing a psychological stressor because of different properties of the CNS

There are subjects who have physiological responses to a stressor that does not activate a response in other subjects. This has led to the concept of stress responders and stress nonresponders (Manuck et al, 1989). Interestingly, an aspect of stress reactivity may be reflected in the hormonal changes induced by exercise. In a recent study of elite athletes, plasma cortisol concentration was measured after exercise (Perna and McDowell, 1995). One cortisol response pattern consisted of a rapid recovery to baseline. Another cortisol response pattern displayed persistence of cortisol elevation for approximately 20 hours. Interestingly, those subjects who reacted with a persistent cortisol elevation reported more stressors in their lives. If persistent cortisol elevation is found to be associated with deleterious effects on the brain, as has been suggested (Lupien et al, 1998), those individuals who exercise and sustain high cortisol elevations may be prone to memory deficits.

It is possible that different neuropeptide patterns within the brain are associated with different behaviors. For example, the stressor-induced change in systolic blood pressure, which would be associated with either sympathetic nervous system activation or decreased parasympathetic nervous system activity, was found to be highest in men who had the characteristics of hostility and defensiveness (Helmers and Krantz, 1996). Could a particular chemical and anatomical structure within the brain be associated with specific types of personalities, with each personality type having characteristic hormonal responses to stress? This has previously been suggested (Kirschbaum et al, 1995).

It is also possible that exercise may not lead to better health but, rather, better health may be associated with the personality type of a person who exercises. Forcing an individual to exercise because "it is good for you" could possibly produce negative effects by becoming an experience that stimulates a hormonal stress response. Beneficial effects of exercise as a buffer of stress may primarily be achieved in those who have an appropriate (but as yet undefined) predisposition to exercise. Telling someone who hates to exercise to do so may be a stressor.

Another consideration regarding whether exercise may have a beneficial effect as a buffer of a stressor on the CNS is how much exercise is appropriate, with regard to intensity and frequency and to duration over time. The subject's background stress level and in utero and neonatal rearing environment may influence this relationship. Whether the subject exercises willingly or is induced to exercise (eg, an animal with a running wheel in its cage can exercise when it wants to, but an animal that is placed onto a treadmill must exercise when demanded to) may influence the buffering effect of stress on immune alteration.

Even characteristics of the stressor may be important in determining whether physical fitness can buffer the hormonal response to the stressor. A novel stressor may produce a different effect than does a stressor that one is familiar with. Working each day in an environment that is a stressor may produce a milder response that could be buffered by being physically fit in comparison with the response generated by going to work and being told that your job is terminated.

The following sections will review the interaction between exercise, the brain, the immune system, and health.

Exercise-Induced Alteration of the Stress Response

There are several ways that exercise could ameliorate the hormone-elevating effects of a psychological stressor. If the areas of the brain that are activated by exercise overlap with the areas of the brain that are activated by a psychological stressor, habituation may occur. When the subject experiences a psychological stressor, habituation would lead to a reduction in the magnitude of activation of the brain areas repeatedly activated by exercise. Alternatively, exercise may produce a sensitization of areas of the brain that would increase the magnitude of their activation when exposed to a psychological stressor. If these areas produce an inhibitory signal to the SNS and HPA axis, attenuation of stressor-induced immune alteration may occur.

Habituation of stressor-induced immune alteration to a repeated stress stimulus has been reported for splenic lymphocytes but not to the peripheral blood lymphocytes of rats (Lysle et al, 1987). Sensitization to repeated stress, as indicated by an accentuated increase of plasma levels of catecholamines, has also been reported (Konarska et al, 1990). As less immune alteration with repeated stress is incompatible with a sensitization of catecholamine release, it is likely that there are very specific aspects of the experimental protocols that influence whether habituation or sensitization occurs. Generalization of these concepts should be avoided.

Another consideration is whether repeated elevations of stress hormones (such as cortisol and catecholamines) lead to a decrease of the receptors for these hormones. If this occurs, regardless of the elevation of the hormone concentration in plasma and/or tissue, there will be a diminished biological effect of the hormones. A decrease of ACTH receptors subsequent to chronic exercise has been suggested in male ultramarathon athletes (Wittert et al, 1996). Although the athletes had significantly higher plasma ACTH concentrations, the concentration of plasma and urinary cortisol were the same in the athletes and control subjects.

Can a regimen of regular exercise modify the response to psychological stress? A meta-analysis was performed of 34 studies that evaluated the interaction between physical fitness and responsiveness to a psychological stressor (Crews and Landers, 1987). The magnitude of the stress response and/or the rate of physiological recovery after a stressor were evaluated in studies comparing physically fit with sedentary subjects. Parameters evaluated in the subjects included stressor-induced heart rate and blood pressure elevations and catecholamine elevations. Analysis of the data suggested that physical fitness was associated with decreased SNS-mediated cardiovascular responses to a psychological stressor. However, the meta-analysis should be considered suggestive, and research should continue to better understand the relationship between fitness and the stress response in individuals of different ages and sex and with different amounts of stress in their lives. A more recent study supports the conclusions of the meta-analysis (Sothmann et al, 1991).

The beneficial effect of physical fitness on buffering stressor-induced hormonal alterations has been reported in elderly subjects (Korkushko et al, 1995). This suggests that beneficial effects of exercise on attenuating the hormonal response to stress may be achieved in older individuals. This is in addition to the cardiovascular and musculoskeletal benefits that elderly individuals receive from exercise.

However, not all studies have found that exercise lowers reactivity to a stressor (Dorheim et al, 1988; Sinyor et al, 1988; De Geus et al, 1993). Highly physically fit individuals have even been reported to have an augmented physiological response to a psychological stressor (Sothmann et al, 1988). It is possible that this augmented response, which produces an elevation of glucocorticoids and catecholamines, suppresses the immune system, leading to an increased susceptibility to infectious disease. Perhaps this is partially responsible for the increased risk of the development of infectious disease in elite athletes (Nieman, 1994a,b). Clearly, more research is needed in this area.

Studies in experimental animals have reported buffering effects of physical fitness on the response to a psychological stressor (Cox et al, 1985a,b; Watanabe et al, 1992).

For example, rats trained to swim or run had less ACTH elevation when doing these tasks than did control rats (Watanabe et al, 1992). In addition, exposure to a novel stressor—cage switching—also had an attenuated ACTH response in trained rats.

Within the brain there are exercise-induced changes in neuropeptides and responses to stress. Rats that exercise on a running wheel and then experience footshock have increased concentrations of norepinephrine in the locus coeruleus and dorsal raphe in comparison with sedentary controls that receive footshock (Dishman et al, 1997). Thus, exercise probably modifies catabolism and synthesis of neuropeptides in various parts of the brain, possibly contributing to sensitization. The associated functional alterations of the identified areas and areas that they regulate need to be further explored to identify how these central changes modify health and immune function.

The importance of the uniqueness of each individual's response to the particular parameters of the exercise regimen needs to be kept in mind. Yet, there is very convincing evidence that exercise does have an effect on some aspects of the autonomic nervous system. For example, physically fit individuals have lower heart rates than do sedentary subjects, possibly related to increased parasympathetic activity (Smith et al, 1989).

Another consideration relates to whether there may be an exercise-related sex hormone effect. An interaction of estrogen with the HPA axis/SNS and exercise and stress would suggest that different exercise-induced stress-buffering effects may be present in males and females. Indeed, an experimental animal model suggests that estradiol increases HPA axis activation in ovariectomized exercise trained rats that experience an acute stressor, in comparison with ovariectomized rats not treated with estradiol (White-Welkley et al, 1996).

Exercise-Induced Alteration of Immune Function

Exercise produces alterations of the plasma concentration of glucocorticoids and catecholamines that are similar to those produced by a psychological stressor. Thus, alterations of immune function would be expected to be produced by exercise. Indeed, that is what happens. However, there are many ramifications of how exercise alters the immune system. The following are likely factors capable of influencing the exercise-related immune alterations:

Intensity of the exercise

Duration of the exercise

Frequency of exercise

Fitness of the subject

Chronic stressors in the subjects life

Acute stressors in the subjects life

Developmental characteristics of the subject

Social support of the subject

We studied the effect of exercise on peripheral blood leukocyte numbers in sedentary and physically fit males and females with a mean age of 25 years (Moyna et al,

1996a). The exercise involved 6-minute incremental increases of stationary bicycle peddling. The resting and exercise-induced leukocytes counts were not related to whether the subjects were physically fit or to their gender, as all subjects had the same changes. Each increment of exercise increased the leukocyte count. Neutrophils, eosinophils, monocytes, and lymphocyte numbers increased. All lymphocyte subpopulations increased with a greater increase of CD8 than CD4 lymphocytes lowering the CD4:CD8 ratio. The number of NK cells demonstrated the largest increase. Plasma catecholamine concentrations also increased significantly. This is similar to the effect of psychological stress on the immune system (Manuck et al, 1991). When we evaluated the function of NK cells, we found an increase of function from baseline, when measured after 6 minutes of exercise, but no further increase in function, even though the numbers continued to increase (Moyna et al, 1996b). The explanation for this discrepancy is unclear. Possibly the cells that were recruited into the blood were immature and less active, or the high concentrations of catecholamines reduced their function. Of course, these results only apply to subjects of the age we studied, as different results might have been obtained with an older age population.

Other studies have reported that physically fit individuals may have more (LaPerriere et al, 1994) or fewer (Nehlsen-Cannarella et al, 1991) numbers of baseline lymphocytes than sedentary subjects. However, the trend of published studies indicates that exercise has an enhancing effect on the quantitative and qualitative components of the immune system. It is possible that regardless of whether exercise increases the ability of an individuals CNS to cope with a stressor, the exercise induced enhancement of immune function would provide more resistance to disease. Or would it?

As I have indicated, it is not merely the number of a particular component of the immune system that is important, but rather it is the function and the interrelationship of components. For example, as cited above, exercise continually increased the number of NK cells in blood over an 18-minute period, but NK function increased only during the first 6 minutes of exercise. Thus, there is a dissociation between function and numbers.

What is the biological significance of a decrease of the CD4:CD8 ratio that is induced by exercise? Is it better to have more CD8 lymphocytes for resistance to viral infections (assuming that newly recruited CD8 lymphocytes function normally)? What does an exercise-induced alteration of the ratio of Th1:Th2 lymphocytes do to cell-mediated immune function? Indeed, exercise has been reported to increase the function of the Th1 lymphocyte population while not altering the function of the Th2 population, as determined by the in vitro production of cytokines by peripheral blood lymphocytes (Moyna et al, 1996c). However, a small study of cytokine gene expression did not find quantitative changes of mRNA for Th1 or Th2 cytokines in subjects undergoing extreme exercise (Natelson et al, 1996). As cytokines are not preformed, but rather synthesis is induced, when proper stimulation of lymphocytes occurs, it is difficult to reconcile these two studies unless different intensities and durations of exercise elicit different hormonal responses with different effects on lymphoid cells. Further, there is not an unequivocal indication that stress increases Th1 activity. A study in humans undergoing the stress of surgery for cholecystectomy has found an increase of Th2 cytokines with a decrease of Th1 cytokines (Decker et al, 1996).

What are the possible consequences of increased CD4 Th1 function relative to CD4 Th2 lymphocytes? The potential benefits of this relationship would be an inhibition of IL-4 production by Th2 lymphocytes and a reduced likelihood of developing an allergic disease. However, could lower concentrations of IgE lead to an increased risk of developing parasitic infections? A relative increase of Th1 lymphocyte function could be beneficial if there is an associated increase of cell mediated immune function that increases resistance to viral and other infections with intracellular pathogens. However, could an increase of Th1 activity increase the risk of developing an organ specific autoimmune disease (Klareskog et al, 1995)?

What are the possible consequences of increased CD4 Th2 function relative to CD4 Th1 lymphocytes? Th2 cytokines produce immunoglobulin heavy chain class switching for production of IgE, IgA, and IgG subclass 4. There is also a decrease in Th1 cytokine production. Thus, an increase in allergic diseases, decreased killing of pathogens by macrophages, increased susceptibility to pyogenic infections, and less organ-specific autoimmune disease may be anticipated. Obviously, the answer to the question regarding whether exercise-induced alteration of immune function would provide increased resistance to disease is not as straightforward as we would like it to be.

A reduction of upper respiratory infections in individuals who engage in moderate amounts of exercise versus an increase in the incidence of upper respiratory infections in individuals who engage in extreme exercise has been reported (Nieman, 1994a). If the clinical outcome is related to optimizing function of the immune system, it is possible that a particular regimen (duration, intensity, frequency) of exercise may contribute to the optimization of immune function. A similar observation has been reported in experimental animal studies (Nieman, 1994a). However, it is likely that there will be no standard of exercise, rather it may have to be determined for each individual. Indeed, different intensities of exercise have been found to have different effects on the immune system (Nieman et al, 1993b, 1994c).

We should not accept a simple conclusion that exercise induced enhanced immune function measured with in vitro assays will be beneficial or detrimental to health. As indicated earlier, when such epidemiological studies have been performed, there does appear to be an association between exercise and improved health. Whether the improvement of health occurs because of an effect on the immune system or because of an increased ability to cope with psychological stressors, has not been determined. Possibly, exercise increases coping abilities for stress as individual who engage in regular exercise have less depression and more feelings of well being than individuals who are sedentary (Stephens, 1988; Camacho et al, 1991).

Can Being Physically Fit Buffer the Effects of a Psychological Stress on Altering Immune Function?

There are studies of NK cell function and lymphocyte nonspecific mitogenic function, performed in rodents, which indicate that stress has a diminished effect on reducing immune function in physically trained animals. NK cell function was determined in rats that had been allowed to run voluntarily on an activity wheel (Dishman et al, 1995). In animals that received footshock, after 6 weeks of running, the NK function of spleen lymphocytes was the same as that of control nonshocked animals. The shocked animals that had not exercised had approximately a 50% reduction of NK function. The percentage of NK cells in the spleens of the shocked exercised and nonexercised animals did not differ.

A similar observation was made with lymphocyte responsiveness to stimulation with Concanavalin A (Con A) (Mahan and Young, 1989). Exercise was achieved by a daily swimming procedure for 10 weeks (2 hr/day). The stressor used was to have the trained rats swim for 4–7 hours. The rats that had not been in an exercise training program were stressed by swimming for 1–3 hours. Although the lymphocyte response to Con A from the trained and untrained rats was significantly lower than the response of control rats that were not stressed, the trained rats exhibited significantly less suppression than did the untrained controls.

The suggestion that exercise may buffer the effects of stress on alteration of immune function will be important to pursue. Could this buffering effect be one of the explanations as to why exercise is beneficial for health?

Is Exercise a Buffer of Disease?

There are several diseases for which exercise has been reported to be a factor in modulating its course. Over the course of a 14-year study, more temporal leisure-time physical activity was associated with a 37% reduction in the development of breast cancer in women aged 20–54 (Thune et al, 1997). Lifelong higher levels of physical activity have also been associated with a reduced risk of developing breast cancer (Bernstein et al, 1994). Parameters associated with the beneficial exercise effect were being premenopausal, younger than age 45, being lean, and exercising at least 4 hours per week. Of course, a mechanism is not obvious. However, consideration must be given to factors such as a healthier (low fat, more fiber) diet of individuals who exercise, greater social interactions (if they exercise with a friend), and enhanced immune function in association with exercise. A similar beneficial effect of leisure time exercise and lean body mass has been found in women in regard to colon cancer (Martinez et al, 1997).

Disappointingly, the association of a reduced risk of developing breast cancer and physical activity has not been found in all studies. Evaluation of more than 100,000 nurses for an association between physical activity during late adolescence and at the time of the study failed to find a reduced risk of breast cancer in those reporting higher levels of physical activity (Rockhill et al, 1998). However, the study did not evaluate lifelong patterns of exercise, which may be more important as a breast cancer risk reducer than are periodic episodes of exercise. Obviously, more work is needed in this important area.

A reduced risk of developing an ischemic stroke has also been associated with a program of regular exercise (Sacco et al, 1998). The more years that an individual exercises may decrease the risk of having a stroke (Shinton and Sagar, 1993). It is possible that a lifelong pattern of exercise may reduce the risk of developing a malignant, cardiovascular, or cerebrovascular disease.

Mortality is also reduced by physical activity (Hakim et al, 1998). In a study of 707 male nonsmokers aged 61–81, walking 2 miles per day was to significantly reduce the risk of dying from cancer, heart disease, and strokes. A total of 208 subjects died during the course of the study; 43% of the subjects who walked less than 1 mile per day died, while 21% of those who walked more than 2 miles per day died.

A study of twins who were discordant for death (usually dying of cardiovascular disease or malignancy) also found a reduced risk of death in association with physical activity. Regardless of whether the same-sex twins were monozygotic or dizygotic, male or female, the twin who died had engaged in significantly less physical activity than did the twin who lived. Exercise is a likely buffer of the deleterious effects of stress on health (Kobasa et al, 1982). The extent of the immune system's contribution to reduced mortality is unknown.

Exercise Has An Effect on the Immune Function of Older Individuals

Maintenance of immune function as an individual ages may contribute to a healthier quality of life with less infectious, autoimmune, and malignant diseases. If exercise can contribute to the maintenance of immune function, it may serve as an important component of preventive medicine. Indeed, there may be a reduction of death rates in older individuals who exercise regularly, as compared with individuals who do not (Fraser and Shavlik, 1997). Whether exercise actually contributes to the reduction of mortality through an effect on the immune system remains to be determined. It is possible that individuals who exercise have other stress-buffering skills not found in sedentary individuals.

Baseline NK function was found to increase after a 16-week aerobic exercise training program in women approximately 72 years old (Crist et al, 1989). When exercised on a treadmill, the trained subjects had a significantly greater increase of NK function than did untrained aged-matched subjects. A question that needs to be addressed relates to *what* was "trained." I doubt that the NK cells were trained to respond with more in vitro cytotoxicity after a 16-week aerobic training program. Rather, it is more likely that there were changes induced within the brain that modified the hormonal milieu of plasma that had an effect on NK function. If the immune system functions in a manner comparable to that usually found in individuals of a younger chronological age, is it possible that the environment in which the immune system is functioning was "made younger" by exercise?

As baseline NK function increased in older individuals who exercised, there may have been changes in (1) the resting hormonal factors that influence NK function, (2) adhesion molecules resulting in different types of NK cells in the blood, (3) release of NK cells from the bone marrow, (4) removal of mature NK cells from the blood, (5) lower baseline concentrations of hormones that suppress NK function, and (6) higher baseline concentrations of hormones that increase NK function. As exercise-induced increases in NK function were greater in the trained subjects, there may have been (1) more rapid release of functional NK cells from endothelial cells, (2) rapid release of functional NK cells from the marrow, (3) less production of hormones that decrease NK function, and (4) increased production of hormones that increase NK function. I suspect that what is being "made younger" by exercise is the hormonal milieu in which the immune system matures, is activated, and functions.

Another study raises questions about the personality and hormonal composition of sedentary versus physically active older individuals (aged 65–85) (Nieman et al, 1993a). Sedentary elderly women failed to show increased NK function or lymphocyte mitogen responsiveness when they exercise. I wonder whether the personality predisposition to be sedentary is related to the lack of alteration of the plasma hormonal milieu by exercise with an associated lack of alteration of immune cell function. Do the brains of individuals who prefer to be sedentary respond differently to exercise than the brains of individuals who enjoy exercising? What are the characteristics of the brain that prefers to be sedentary? What are the characteristics of the brain that prefers to be physically active?

Another study of exercise in elderly subjects failed to find exercise-induced alteration of lymphocyte subsets, cytokine production, or in vivo delayed hypersensitivity skin-test reactivity (Rall et al, 1996). However, a study of elderly women (aged 60–98) self-rated as having an active or an inactive lifestyle found significantly enhanced immune function in those rating themselves as active (Gueldner et al, 1997). Interestingly, the incidence of upper respiratory infections was significantly lower in physically fit elderly subjects than in the other subjects (Gueldner et al, 1997). More studies are needed to obtain a better understanding of the reasons for the variability of the reported studies.

The question must be considered as to whether exercise will be of benefit to enhancing immune function in all individuals or only in a subset. That question also redirects attention to what it is about exercise that has an influence on the function of the immune system. However, to know that, we must have a better understanding of the effect of various hormones on immune cell function. This will require more basic science research.

Regardless of the mechanism, the fact that fewer infections are found in physically fit subjects is encouraging. However, if exercise does not change immune function in some subjects, the benefits of exercise on resistance to infectious disease may not occur in all individuals, even though they may benefit with regard to reduced risk of atherosclerotic heart disease and stroke.

Is it likely that a factor in longevity is exercise and for many individuals engaging in a lifelong behavior of exercise is easier to do than for other subjects. Is there something that occurs during in utero developmental, preadolescent and adolescent development, and during mid-life that contributes to a pattern of exercise involvement? If engaging in this behavior is easier for some than for others, we need to determine how to optimize involvement in exercise programs for those that find difficulty in exercising more. However, it must still be remembered that it is unlikely that all individuals will receive benefit to immune system function by regular exercise.

INTIMACY

As I have indicated, finding a means to cope with stress—regardless of whether the coping is achieved through friends, exercise, hobbies, meditation, religion, or whatever works for you—will promote a better quality of health. Another contributing element in stress reduction and coping capabilities is an emotionally satisfying sex life.

A common emotional after-effect of sexual fulfillment is a feeling of relaxation and peace. The problems one is having with the world and the people in it disappear, for a short time. Contrary to this, the lack of emotionally fulfilling sexual interactions may have an effect that is the opposite of emotional peace. The lack of an emotionally fulfilling sexual life may have an association with anxiety, hostility, or even violence.

How strong is the desire for the emotional satisfaction that is derived from satisfying sexual activity? Obviously, quite strong, as exemplified by its reaching into the pillar of power known as the White House. As we look back through the presidents of the United States, individuals who have been president and who must have achieved a sense of satisfaction by being elected to represent the United States as its president still needed extracurricular fulfillment in the sexual arena. This may indicate that the need for sexual gratification is separate from, and not influenced by, other gratifications and, as such, probably has a mind of its own. If some presidents of the United States had this need for sexual gratification, it is likely that many who are not president have the same need.

I do not want to falsely represent myself as a sex therapist or as a psychologist who has an intimate understanding of the emotional subtleties of sex counseling, sex cravings, sexual function, or sex practices. What I do claim to have is some common sense associated with practical experience.

Acknowledging that many are not satisfied with the quantity or quality of their sexual activity, and that sexual satisfaction can produce a state of mind that is happier than the state of mind associated with sexual dissatisfaction, the question that arises is what can be done to improve one's situation. This is especially important if, as we believe, one's state of mind can influence the hormonal composition of blood and this hormonal milieu influences the function of the immune system and, as a result, one's health.

The obvious answer regarding what can be done is "nothing easy." If it were easy, it would have been done by now. Possibly Viagra is a step in the right direction. Clearly, there will be no consensus regarding how to deal with the sexual needs of various age groups, religious groups, ethnic groups, political liberal groups, political conservative groups, males, females, those who are physically fit, those who are physically handicapped, those with high blood pressure, those with impotency, and so on. How effective comfortable, emotionally satisfying sex, with a supportive partner and a relationship in which each feels loved and cared about, will be in the lessening of sexual tensions, increasing relaxation, providing greater abilities to cope with stress, and as a result better health, needs to be determined.

How does one deal with the emotional disruption when their partner tells them that they are not finding fulfillment in their sex life? Does our educational process prepare us for this? Indeed, does scholastic education teach us how to negotiate buying a house, evaluate the capabilities of a plumber, control our anger when we get angry, raise children, interact with one's in-laws, or practice emotionally fulfilling sex? We may learn about Shakespearean sonnets and the history of our country, as well as how the DNA molecule replicates, but there may be a few things that are not included in a standard education. Do we invest as much time planning for our financial retirement as for our need to deal with emotional disruptions? Clearly, the brain can modify our immune function. It is hoped that psychologists, psychiatrists, nurses, family practice physicians, medical practice specialists, dentists, and each individual will learn of the importance of mutual support for the benefit it can bring to each of us as well as others.

I believe that an improved quality of mental, emotional, and physical health can be achieved by those who are comfortable, joyful, and satisfied with sexual interactions. If we are to develop a means of achieving our goal of an improved quality of health and less dependency on the health care system, attention must be paid to the role of sex in an individual's life and in the life of a couple, in the lives of residents of elder care facilities, and in the life of the physically disabled—indeed, in each living human being.

SUMMARY

This chapter has discussed the importance of social interactions, belief systems, intimacy, and exercise, as modalities and behaviors that may ameliorate a negative impact of psychological stress on the immune system and health and that may also contribute to the maintenance of health during the aging process. Their influence is likely through effects within the brain that suppress activation of the areas of the brain responsible for altering immune function. Other behaviors, such as being optimistic, having a sense of humor, or merely believing that one will be healthy may contribute to buffering the alteration of immune function by stress. In this regard, it is likely that the most important host factor is believing that the activity that one is using as a stress buffer will work for them. Each individual may respond differently to social interactions, belief systems, and exercise. Their response may be influenced by factors as diverse as their in utero environment to the happiness of their marriage.

It is also possible that there are fluctuations that occur in the neuroanatomy of the brain during life. Certainly, Alzheimer's disease is an example. Other changes may be more subtle. For example, severe acute stress may change the size of the hippocampus (Gurvits et al, 1996), as may high levels of chronic stress (Bremner et al, 1997). Chronic elevation of glucocorticoids, possibly induced by stress, may produce anatomical and functional alterations of the hippocampal neurons (Sapolsky, 1996). The glucocorticoid response to stress may be influenced by physical contact between young offspring and the mother (Liu et al, 1997), reemphasizing the multitude of environmental factors that influence the eventual interrelationship between the mind and health.

In addition, glucocorticoids may contribute to cognitive function, with decreased cognitive function associated with higher glucocorticoid levels (Lupien et al, 1994). Of course, other areas of the brain may also become altered by stress. Unless someone seeks to find such changes, they may go undetected. However, the hormonally induced changes that are known to occur within the brain may influence changes in responsiveness to stress buffering at different stages of aging. Thus, once again, it is important to emphasize that generalization must be avoided when discussing behaviors that will buffer the effect of stress on the immune system and health.

REFERENCES

Bartrop RW, Luckhurst E, Lazarus L, Kiloh LG, Penny R. Depressed lymphocyte function after bereavement. Lancet. 1: 834–836, 1977.

Berk LS, Tan SA, Napier BJ, Lee JW, Hubbard RW, Lewis JE, Eby WC. Neuroendocrine and stress hormone changes during mirthful laughter. American Journal of the Medical Sciences. 298: 390–396, 1989.

Berkel J, DeWaard F. Mortality pattern and life expectancy of Seventh Day Adventists in the Netherlands. International Journal of Epidemiology. 12: 455–459, 1983.

Berkman LF, Syme SL. Social networks, host resistance, and mortality: A nine-year follow-up study of Alameda county residents. American Journal of Epidemiology. 109: 186–204, 1979.

Berkman LF. The role of social relations in health promotion. Psychosomatic Medicine. 57: 245–254, 1995.

Bernstein L, Henderson BE, Hanisch R, Sullivan-Halley J, Ross PK. Physical exercise and reduced risk of breast cancer in young women. Journal of the National Cancer Institute. 86: 1403–1408, 1994.

Blazer D, Palmore E. Religion and aging in a longitudinal panel. Gerontologist. 16: 82–85, 1976.

Blazer DG. Social support and mortality in an elderly community population. American Journal of Epidemiology. 115: 684–694, 1982.

Boccia ML, Scanlan JM, Laudenslager ML, Berger CL, Hijazi AS, Reite ML. Juvenile friends, behavior, and immune responses to separation in bonnet macaque infants. Physiology and Behavior. 61: 191–198, 1997.

Bremner JD, Randall P, Vermetten E, Staib L, Bronen RA, Mazure C, Capelli S, McCarthy G, Innis RB, Charney DS. Magnetic resonance imaging-based measurement of hippocampal volume in posttraumatic stress disorder related to childhood physical and sexual abuse—A preliminary report. Biological Psychiatry. 41: 23–32, 1997.

Camacho TC, Roberts RE, Lazarus NB, Kaplan GA, Cohen RD. Physical activity and depression: Evidence from the Alameda County study. American Journal of Epidemiology. 134: 220–231, 1991.

Cassel J. The contribution of the social environment to host resistance. American Journal of Epidemiology. 104: 107–123, 1976.

Cerhan JR, Wallace RB. Change in social ties and subsequent mortality in rural elders Epidemiology. 8: 475–481, 1997.

Christenfeld N, Gerin W, Linden W, Sanders M, Mathur J, Deich JD, Pickering T. Social support effects on cardiovascular reactivity: Is a stranger as effective as a friend? Psychosomatic Medicine. 59: 388–398, 1997.

Claytor RP, Cox RH, Howley ET, Lawler KA, Lawler JA. Aerobic power and cardiovascular response to stress. Journal of Applied Physiology. 65: 1416–1423, 1988.

Cobb S. Social support as mediator of life stress. Psychosomatic Medicine. 38: 300–314, 1976.

Cohen S, Doyle WJ, Skoner DP, Rabin BS, Gwaltney JM. Social ties and susceptibility to the common cold. Journal of the American Medical Association. 277: 1940–1944, 1997.

Colantonio A, Kasl SV, Ostfeld AM, Berkman LF. Psychosocial predictors of stroke outcomes in an elderly population. Journal of Gerontology: Social Sciences. 48: S261–S268, 1993.

Comstock GW, Partridge KB. Church attendance and health. Journal of Chronic Diseases. 25: 665–672, 1972.

Cooper R, Joffe BI, Lamprey JM, Botha A, Shires R, Baker SG, Seftel HC. Hormonal and biochemical responses to transcendental meditation. Postgraduate Medical Journal. 61: 301–304, 1985.

Cousins N. Anatomy of an Illness. Bantam Doubleday Dell, New York, 1991.

Cox RH, Hubbard JW, Lawler JE, Sanders BJ, Mitchell VP. Exercise training attenuates stress-induced hypertension in the rat. Hypertension. 7: 747–751, 1985a.

Cox RH, Hubbard JW, Lawler JE, Sanders BJ, Mitchell VP. Cardiovascular and sympatho-adrenal responses to stress in swim trained rats. Journal of Applied Physiology. 58: 1207–1214, 1985b.

Crews DJ, Landers DM. A meta-analytic review of aerobic fitness and reactivity to psychosocial stressors. Medicine and Science in Sports and Exercise. 19: S114–S120, 1987.

Crist DM, MacKinnon LT, Thompson RF, Atterborn HA, Egan PA. Physical exercise increases natural cellular-mediated tumor cytotoxicity in elderly women. Gerontology. 35: 66–71, 1989.

Cunnick JE, Cohen S, Rabin BS, Carpenter AB, Manuck SB, Kaplan JR. Alterations in specific antibody production due to rank and social instability. Brain, Behavior, and Immunity. 5: 357–369, 1991.

De Geus EJC, van Doornen JP, Orlebeke JF. Regular exercise and aerobic fitness in relation to psychological make-up and physiological stress reactivity. Psychosomatic Medicine. 55: 347–363, 1993.

Decker D, Schondorf M, Bidlingmaier F, Hirner A, Vonruecker AA. Surgical stress induces a shift in the type-1/type-2 T-helper cell balance, suggesting down regulation of cell-mediated and up-regulation of antibody-mediated immunity commensurate to the trauma. Surgery. 119: 316–325, 1996.

Dillon KM, Minchoff B, Baker KH. Positive emotional states and enhancement of the immune system. International Journal of Psychiatry in Medicine. 15: 13–18, 1985.

Dishman RK, Warren JM, Youngstedt SD, Yoo H, Bunnell BN, Mougey EH, Meyerhoff JL, Jaso-Friedmann L, Evans DL. Activity-wheel running attenuates suppression of natural killer cell activity after footshock. Journal of Applied Physiology. 78: 1547–1554, 1995.

Dishman RK, Renner KJ, Youngstedt SD, Reigle TG, Bunnell BN, Burke KA, Yoo HS, Mougey EH, Meyerhof JL. Activity wheel running reduces escape latency and alters brain monoamine levels after footshock. Brain Research Bulletin. 42: 399–406, 1997.

Dorheim TA, Ruddel JC, Eliot RS. Cardiovascular response of marathoners to mental challenge. Journal of Cardiac Rehabilitation. 4: 476–480, 1984.

Ellison CG. Religious involvement and subjective well-being. Journal of Health and Social Behavior. 32: 80–99, 1991.

Esterling BA, Kiecolt-Glaser JK, Glaser R. Psychosocial modulation of cytokine-induced natural killer cell activity in older adults. Psychosomatic Medicine. 58: 264–272, 1996.

Francis RC, Kiran S, Fernald RD. Social regulation of the brain-pituitary axis. Proceedings of the National Academy of Science USA. 90: 7794–7798, 1993.

Fraser GE, Shavlik DJ. Risk factors for all-cause and coronary heart disease mortality in the oldest-old. The Adventist Health Study. Archives of Internal Medicine. 157: 2249–2258, 1997.

Fried I, Wilson CL, MacDonald KA, Behnke EJ. Electric current stimulates laughter (Letter). Nature. 391: 650, 1998.

Friedman HS, Tucker JS, Schwartz JE, Tomlinson-Keasey C, Martin LR, Wingard DL, Criqui MH. Psychosocial and behavioral predictors of longevity. The aging and death of the "termites." American Psychologist. 50: 69–78, 1995.

Gannon GA, Rhind SG, Suzui M, Shek PN, Shephard RJ. Circulating levels of peripheral blood leukocytes and cytokines following competitive cycling. Canadian Journal of Applied Physiology. 22: 133–147, 1997.

Glaser R, Kiecolt-Glaser JK, Speicher CE, Holliday JE. Stress, loneliness, and changes in herpesvirus latency. Journal of Behavioral Medicine. 8: 249–260, 1985.

Glass TA, Matchar DB, Belyea M, Feussner JR. Impact of social support on outcome in first stroke. Stroke. 24: 64–70, 1993.

Gradner JW, Lyon JL. Cancer in Utah Mormon men by church activity level. American Journal of Epidemiology. 116: 243–257, 1982.

Gueldner SH, Poon LW, La Via M, Virella G, Michel Y, Bramlett MH, Noble CA, Paulling E. Long-term exercise patterns and immune function in healthy older women. A report of preliminary findings. Mechanisms of Aging and Development. 93: 215–222, 1997.

Gust DA, Gordon TP, Brodie AR, McClure HM. Effect of companions in modulating stress associated with new group formation in juvenile rhesus macaques. Physiology and Behavior. 59: 941–945, 1996.

Gurvits TV, Shenton ME, Hokama H, Ohta H, Lasko NB, Gilbertson MW, Orr SP, Kikinis R, Jolesz FA, McCarley RW, Pitman RK. Magnetic resonance imaging study of hippocampal volume in chronic, combat-related posttraumatic stress disorder. Biological Psychiatry. 40: 1091–1099, 1996.

Hakim AA, Petrovitch H, Burchfiel CM, Ross GW, Rodriguez BL, White LR, Yano K, Curb JD, Abbott RD. Effects of walking on mortality among nonsmoking retired men. New England Journal of Medicine. 338: 94–99, 1998.

Hallberg H. Life after divorce—A five year follow-up study of divorced middle-aged men in Sweden. Family Practice. 9: 49–56, 1992.

Helmers KF, Krantz DS. Defensive hostility, gender and cardiovascular levels and responses to stress. Annals of Behavioral Medicine. 18: 246–254, 1996.

Hisano S, Sakamoto K, Ishiko T, Kamohara T, Ogawa M. IL-6 and IL-6 receptor levels change differently after surgery both in the blood and in the operative field. Cytokine. 9: 447–452, 1997.

Hoffman JW, Benson H, Arns PA, Stainbrook GL, Landsberg L, Young JB, Gill A. Reduced sympathetic nervous system responsivity associated with the relaxation response. Science. 215: 190–192, 1982.

House JS, Landis KR, Umberson D. Social relationships and health. Science. 241: 540–545, 1988.

House JS, Robbins C, Metzner HL. The association of social relationships and activities with mortality: Prospective evidence from the Tecumseh community health study. American Journal of Epidemiology. 116: 123–140, 1982.

Idler EL, Kasl S. Health perceptions and survival: Do global evaluations of health status really predict mortality? Journal of Gerontology. 46: S55–S65, 1991.

Kamarck T, Manuck SB, Jennings JR. Social support reduces cardiovascular reactivity to psychological challenge: A laboratory model. Psychosomatic Medicine. 52: 42–58, 1990.

Kaplan JR, Heise ER, Manuck SB, Shively CA, Cohen S, Rabin BS, Kasprowics AL. The relationship of agonistic and affiliative behavior patterns to cellular immune function among Cynomolgus monkeys (*Macaca fascicularis*) living in stable and unstable social groups. American Journal of Primatology. 25: 157–173, 1991a.

Kaplan JR, Petersson K, Manuck SB, Olsson G. Role of sympathoadrenal medullary activation in the initiation and progression of atherosclerosis. Circulation. 84(suppl 6): 23–32, 1991b.

Kark JD, Carmel S, Sinnreich R, Goldberger N, Friedlander Y. Psychosocial factors among members of religious and secular kibbutzim. Israel Journal of Medical Sciences. 32: 185–194, 1996.

Kemp VH, Hatmaker DD. Stress and social support in high-risk pregnancy. Research in Nursing Health. 12: 331–336, 1989.

Kiecolt-Glaser JK, Glaser R, Shuttleworth EC, Dyer CS, Ogrocki P, Speicher, CE. Chronic stress and immunity in family caregivers of Alzheimer's disease victims. Psychosomatic Medicine. 49: 523–535, 1987.

Kiecolt-Glaser JK, Kennedy S, Malkoff S, Fisher L, Speicher CE, Glaser R. Marital discord and immunity in males. Psychosomatic Medicine. 50: 213–229, 1988.

Kirschbaum C, Prussner JC, Stone AA, Federenko I, Gaab J, Lintz D, Schommer N, Hellhammer DH. Persistent high cortisol responses to repeated psychological stress in a subpopulation of healthy men. Psychosomatic Medicine. 57: 468–474, 1995.

Klareskog L, Ronnelid J, Holm G. Immunopathogenesis and immunotherapy in rheumatoid arthritis: An area in transition. Journal of Internal Medicine. 238: 191–206, 1995.

Kobasa SC, Maddi SR, Puccetti MC. Personality and exercise as buffers in the stress–illness relationship. Journal of Behavioral Medicine. 5: 391–404, 1982.

Koenig HG, Cohen HJ, George LK, Hays JC, Larson DB, Blazer DG. Attendance at religious services, interleukin-6, and other biological parameters of immune function in older adults. International Journal of Psychiatry in Medicine. 27: 233–250, 1997a.

Koenig HG, Hays JC, George LK, Blazer DG, Larson DB, Landerman LR. Modeling the cross-sectional relationships between religion, physical health, social support, and depressive symptoms. American Journal of Geriatric Psychiatry. 5: 131–144, 1997b.

Konarska M, Stewart RE, McCarty R. Habituation and sensitization of plasma catecholamine responses to chronic intermittent stress: Effects of stressor intensity. Physiology and Behavior. 47: 647–652, 1990.

Korkushko OV, Frolkis MV, Shatilo VB. Reaction of pituitary-adrenal and autonomic nervous systems to stress in trained and untrained elderly people. Journal of the Autonomic Nervous System. 54: 27–32, 1995.

LaPerriere A, Antoni MH, Ironson G, Perry A, McCabe P, Klimas N, Helder L, Schneiderman N, Fletcher MA. Effects of aerobic exercise training on lymphocyte subpopulations. International Journal of Sports Medicine. 15: S127–S130, 1994.

Laudenslager ML, Boccia ML. Some observations on psychosocial stressors, immunity, and individual differences in nonhuman primates. American Journal of Primatology. 39: 205–221, 1996.

Levin JS. Religion and health: Is there an association, is it valid, and is it causal? Social Science and Medicine. 38: 1475–1482, 1994.

Levin JS, Vanderpool HY. Is religion therapeutically significant for hypertension? Social Science and Medicine. 29: 69–78, 1989.

Liu D, Diorio J, Tannenbaum B, Caldji C, Francis D, Freedman A, Sharma S, Pearson D, Plotsky PM, Meaney MJ. Maternal care, hippocampal glucocorticoid receptors, and hypothalamic-pituitary-adrenal responses to stress. Science. 277: 1659–1662, 1997.

Lupien S, Lecours AR, Lussier I, Schwartz G, Nair NP. Basal cortisol levels and cognitive deficits in human aging. Journal of Neuroscience. 14: 2893–2903, 1994.

Lupien S, de Leon M, de Santi S, Convit A, Chaim T, Nair NPV, Thakur M, McEwen BS, Hauger RL, Meaney MJ. Cortisol levels during human aging predict hippocampal atrophy and memory deficits. Nature Neuroscience. 1: 69–73, 1998.

Lupoarello T, Leist N, Lourie CH, Sweet P. The interaction of psychologic stimuli and pharmacologic agents on airway reactivity in asthmatic subjects. Psychosomatic Medicine. 32: 509–513, 1970.

Lysle DT, Lyte M, Fowler H, Rabin BS. Shock-induced modulation of lymphocyte reactivity: Suppression, habituation, and recovery. Life Sciences. 41: 1805–1814, 1987.

Mahan MP, Young MR. Immune parameters of untrained or exercise-trained rats after exhaustive exercise. Journal of Applied Physiology. 66: 282–287, 1989.

Manuck SB, Cohen S, Rabin BS, Muldoon MF, Bachen EA. Individual differences in cellular immune response to stress. Psychological Science. 2 : 1–5, 1991.

Manuck SB, Kasprowicz AL, Monroe SM, Larkin KT, Kaplan JR. Psychologic reactivity as a dimension of individual differences. In Handbook of Research Methods in Cardiovascular Behavior Medicine. Schneiderman N, Weiss SM, Kaufmann PG (eds). Plenum Press, New York, 1989, pp 365–382.

Marmot MG, Shipley MJ, Rose G. Inequalities in death—Specific explanations of a general pattern? Lancet 1: 1003–1006, 1984.

Marmot MG, Bosma H, Hemingway H, Brunner E, Stansfeld S. Contribution of job control and other risk factors to social variations in coronary heart disease incidence. Lancet. 350: 235–239, 1997.

Martinez ME, Giovannucci E, Spiegelman D, Hunter DJ, Willett WC, Colditz GA. Leisure-time physical activity, body size, and colon cancer in women. Nurses' Health Study Research Group. Journal of the National Cancer Institute. 89: 948–955, 1997.

Mendes de Leon CF, Seeman TE, Baker DI, Richardson ED, Tinetti ME. Self-efficacy, physical decline, and change in functioning in community-living elders: A prospective study. Journals of Gerontology. 51: S183–S190, 1996.

Mossey JM, Shapiro E. Self-rated health: A predictor of mortality among the elderly. American Journal of Public Health. 72: 800–807, 1982.

Moyna NM, Acker GR, Weber KM, Fulton JR, Goss FL, Robertson RJ, Rabin BS. The effects of incremental submaximal exercise on circulating leukocytes in physically active and sedentary males and females. European Journal of Applied Physiology. 74: 211–218, 1996a.

Moyna NM, Acker GR, Weber KM, Fulton JR, Goss FL, Robertson RJ, and Rabin BS. Exercise-induced alterations in natural killer cell number and function. European Journal of Applied Physiology. 74: 227–233, 1996b.

Moyna NM, Acker GR, Fulton JR, Weber KM, Goss FL, Robertson RJ, Tollerud DJ, Rabin BS. Lymphocyte function and cytokine production during incremental exercise in active and sedentary males and females. International Journal of Sports Medicine. 17: 585–591, 1996c.

Natelson BH, Zhou X, Ottenweller JE, Bergen MT, Sisto SA, Drastal S, Tapp WN, Gause WL. Effect of acute exhausting exercise on cytokine gene expression in men. International Journal of Sports Medicine. 17: 299 302, 1996.

Nehlsen-Cannarella SL, Nieman DC, Balk-Lamberton AJ, Markoff PA, Chritton DWB, Gusewitch G, Lee JW. The effect of moderate exercise on immune response. Medicine and Science in Sports and Exercise. 23: 64–70, 1991.

Newman MG, Stone AA. Does humor moderate the effects of experimentally-induced stress? Annals of Behavioral Medicine. 18: 101–109, 1996.

Nieman DC, Henson DA, Gusewitch G, Warren BJ, Dotson RC, Butterworth DE, Nehlsen-Cannarella SL. Physical activity and immune function in elderly women. Medicine and Science in Sports and Exercise. 25: 823–831, 1993a.

Nieman DC, Miller AR, Henson DA, Warren BJ, Gusewitch G, Johnson RL, Davis JM, Butterworth DE, Nehlsen-Cannarella SL. Effects of high-vs moderate-intensity exercise on natural killer cell activity. Medicine and Science in Sports and Exercise. 25: 1126–1134, 1993b.

Nieman DC. Exercise, upper respiratory tract infection, and the immune system. Medicine and Science in Sports and Exercise. 26: 128–139, 1994a.

Nieman DC. Exercise, infection, and immunity. International Journal of Sports Medicine. 15(suppl 3): S131–S141, 1994b.

Nieman DC, Miller AR, Henson DA, Warren BJ, Gusewitch G, Johnson RL, Davis JM, Butterworth DE, Herring JL, Nehlsen-Cannarella SL. Effect of high-versus moderate-intensity exercise on lymphocyte subpopulations and proliferative response. International Journal of Sports Medicine.15: 199–206, 1994c.

Orme-Johnson D. Medical care utilization and the transcendental meditation program. Psychosomatic Medicine. 49: 493–507, 1983.

Penninx BW, van Tilburg T, Kriegsman DM, Deeg DJ, Boeke AJ, van Eijk JT. Effects of social support and personal coping resources on mortality in older age: The Longitudinal Aging Study Amsterdam. American Journal of Epidemiology. 146: 510–519, 1997.

Perna FM, McDowell SL. Role of psychological stress in cortisol recovery from exhaustive exercise among elite athletes. International Journal of Behavioral Medicine. 2: 13–26, 1995.

Pike JL, Smith TL, Hauger RL, Nicassio PM, Patterson TL, McClintick BS, Costlow C, Irwin MR. Chronic life stress alters sympathetic, neuroendocrine, and immune responsivity to an acute psychological stressor in humans. Psychosomatic Medicine. 59: 447–457, 1997.

Rall LC, Roubenoff R, Cannon JG, Abad LW, Dinarello CA, Meydani SN. Effects of progressive resistance training on immune response in aging and chronic inflammation. Medicine and Science in Sports and Exercise. 28: 1356–1365, 1996.

Reifman A. Social relationships, recovery from illness, and survival: A literature review. Annals of Behavioral Medicine. 17: 124–131, 1995.

Roberts AH. The powerful placebo revisited: Magnitude of nonspecific effects. Mind/Body Medicine. 1: 35–43, 1995.

Russek LG, Schwartz GE. Perceptions of parental caring predict health status in midlife: A 35-year follow-up of the Harvard mastery of stress study. Psychosomatic Medicine. 59: 144–149, 1997.

Sacco RL, Gan R, Boden-Albala B, Lin I-F, Kargman DE, Hauser WA, Shea S, Paik MC. Leisure-time physical activity and ischemic stroke risk. Stroke. 29: 380–387, 1998.

Sapolsky RM. Endocrine aspects of social instability in the Olive Baboon (*Papio anubis*). American Journal of Primatology. 5: 365–379, 1983.

Sapolsky RM. Hypercortisolism among socially subordinate wild baboons originates at the CNS level. Archives of General Psychiatry. 46: 1047–1051, 1989.

Sapolsky RM. Stress, glucocorticoids, and damage to the nervous system: The current state of confusion. Stress. 1: 1–19, 1996.

Sarason IG, Sarason BR, Potter EH, Antoni MH. Life events, social support, and illness. Psychosomatic Medicine. 47: 156–163, 1985.

Scheier MF, Bridges MW. Person variables and health: Personality predispositions and acute psychological states as shared determinants for disease. Psychosomatic Medicine. 57: 255–268, 1995.

Schoenbach VJ, Kaplan BH, Fredman L, Kleinbaum DG. Social ties and mortality in Evans County, Georgia. American Journal of Epidemiology.123: 577–591, 1986.

Schoenfeld DE, Malmrose LC, Blazer DG, Gold DT, Seeman TE. Self-rated health and mortality in the high-functioning elderly—A closer look at healthy individuals: MacArthur field study of successful aging. Journal of Gerontology. 49: M109–115, 1994.

Schwartz JE, Friedman HS, Tucker JS, Tomlinson-Keasey C, Wingard DL, Criqui MH. Childhood sociodemographic and psychosocial factors as predictors of longevity across the lifespan. American Journal of Public Health. 85: 1237–1245, 1995.

Seeman TE, McEwen BS. Impact of social environment characteristics on neuroendocrine regulation. Psychosomatic Medicine. 58: 459–471, 1996.

Seeman TE, Berkman LF, Kohout F, Lacroix A, Glynn R, Blazer D. Intercommunity variations in the association between social ties and mortality in the elderly. A comparative analysis of three communities. Annals of Epidemiology. 3: 325–335, 1993.

Seeman TE, Berkman LF, Blazer D, Rowe JW. Social ties and support and neuroendocrine function. MacArthur studies of successful aging. Annals of Behavioral Medicine. 16: 95–106, 1994.

Seeman TE, Berkman LF, Charpentier PA, Blazer DG, Albert MS, Tinetti ME. Behavioral and psychosocial predictors of physical performance: MacArthur studies of successful aging. Journal of Gerontology. 50: M177–183, 1995.

Segerstrom SC, Taylor SE, Kemeny ME, Fahey JL. Optimism is associated with mood, coping, and immune change in response to stress. Journal of Personality and Social Psychology. 74: 1646–1655, 1998.

Shinton R, Sagar G. Lifelong exercise and stroke. British Medical Journal. 307: 231–234, 1993.

Simons RL, West GE. Life changes, coping resources, and health among the elderly. Journal of Psychiatric Treatment and Evaluation. 4: 403–408, 1985.

Sinyor D, Peronnet F, Brisson G, Seraganian P. Failure to alter sympathoadrenal response to physiological stress following aerobic training. Physiology and Behavior. 42: 293–296, 1988.

Smith CE, Fernengel K, Holcroft C, Gerald K, Marien L. Meta-analysis of the associations between social support and health outcomes. Annals of Behavioral Medicine. 16: 352–362, 1994.

Smith ML, Hudson DL, Graitzer HM, Raven PB. Exercise training bradycardia: The role of autonomic balance. Medicine and Science in Sports and Exercise. 21: 40–44, 1989.

Sothmann MS, Gustafson AB, Garthwaite TL, Horn TS, Hart BA. Cardiovascular fitness and selected adrenal hormone responses to cognitive stress. Endocrine Research. 14: 59–69, 1988.

Sothmann MS, Horn TS, Hart BA. Plasma catecholamine response to acute psychological stress in humans: Relation to aerobic fitness and exercise training. Medicine and Science in Sports and Exercise. 23: 860–867, 1991.

Stephens T. Physical activity and mental health in the United states and Canada: Evidence from four population surveys. Preventive Medicine. 17: 35 47, 1988.

Strawbridge WJ, Cohen RD, Shema SJ, Kaplan GA. Frequent attendance at religious services and mortality over 28 years. American Journal of Public Health. 87: 957–961, 1997.

Thune I, Brenn T, Lund E, Gaard M. Physical activity and the risk of breast cancer. New England Journal of Medicine. 336: 1269–1275, 1997.

Vogt T, Pope C, Mullooly J, Hollis J. Mental health status as a predictor of morbidity and mortlaity: A 15 year follow-up of members of a health maintanence organization. American Journal of Public Health. 84: 227–231, 1994.

Wallace PK, Silver J, Mills PJ, Dillbeck MC, Wagoner DE. Systolic blood pressure and long-term practice of transcendental meditation and TM-Sidhi program: Effects of TM on systolic blood pressure. Psychosomatic Medicine. 45: 41–46, 1983.

Watanabe T, Morimoto A, Sakata Y, Tan N, Morimoto K, Murakami N. Running training attenuates the ACTH responses in rats to swimming and cage-switch stress. Journal of Applied Physiology. 73: 2452–2456, 1992.

Welin L, Tibblin G, Svardsudd K, Tibblin B, Ander-Peçiva S, Larsson B, Wilhelmsen L. Prospective study of social influences on mortality. Lancet. 1: 915–918, 1985.

White-Welkley JE, Warren GL, Bunnell BN, Mougey EH, Meyerhoff JL, Dishman RK. Treadmill exercise training and estradiol increase plasma ACTH and prolactin after novel footshock. Journal of Applied Physiology. 80: 931–939, 1996.

Wittert GA, Livesey JH, Espiner EA, Donald RA. Adaptation of the hypothalamopituitary adrenal axis to chronic exercise stress in humans. Medicine and Science in Sports and Exercise. 28: 1015–1019, 1996.

Yasuda N, Zimmerman SI, Hawkes W, Fredman L, Hebel JR, Magaziner J. Relation of social network characteristics to 5-year mortality among young-old versus old-old white women in an urban community. American Journal of Epidemiology. 145: 516–523, 1997.

Zhou D, Kusnecov AW, Shurin MR, DePaoli M, and Rabin BS. Exposure to physical and psychological stressors elevates plasma interleukin 6: Relationship to the activation of hypothalamic-pituitary-adrenal axis. Endocrinology. 133: 2523–2530, 1993.

8

Effect of Maternal Stress on the Offspring

A difficult question to answer in regard to many biologic parameters is "What is normal?" An important concern is how one establishes a normal baseline for evaluating the immune system. Is it established by taking a blood specimen from a subject who is receiving no medications that can affect the immune system, who has no diseases that can affect the immune system, and who is at rest having experienced no recent psychological or physical stressors? However, even trying to achieve this, the range of normal for immune parameters is very broad. We have done studies of collecting blood specimens from normal individuals and evaluating immune components for several months and found the data from each individual to vary over a wide range. Thus, when studying the immune system, it is difficult to assign an absolute value to "normal." With regard to the immune system, normal varies over time both within an individual and between individuals.

What influences baseline measurements immune function and behavior? I link immune function and behavior together because, as has been described, behavior can influence quantitative and qualitative measurements of immune function. How early in development does the relationship between behavior and immune function begin? Can a pregnant mother's behavior influence the immune function and the behavior of the offspring?

An interaction between the release of neuropeptide mediators in the brain and their binding to specific receptors influences central nervous system (CNS) activity and subsequently the hormonal milieu in the body in which the immune system resides and functions. It is unlikely that every interaction between a ligand and a receptor always produces the same outcome. The concentration of ligand, the concentration of receptor, and the presence of other ligands and receptors that modify the functional activity of the first set of interactions influence the net effect of the interaction. Therefore, if the hormonal milieu of different individuals is influenced by different "baseline" concentrations of a neuropeptide, or the receptor for that neuropeptide, or of another neuropeptide that modifies the functional activity of the first system, different measurements of baseline immune function would be anticipated, as well as different stressor-induced alterations of immune function.

The baseline (resting) immune function of each individual will be unique to that individual. If the baseline is suboptimal or weakened (a weak defensive line), it may bend and allow offensive materials to become more readily established—sounds like a football game! Actually, the analogy may not be facetious, as the immune system constitutes a major defense against invaders. Just as many football coaches believe that they win with a strong defense, we will achieve better health by building a strong immune defense. To build a strong football defense requires strong players. Having a strong immune defense requires a strong baseline immune system. The development of the strong baseline immune system probably begins in utero.

Different experimental treatments of pregnant animals have been used to determine whether hormones that are present in the maternal circulation can alter, either short-term or long-term, the behavior, behavioral response to stress, and immune function of the offspring. These studies are of public health concern. If immune function of a fetus is altered in a manner that will predispose the offspring to infectious diseases, autoimmune diseases, or malignant disease, health care resources will be required to provide appropriate care for these individuals. Therefore, learning about environmental factors that can affect a pregnant individual and subsequently a fetus is an important component of mind–body–health medicine.

IN UTERO ENVIRONMENT AND THE OFFSPRING

Can the long-term functioning of the immune system be influenced by the mother's psychological reactions during pregnancy? Two factors need to be considered in regard to whether soluble substances in the plasma of a pregnant mother can cross the placenta to the fetus and influence the behavior and immune function of the fetus. The two factors are hormones produced in response to stress (glucocorticoid and neuropeptides) and soluble products of an activated immune system (cytokines). If hormones or cytokines cross the placenta and enter the fetal circulation, they will bind to their appropriate receptor if the receptors are concurrently expressed at gestation. This will activate second messenger systems associated with the receptor. Whether this early binding and activation leaves a permanent alteration in subsequent interactions between the ligand and receptor and on second messenger activation is important, as it can have significant effects on CNS function and, subsequently, immune function.

Effect of In Utero Environment on Receptors in the Brain

As an example that receptor hormone alterations occur during pregnancy, rats were stressed at different times of gestation and an assessment of the concentration of μ

opioid receptors determined in the brain (Sanchez et al, 1996). The data showed that, in regard to μ opioid receptor measurements, there was a specific time of gestation when stressing the mother decreased μ receptor concentration in several areas of the brain of the offspring. Thus, there may be a window of time for alteration of receptors, and this may or may not be identical for each type of hormone receptor.

Alterations in the concentration of glucocorticoid receptors induced in the brains of offspring of stressed rodent mothers have been reported (McCormick et al, 1995). The alteration was not present in all areas of the brain; it was found to be sex related. Glucocorticoid receptor density was not altered by prenatal stress in the hypothalamus and hippocampus. In the frontal cortex of males, but not that of females, prenatal stress significantly decreased the concentration of receptors. In the septum, prenatal stress increased the concentration of glucocorticoid receptors in males. In the amygdala, prenatal stress increased glucocorticoid receptors in both males and females. Measurements of the adrenocorticotropic hormone (ACTH) and corticosterone response to restraint stress were also performed in the experimental animals. Preterm stress was associated with a significant increase of restraint stress-induced ACTH and corticosterone production in female, but not in male, rats. Thus, it is possible that an interaction with sex hormones modifies the stress-induced response of the offspring of mothers who had been stressed during pregnancy.

Effect of In Utero Environment on Hormones in the Brain

Prenatal stress can affect the concentration of hormones in the fetal brain. In a representative study, the content and release of corticotropin-releasing hormone (CRH) from the amygdala of adult rats born to mothers who had been stressed during pregnancy was significantly greater in comparison with matched control rats (Cratty et al, 1995). Even structural alterations in the newborn brain have been reported to be induced by prenatal stress (Jones et al, 1997).

Alteration of the hypothalamic pituitary adrenal (HPA) axis in adult offspring of rodent mothers that were stressed by repeated restraint during pregnancy has been shown to be due to corticosterone elevation in the mother (Barbazanges et al, 1996). Adrenalectomized mothers that were stressed did not produce offspring that had altered HPA responses to stress. Thus, it is likely that transplacental passage of corticosterone is the mediator of the change in the fetus and directs attention to the maternal hormonal environment as a modifier of important CNS pathways of the fetus and, depending on the duration of the effect, adults.

Effect of In Utero Environment on Behavior

In a study of behavior, adult rats, whose mothers had been stressed during the last week of gestation, were compared with control rats whose mothers had not been stressed (Vallee et al, 1997). High anxiety behaviors were found in the offspring of stressed mothers, but these animals did not differ in their learning ability in comparison with controls. Similar results have been reported using different stressors and assays (Poltyrev et al, 1996). The data indicate that emotional behaviors of adults may be influenced by events that occur during ontogeny. However, whether learning ability is affected will require additional studies, as stressing at different times of gestation or intensities of stress may be found to alter learning ability.

A study conducted in rats reported an association between CNS neuropeptide concentrations that were altered in adults by prenatal stress and behavior (Takahashi et al, 1992). The adult rats born to mothers that had been stressed during pregnancy responded differently to an electric shock stressor than did rats born to mothers not stressed during pregnancy. Although HPA axis activity was the same in both groups, there were significant differences in catecholamine metabolism in the cerebral cortex and locus coeruleus, with increased metabolism present in the offspring of stressed mothers.

Studies of nonhuman primates have been reported that indicate that the endocrine response, behavior, and immune function of monkeys born to mothers stressed during pregnancy are altered as a consequence of the maternal stress (Schneider et al, 1992; Schneider et al, 1993; Clarke and Schneider, 1993). The same effects are obtained if, as a means of mimicking the hormonal response to stress, monkeys were injected with ACTH to elevate plasma cortisol.

Thus, the question of baseline and the problem of defining what comprises a normal baseline can be better understood. As behavior, hormone concentrations, and the immune response may permanently be influenced by hormones that are present during gestation, predictions regarding how stress will affect an individual's health and behavior may have to be highly personalized. What is defined as baseline for one individual may not be baseline for another.

Effect of In Utero Environment on Immune Function

The immune response of adult rats born to mothers that were stressed or not stressed has been studied (Klein and Rager, 1995). In rats immunized with a protein antigen (keyhole limpet hemocyanin), the antibody response was found to be significantly higher in the offspring of mothers that had been stressed during pregnancy. Interestingly, studies using lymphocyte responsiveness to mitogens as an indication of immune alteration find a decrease of lymphocyte function of animals born to mothers that had been stressed during pregnancy.

Limited studies have been done regarding stress hormones during the prenatal stage and immune function in humans (Kauppila et al, 1983). Offspring of pregnant mothers who were treated with glucocorticoids to promote lung maturity were studied at 3–10 years after delivery. No deficiencies of in vitro lymphocyte function were detected. As lymphocyte proliferation has an extremely wide range of results, this study should be considered preliminary data and does not conclusively indicate that maternal stress does, or does not, modify the fetal immune system. Studies of several aspects of the immune system are needed. These should include antibody production to immunization and delayed hypersensitivity skin testing.

A 2-week course of ACTH injection into pregnant nonhuman primates at 1 month before birth produced suppression of immune function in the offspring that persisted for a minimum of 6 months (Coe et al, 1996). Immune function parameters measured included mixed lymphocyte culture responsiveness (a measure of T-cell antigen recognition capabilities), lymphocyte responsiveness to stimulation with nonspecific mitogens, and the ability to kill target cells (a likely measurement of the function of natural killer [NK] cells). It is unclear whether the assays measured baseline immune function (immune function occurring without activation of the HPA axis or the sympathetic nervous system [SNS]) or the response of the lymphocytes to stress. This is because collection of the blood from the infants required separations from the mother and handling of the infant which is a stressor. Regardless, there were significant differences between infants of saline- and ACTH-injected mothers.

There is evidence from studies in mice that alteration of HPA axis function occurs subsequent to neonatal exposure of interleukin-1 (IL-1) (Del Rey et al, 1996). The importance of this observation relates to the production of IL-1 in association with an immune response occurring in the mother. An infection or autoimmune process may increase the concentration of IL-1 in the maternal plasma, which may cross the placenta to the fetus. Although the study was performed in neonatal animals, it was demonstrated that IL-1 administered during the first 5 days of life produces a long-term, possibly permanent, effect on the adult HPA axis. When the experimental animals reach adulthood, they have a reduced morning corticosterone concentration, with increased concentration of ACTH, suggesting an altered responsivity of the adrenal to ACTH. This study adds to the information regarding potential alteration of both endocrine and immune function by environmental factors early in life.

EFFECT OF NEONATAL STRESS ON INFANT AND ADULT BEHAVIOR AND IMMUNE FUNCTION

After birth (and it is unclear as to how much of a stressor birth is itself), stressors that the infant, or possibly the young child, are exposed to may have the capability of altering immune function and behavior. These changes may have longlasting, possibly permanent, effects on the response to stress both of behavior and of immune function.

Of course, the importance of the background on which stress is imposed must always be considered (reemphasizing our concern of how to define baseline and the effect of baseline parameters on stressor-induced immune alteration). For example, it has been reported that clinical depression in patients who become depressed without a preceding stress in their lives have lower concentrations of a serotonin and dopamine metabolite than levels in patients who become depressed after sustaining a stress (Roy et al, 1986). Separation of newborn rhesus monkeys from their mothers and rearing them in peer groups results in a lower level of 5-HIAA, a serotonin metabolic product, in the separated monkeys at 6 months of age, in comparison with mother-reared controls (Higley et al, 1992). The separated monkeys were later found to be more aggressive and to display less affiliative behaviors than the mother-reared monkeys. There is also an indication that genetic factors may contribute to baseline hormone levels within the CNS (Higley et al, 1993).

An alteration of the hormonal response to stress has been shown to occur in adult rats that were isolated from their mothers for 6 hours a day on days 2–20 after birth

(Ladd et al, 1996). When stressed by electric footshock at 3 months of age, the rats that had been isolated had a greater increase of plasma ACTH than was found in the rats that were stressed but that had not been isolated from their mothers. Interestingly, these rats also had a higher resting plasma ACTH concentration than that of the controls. A reduction in the number of receptors for corticotropin-releasing factor (CRF) was detected in the anterior pituitary and the raphe nucleus and an increase in the concentration of CRF was present in the parabrachial nucleus and median eminence of the rats who were isolated from their mothers. As these studies were performed approximately 2 months after maternal isolation, the induced changes are long term. The significance with regard to the response of an adult to stress is obvious. Early life events can influence later hormonal responses to stress and may also influence the resting level of hormones and receptors in the brain. Indeed, glucocorticoid receptor mRNA is reduced in the brains of rats that have been separated from their mothers (van Oers et al, 1997). It is not surprising, therefore, that different individuals respond with different hormone and immune alterations to stress.

A study was performed in rats that suggests that corticosterone entering the newborn's circulation during lactation may have a long-term effect on the HPA axis (Catalani et al, 1993). As long as 3 months after birth, the pups of mothers ingesting corticosterone in their drinking water (elevating the mothers plasma corticosterone to the level induced by psychological stress) had a lower resting plasma concentration of ACTH and corticosterone and lower levels after a restraint stress than that of control animals.

Neonatal rats separated from their mothers daily for 15 minutes from birth to the time of weaning have significantly lower levels of CRF mRNA in the hypothalamus as adults than do rats that were not separated for these brief periods (Plotsky and Meaney, 1993). This finding indicates that the synthesis of CRF in the brain is affected by early life experiences. When the adults that had been separated as neonates were stressed by physical restraint, the plasma corticosterone concentration was significantly higher in rats that had not been separated from their mothers in comparison with the rats that had been separated.

Whether or not early life events can produce long-term alterations in hormone levels with subsequent behavioral effects needs to be carefully evaluated. If an effect is found to have a negative impact on behavior, health, and learning ability, public health measures that address this concern may have to be upgraded. Pregnant mothers, living under highly stressful conditions, and not having support during the early months of caring for a child, may possibly contribute to the behavioral and health problems that the child will have to endure.

Separation from the mother is a stressor for infants. The perceived loss of the mother initiates psychological responses that will influence the behavior of the child. In addition, the hormonal response associated with activation of discrete areas of the brain will modify the function of the immune system and health. The effect of stress on infants differs from the effects of maternal stress on the fetus. The changes that occur in the fetus are passive changes produced by hormones or cytokines crossing the placenta to the fetal circulation. In the infant, the behavioral and immune changes are active, as they are produced as a result of activation of the brain and require that infant be aware of stress-related events in its environment. Some of the effects on the immune system will be described.

Early Environmental Effects on Antibody Production

Subjecting juvenile monkeys to 4 weeks of stress, followed by immunization with bovine serum albumin (BSA) produces a significantly lower antibody level than that produced by nonstressed juvenile monkeys (Hill et al, 1967). Although measuring antibody levels, as done in this study, does not identify whether a single or multiple components of the immune system have been altered, it does provide a measurement of an important protective aspect of the immune system. Antibody responses in monkeys are susceptible to modification by stress, but this study did not determine the duration of the effect. Measurement of specific components of the immune system will only provide information regarding what component is actually measured. Thus, both approaches are useful and provide different information.

Another study of antibody to tetanus toxoid immunization was performed in free-ranging rhesus monkeys approximately 1 year of age (Laudenslager et al, 1993). When the monkeys were captured for immunization, several measures were performed that were found to be related to the level of antibody produced. The highest antibody levels were in the monkeys that had the highest heart rate. The significance of this observation is difficult to interpret as the increase of heart rate could have been due to either activation of the SNS (which has been shown to be associated with decrease of some immune functions) or decrease of the vagal activity innervating the heart (which would not be associated with immune alteration). Catecholamine measurements, as an indicator of SNS activation, were not done. Measures of the HPA axis (ACTH and cortisol) were not related to antibody levels. Interestingly, the lowest antibody responses were found in monkeys who showed the highest level of distress when their mothers resumed their normal mating practices. This behavior may indicate a specific type of personality pattern that is associated with a hormonal environment in the monkey that prevents a vigorous antibody response.

Early Environmental Effects on Lymphocyte Function

The effect of brief stress produced through separation from a mother has been studied in monkeys, using either lymphocyte responsiveness to nonspecific mitogens (Laudenslager et al, 1984; Coe et al, 1989; Lubach et al, 1995) or alteration of natural killer cell activity (Laudenslager et al, 1996). There are long lasting changes in lymphocyte proliferative function in comparison to control monkeys that are not separated from their mothers. Reduced responses of lymphocytes to stimulation with mitogens were noted. With regard to NK function, no changes of NK function occurred rapidly, but eventually the separated monkeys had higher NK function than that of the controls. The monkeys were followed for several months and for as long as 4 years. Monkeys that were nursery reared, as opposed to maternally reared, were found to have lower levels of NK function and higher levels of mitogenic function (Lubach et al, 1995). The monkeys were studied for 2 years.

SOCIAL INTERACTIONS IN YOUNG MONKEYS BUFFER THE IMMUNE CHANGES INDUCED BY SEPARATION

Chapter 7 described the effect of buffering activities, such as friendship or moderate exercise, on ameliorating the effects of stress on altering immune system function. Interestingly, similar buffering effects have been reported in infant monkeys. Separation of 7-month-old monkeys from their mothers for 2 weeks produces the behavioral changes of reduced motor activity, increased vocalization, and a slouched posture (Laudenslager et al, 1990). Some, but not all, of the separated monkeys were found to have decreased responsiveness of lymphocytes to nonspecific mitogenic stimulation. Those infants that displayed the highest levels of vocalizations and slouched posture were the ones with the greatest depression of mitogenic responsiveness. It can be hypothesized that the monkeys with the greatest behavioral changes had the most marked activation of the SNS which resulted in greater immune function change.

The specific effect of friends as buffers against the effects of separation from the mother and peers on immune alteration has been studied in monkeys (Boccia et al, 1997). Separation of 4- to 6-month-old monkeys from their social group led to a suppression of T-lymphocyte responsiveness to nonspecific mitogen proliferation and NK function. However, if the infant monkey was provided with social support from a 18- to 24-month-old monkey, the alteration of immune function was attenuated. Thus, there is a clear suggestion that social interaction may have significant health benefits for infants who experience stressors in their lives. It is never too early to learn to make friends.

MODIFICATION OF BEHAVIOR AND RESPONSE TO STRESS BY ENVIRONMENTAL MANIPULATION OF NEONATES

A final area of interest regarding how an individual responds to stress is whether there are maternal interactions that can influence the reactivity of the offspring. For example, rats that are handled from birth to the time of weaning secrete less glucocorticoids when stressed as adults, than do nonhandled rats (Meaney et al, 1988). Handled rats have lower resting glucocorticoid plasma concentrations than those of nonhandled rats.

The influence of handling of neonatal rats on the development of autoimmune disease (experimental allergic encephalomyelitis [EAE]) has been investigated (Laban et al, 1995). Neonatal rats were separated from their mothers for brief times and either left alone or gently handled while separated before being reunited with the mothers. Controls consisted of rats that were left with their mothers. Following immunization with spinal cord antigen handled rats were more likely to develop EAE, and the severity was greater than in the nonhandled control rats. The severity of the disease was greater in male rats.

The immune and neuroendocrine mechanisms responsible for the increased severity of the disease are not established. However, there is ample evidence that associates the development of EAE in rats with a decreased concentration of plasma gluco-corticoids (Sternberg et al, 1992). Possibly, the severity of disease in the handled rat was related to a decreased concentration of corticosterone production which allowed a more intense inflammatory response. Until appropriate studies are performed, the mechanisms will remain unexplained.

CONCLUSION

Of primary importance to the theme of this book is whether there is an effect of maternal stress on the emotional behavior and immune function of the offspring and, if there is an effect, whether it is permanent. If the hormonal response to stress of an adolescent, a young adult, a middle-aged adult, or an elderly adult can modify the function of the immune system and the person's health, developmental factors that are found capable of influencing an individual's mental responsiveness to stressful situations must become of concern to health care planners.

When a building is constructed, architects can select any type of covering to hide the framework. This will give the outward appearance that the architects want to be seen. However, the structure is the same, regardless of how the building looks on the outside. If an earthquake occurs, the building will react as was determined by its structure, not its appearance. If the construction workers did not do their job properly and left a weak spot, the earthquake-induced collapse of the building is likely to occur more readily, and with greater devastation. The analogy I am using relates to the formation of the core structure of the human and developing an appreciation of what influences the construction.

Although it may be inconsistent with the character of this book, which is intended to inform and educate professionals about the interactions between the brain, the immune system, and health, I must pause for a brief editorial comment. It is essential that increased attention be paid to the influence of the maternal hormonal environment on the subsequent behavioral activities of children. Frequently, when I give a talk on the subject of mind–body medicine, a pediatrician or a primary schoolteacher will tell me about the changing pattern of behavior that they have observed in young children. It is never in a positive direction. Rather, the comments invariably reflect on decreased attention to academic subjects, decreased ability to interact with peers, increased hostility, anger, and violent behaviors. A variety of social and environmental factors experienced after birth may contribute to the behavior of children. However, as is now apparent, the in utero environment can also effect children's behavior.

It is important to note that biological consequences of hormonal alterations during development cannot be determined unless appropriate studies are done. Changes in numbers of receptors or hormones and neuropeptides in the brain can only be shown to influence immune function and behavior if well-designed experimental studies are conducted. However, it would not be surprising to find that alteration of receptor numbers and hormone production is associated with altered biological functions related to that specific receptor and its ligand. Although specific correlations cannot be made between an alteration of hormone receptor numbers and behavior or altered immune function in the offspring of mothers who are stressed during pregnancy, there are numerous studies reporting associations between prenatal stress and behavior and between prenatal stress and immune function alterations. Mechanistic studies are still needed.

These studies reflect on the question of how to define baseline normal behavior. If behavior is susceptible to the transplacental passage of hormones to the fetus, there may be no proper definition of normal behavior. All behavior may be a partial representation of genetic factors that determine hormone and hormone receptor concentrations and the influence of maternal hormones on modifying the relationship of hormones to receptors or second-messenger activation. This does not imply an adverse effect on behavior. However, if future studies determine that a child born to a mother who has high levels of stress hormones during pregnancy has an impaired ability to cope with stress, and to adjust to anxiety-producing situations, interventions designed to help the child in coping with aversive situations may be found to be beneficial.

REFERENCES

Barbazanges A, Piazza PV, Lemoal M, Maccari S. Maternal glucocorticoid secretion mediates long-term effects of prenatal stress. Journal of Neuroscience. 16: 3943–3949, 1996.

Boccia ML, Scanlan JM, Laudenslager ML, Berger CL, Hijazi AS, Reite ML. Juvenile friends, behavior, and immune responses to separation in bonnet macaque infants. Physiology and Behavior. 61: 191–198, 1997.

Catalani A, Marinelli M, Scaccianoce S, Nicolai R, Muscolo LA, Porcu A, Koranyi L, Piazza PV, Angelussi L. Progeny of mothers drinking corticosterone during lactation has lower stress-induced corticosterone and better cognitive performance. Brain Research. 624: 209–215, 1993.

Clarke AS, Schneider ML. Prenatal stress has long-term effects on behavioral responses to stress in juvenile rhesus monkeys. Developmental Psychobiology. 26: 293–304, 1993.

Coe CL, Lubach GR, Erschler WB, Klopp RG. Influence of early rearing on lymphocyte proliferation responses in juvenile rhesus monkeys. Brain, Behavior, and Immunity. 3: 47–60, 1989.

Coe CL, Lubach GR, Karaszewski JW, Erschler WB. Prenatal endocrine activation alters postnatal cellular immunity in infant monkeys. Brain, Behavior, and Immunity. 10: 221–234, 1996.

Cratty MS, Ward HE, Johnson EA, Azzaro AJ, Birkle DL. Prenatal stress increases corticotropin releasing factor content and release in rat amygdala minces. Brain Research. 675: 297–302, 1995.

Del Rey A, Furukawa H, Monge-Arditi G, Kabiersch A, Voigt K-H. Alterations in the pituitary-adrenal axis of adult mice following neonatal exposure to interleukin-1. Brain, Behavior, and Immunity. 10: 235–248, 1996.

Higley JD, Suomi SJ, Linnoila M. A longitudinal assessment of CSF monoamine metabolites and plasma cortisol concentrations in young rhesus monkeys. Biological Psychiatry. 32: 127–145, 1992.

Higley JD, Thompson WW, Champoux M, Goldman D, Hasert MF, Kraemer GW, Scanlan JM, Suomi SJ, Linnoila M. Paternal and maternal genetic and environmental contributions to cerebrospinal fluid monoamine metabolites in rhesus monkeys (*Macaca mulatta*). Archives of General Psychiatry. 50: 615–23, 1993.

Hill CW, Greer WE, Felsenfeld O. Psychological stress, early response to foreign protein and blood cortisol level in vervets. Psychosomatic Medicine. 24: 279–283, 1967.

Jones HE, Ruscio MA, Keyser LA, Gonzalez C, Billack B, Rowe R, Hancock C, Lambert KG, Kinsley CH. Prenatal stress alters the size of the rostral anterior commisure in rats. Brain Research Bulletin. 42: 341–346, 1997.

Kauppila A, Hartikainen-Sorri AL, Koivisto M, Ryhanen P. Cell-mediated immunocompetence of children exposed in utero to short- or long-term glucocorticoids. Gynecological and Obstetrics Investigation. 15: 41–48, 1983.

Klein SL, Rager DR. Prenatal stress alters immune function in the offspring of rats. Developmental Psychobiology. 28: 321–326, 1995.

Laban O, Dimitrijevic M, Vonhoersten S, Markovic BM, Jankovic BD. Experimental allergic encephalomyelitis in adult DA rats subjected to neonatal handling or gentling. Brain Research. 676: 133–140, 1995.

Ladd CO, Owens MJ, Nemeroff CB. Persistent changes in corticotropin-releasing factor neuronal systems induced by maternal deprivation. Endocrinology. 137: 1212–1218, 1996.

Laudenslager ML, Capitanio JPC, Reite ML. Possible effects of early separation on subsequent immune function in macaque monkeys. American Journal of Psychiatry. 142: 862–864, 1984.

Laudenslager ML, Held PE, Boccia ML, Reite ML, Cohen JJ. Behavioral and immunological consequences of brief mother–infant separation: A species comparison. Developmental Psychobiology. 23: 247–264, 1990.

Laudenslager ML, Rasmussen KLR, Berman CM, Suomi SJ, Berger CB. Specific antibody levels in free-ranging rhesus monkeys: Relationships to plasma hormones, cardiac parameters, and early behavior. Developmental Psychobiology. 26: 407–420, 1993.

Laudenslager ML, Berger CL, Boccia ML, Reite ML. Natural cytotoxicity toward K562 cells by Macaque lymphocytes from infancy through puberty: Effects of early social challenge. Brain, Behavior, and Immunity. 10: 275–287, 1996.

Lubach GR, Coe CL, Erschler WB. Effects of early rearing environment on immune responses in infant rhesus monkeys. Brain, Behavior, and Immunity. 9: 31–46, 1995.

McCormick CM, Smythe JW, Sharma S, Meaney MJ. Sex-specific effects of prenatal stress on hypothalamic–pituitary–adrenal responses to stress and brain glucocorticoid receptor density in adult rats. Developmental Brain Research. 84: 55–61, 1995.

Meaney MJ, Aitken DH, van Berkel C, Bhatangar S, Sapolsky RM. Effect of neonatal handling on age-related impairments associated with the hippocampus. Science. 239: 766–768, 1988.

Plotsky PM, Meaney MJ. Early, postnatal experience alters hypothalamic corticotropin-releasing factor (CRF) mRNA, median eminence CRF content and stress induced release in adult rats. Brain Research. Molecular Brain Research. 18: 195–200, 1993.

Poltyrev T, Keshet GI, Kay G, Weinstock M. Role of experimental conditions in determining differences in exploratory behavior of prenatally stressed rats. Developmental Psychobiology. 29: 453–462, 1996.

Roy A, Pickar D, Linnoila M, Doran AR, Paul SM. Cerebrospinal fluid monoamine and monoamine metabolite levels and the dexamethasone suppression test in depression: Relationship to life events. Archives of General Psychiatry. 43: 356–360, 1986.

Sanchez MD, Milanes MV, Pazos A, Diaz A, Laorden ML. Autoradiographic evidence of mu opioid receptor down-regulation after prenatal stress in offspring rat brain. Developmental Brain Research. 94: 14–21, 1996.

Schneider ML, Coe CL, Lubach GR. Endocrine activation mimics the adverse effects of prenatal stress on neuromotor development of the infant primate. Developmental Psychobiology. 25: 427–439, 1992.

Schneider ML, Coe CL. Repeated social stress during pregnancy impairs neuromotor development of the primate infant. Journal of Developmental Behavioral Pediatrics. 14: 81–87, 1993.

Sternberg EM, Chrousos GP, Wilder RL, Gold PW. The stress response and the regulation of inflammatory disease. Annals of Internal Medicine. 117: 854–866, 1992.

Takahashi LK, Turner JG, Kalin NH. Prenatal stress alters brain catecholaminergic activity and potentiates stress-induced behavior in adult rats. Brain Research. 574: 131–137, 1992.

Vallee M, Mayo M, LeMoal M, Simon H, Maccari S. Prenatal stress induces high anxiety and postnatal handling induces low anxiety in adult offspring: Correlation with stress induced corticosterone secretion. Journal of Neuroscience. 17: 2626–2636, 1997.

van Oers HJJ, de Kloet ER, Levine S. Persistent, but paradoxical effects on HPA regulation of infants maternally deprived at different ages. Stress. 1: 249–261, 1997.

9

Psychoneuroimmunology and the Elderly

An important goal of psychoneuroimmunology is to contribute to the maintenance of the function of the immune system and resultant good health during aging. As a result of changes in the immune system which reduce its function during aging, individuals become more susceptible to infectious diseases, autoimmune diseases, and, possibly, malignant diseases.

However, it is unclear whether the changes that occur in immunity as we age are irreversibly programmed into lymphocytes or whether behaviors can be adopted that modify the age-related changes of immune function. Possibly the lifelong effects of glucocorticoids, catecholamines, and other hormones whose plasma and tissue concentration is increased by stress will lead to an eventual decline of immune function by an effect on the development of mature lymphocytes from progenitor cells in the bone marrow and effector lymphocytes from naive lymphocytes. Those individuals who maintain higher concentrations of stress hormones for prolonged periods may have a less efficient immune function in comparison with those who have consistently lower concentrations of stress hormones.

AGING AND AUTOIMMUNITY

Autoimmunity provides an example of an interaction between the immune system, health, and aging. As individuals age, there is an increased incidence of autoimmune diseases and autoantibody formation. There is an association between the presence of an autoimmune response and life span. Strains of animals that spontaneously develop autoimmune diseases have significantly shorter life spans than are enjoyed by strains of animals that do not develop autoimmunity. Thus, those individuals who do not develop autoantibodies during the aging process may have the potential of having a longer life span than individuals who develop autoantibodies.

As an example, the prevalence of autoantibodies to thyroid antigens was measured in 34 centenarians (Mariotti et al, 1992). The prevalence of autoantibodies was significantly greater in subjects aged 70–85 than in subjects less than 50 years of age. The prevalence of autoantibodies in the centenarians was the same as in the less than 50 age group. Other studies have reported similar findings that indicate that healthy older subjects are less likely to have autoantibodies in their serum than are older individuals who are ill, and that the titer of autoantibodies, when present in older individuals, is low (Hijmans et al, 1984; Moulias et al, 1984). It is likely that autoantibodies have an association with disease when their titer is high, while low levels of antibody may have no influence on health.

If humans, as do animals that spontaneously develop autoimmunity, tend to have shortened life spans, preventive medicine procedures to maintain immune function in a manner that attenuates the development of autoimmunity would be of enormous public health benefit.

The mechanism for an alteration of life span based on autoimmune processes may relate to the presence of autoantibodies to physiologically relevant proteins. For example, if antibodies directed to the adrenergic receptors, endocrine hormone receptors, or transport proteins are produced by some individuals as they age, an alteration of the normal activity of tissues and cells may occur (Reichlin, 1998). Thus, decreased functional activity of tissue, which occurs during aging, may not merely be a passive wearing out of the tissue. Rather, decreases of tissue and organ function may be partially due to an active process brought about by an autoimmune response. If it is confirmed through appropriate studies of large populations that are followed for the presence of autoantibodies and the correlation of the autoantibodies with morbidity and mortality that autoimmune responses are associated with a shortening of life span, a means of preventing this increase in immunological autoreactivity should be sought. Possibly stress reduction and enhanced abilities to cope with stress, as reviewed in Chapter 7, may contribute to this goal.

There are families that are known to have longevity as a characteristic. The immunological characteristics of the longevity needs to be determined. Maintaining a high level of immune system function (as is found in most healthy young individuals) may be found to contribute to longevity. Thus, a means of keeping the immune system functioning at a level that will prevent diseases associated with aging may contribute to maintaining an optimal quality of health during aging.

We should not accept the concept that an individual who is living a long life does so because he or she comes from a family of long-lived people. Indeed, that may be true, but there are reasons why longevity runs in families, and such reasons need to be determined. It is in this regard that a better understanding of immunological aging and the factors that influence immunological aging needs to be achieved so that we can develop behaviors that will allow us to remain healthy as we age.

It is important to remember that there are significant differences between how different individuals will age. Some of these factors may not be susceptible to alteration, such as the presence of male or female hormones and their effect on physiological function. What will be important for a successful aging process is to identify those age-inducing factors that can be influenced by our behaviors and to do all that we can, within the bounds of maintaining a life that is pleasant and comfortable, to help ourselves age in a healthy fashion. It would be ridiculous to propose the adoption of behaviors that would make one unhappy just because such behaviors were believed to maintain health during aging. Overly restrictive diets that are difficult to maintain and the cause a high level of frustration as a result are an example of taking things too far. Who wants to be a healthy old person who is being made unhappy by the behaviors that they adopt in order to stay alive?

THE VARIABILITY OF THE COMPOSITION OF GROUPS OF OLDER SUBJECTS

The study of immune function of different age groups requires careful planning as the population of subjects with a stated chronological age will contain many variables. Examples of obvious population variables include:

Economic status
Quality of the diet
Whether the subject is physically fit or sedentary
Whether the subject has an autoimmune disease

In addition, other variables that are not often considered include:

Whether the subject is HLA-B8 and/or HLA-DR3 positive
Whether the subject's mother experienced high levels of stress during the pregnancy
The coping skills of the subject, including social support, sense of humor, and belief systems
Job satisfaction of the individual if employed (where in the hierarchy are they and do they have any control over the workplace)

When studying a population of subjects who are of a given age, there will be some subjects who have in vitro immune measures that are above or below the mean. Assuming that these are stable aspects of immune function for each individual, the question can be asked whether there is a biological significance to the characteristics of immune function in a subject. There has been the suggestion that in elderly individuals older than 70 years of age, significantly suppressed responsiveness of lymphocytes to stimulation with nonspecific mitogens is associated with a shortened duration of life, in comparison with elderly individuals who have a higher mitogenic responsiveness (Murasko et al, 1988).

Another study followed 102 individuals aged 86–92, to determine whether there were immune parameters associated with mortality (Ferguson et al, 1995). Two years after collecting baseline immune data, 27 of the subjects had died. The combination of low CD4, high CD8, and low B-cell percentages with low nonspecific mitogen re-activity was significantly associated with mortality.

It is logical to suggest that those individuals who maintain better immune function will have increased longevity. If this actually happens, the population of older sub-jects available for study of immune function will change with increasing age. As those whose immune function is less capable of maintaining health die, the older pool of subjects will have better immune function. Associated with the better im-mune function should be a decreased rate of mortality as the population ages, as has been found for the med-fly (Carey et al, 1992). The rate of mortality decreases after the early death of most med-flies housed together in a large population. Apparently, the surviving med-flys differ biologically from the others and die at a slower rate.

Another way in which the population changes with age relates to some of the vari-able characteristics of the population. For example, if individuals who lack of a social support system have shorter longevity, the remaining population will consist of those with who are better able to buffer the effects of stress on the alteration of immune function. This personality characteristic may slow their rate of mortality. Similar ar-guments can be proposed for individuals who actively engage in religious practices. This would suggest that the older groups of individuals will have better immune function in comparison to those less old. For example, a group who has achieved the age of 100 may have better average immune function than a group in their 80s.

An additional concern relates to selection of subjects for studies of immune func-tion. If subjects are excluded who have high blood pressure, are obese, lack social support systems, or have endocrine or autoimmune diseases, the resultant population selected for study will likely represent the level of immune function that is attainable. However, selection of subjects who were ill, may provide different values for the im-mune parameters measured. Thus, the study of immune function in older individuals is difficult because of the variability of the population.

IMMUNE FUNCTION IN THE ELDERLY

The study of centenarians provides a more homogeneous population for study. In-volvement in activities associated with religion, low tension and high extraversion, use of cognitive abilities, but low social resources were found to be characteristic of this population (Courtenay et al, 1992; Poon et al, 1992; Adkins et al, 1996; et al, 1996). Study of immune function in a carefully selected population of centenarians found a decrease of CD4 lymphocytes with no change of CD8 and an increase of nat-ural killer (NK) cell numbers (Thompson et al, 1984). Lymphocyte responsiveness to nonspecific mitogen and IL-2 production was decreased. It is possible to explain the results on the basis of decreased CD4 lymphocyte numbers. The decreased mitogenic response and IL-2 production could reflect a decrease of the cells producing IL-2 and being induced into mitotic division by the mitogens. Thus, assuming that the centenarians were healthy, decreased immune function does occur with aging. However, comparison of the immune function of sick with healthy centenarians may demonstrate that the sick centenarians had significantly reduced immune function relative to that of the healthy centenarians. The other concern relates to how much immune function is needed to maintain health. As discussed in Chapter 2, we do not know how much of an in vitro response to phytohemagglutinin (PHA), or how many CD4 or CD8 or NK or how much IL-2 or IL-4 is needed to maintain immune function at a level that resists infectious disease. Remember, there are big differences between the statistical normal range for IgG in plasma and the amount of IgG that is needed to resist pyogenic infections.

Stress has been found to decrease the amount of antibody produced in response to immunization to influenza vaccine in older individuals (Kiecolt-Glaser et al, 1996). Measuring the amount of antibody produced following immunization is an in vivo reflection of all of the steps required for antibody formation. Obviously, stress reduces the function of one or many of the factors that must interact for normal antibody production to occur. Even though the elderly individuals who are experiencing stress have more upper respiratory infections than do the elderly who are experiencing less stress, and produce greater amounts of antibody, this does not mean that the increased risk of infection is attributable to the lower amounts of antibody. Viral attachment to its specific receptor, viral replication within the cell, mucous production, interferon-α and interferon-β production, may all influence the manifestation of a viral infection. Careful attention must be directed to differences between association and linkages. Just because two events are associated (reduced antibody levels and increased infections) does not mean that there is linkage (cause and effect).

Another in vivo measure of immune function is the delayed hypersensitivity (DTH) skin test response (described in Chapter 2). Decreased DTH was found in the elderly (Goodwin et al, 1982; Bartoloni et al, 1991). However, linkage of the reduction of the DTH response to an increased risk of infectious disease cannot be reliably done. It can be hypothesized, but not proved, until a determination is made regarding how much DTH is enough for biological resistance to infectious agents.

CONCLUSION

From conception through becoming a senior citizen, our immune function and our health are influenced by the hormonal milieu present in our bodies at the direction of our mind. Psychoneuroimmunology is an embryonic science, just beginning to provide an understanding of the mind–body–health connection. The contributions of psychologists, physiologists, immunologists, pharmacologists, psychiatrists, neuroanatomists, endocrinologoists, and all who are involved in clinical care, will be required to further develop our understanding of the mechanisms which are operative in the mind–body–health connection and how to best apply the knowledge to maintaining mental and physical health as we age. There is a long way to go but, with the dedication of the scientists who are currently working in the discipline, and those who are being attracted to it, progress will continue to be achieved to the benefit of all.

REFERENCES

Adkins G, Martin P, Poon LW. Personality traits and states as predictors of subjective well-being in centenarians, octogenarians, and sexagenians. Psychology and Aging. 11: 408–416, 1996.

Bartoloni C, Guidi L, Frasca D, Antico L, Pili R, Cursi F, DiGiovanni A, Rumi C, Menini E, Carbonin P, Doria G, Gambassi G. Immune parameters in a population of institutionalized elderly subjects: Influence of depressive disorders and endocrinological correlations. Mechanisms of Aging and Development. 60: 1–12, 1991.

Carey JR, Liedo P, Orozco D, Vaupel JW. Slowing of mortality rates at older ages in large med-fly cohorts. Science. 258: 457–461, 1992.

Courtenay BC, Poon LW, Martin P, Clayton GM, Johnson MA. Religiosity and adaptation in the oldest-old. International Journal of Aging and Human Development. 34: 47–56, 1992.

Ferguson FG, Wikby A, Maxson P, Olsson J, Johansson B. Immune parameters in a longitudinal study of a very old population of Swedish people: A comparison between survivors and nonsurvivors. Journal of Gerontology. 50A: B378–B382, 1995.

Goodwin JS, Searles RP, Tung KSK. Immunological responses of a healthy elderly population. Clinical and Experimental Immunology. 48: 403–410, 1982.

Hijmans W, Radl J, Bottazzo GF, Doniach D. Autoantibodies in highly aged humans. Mechanisms of Aging and Development. 26: 83–89, 1984.

Kiecolt-Glaser JK, Glaser R, Gravenstein S, Malarkey W, Sheridan J. Chronic stress alters the immune response to influenza virus vaccine in older adults. Proceedings of the National Academy of Sciences USA. 93: 3043–3047, 1996.

Mariotti S, Sansoni P, Barbesino G, Caturegli P, Monti D, Cossarizza A, Giacomelli T, Passeri G, Fagiolo U, Pinchera A, Franceshi C. Thyroid and other organ-specific autoantibodies in healthy centenarians. Lancet. 339: 1506–1508, 1992.

Martin P, Poon LW, Kim E, Johnsin MA. Social and psychological resources in the oldest old. Experimental Aging Research. 22: 121–139, 1996.

Moulias R, Proust J, Wang A, Congy F, Marescot MR, Chabrolle A, Hamelin A, Lesourd B. Age related increase in autoantibodies. Lancet. 1: 1128–1129, 1984.

Murasko DM, Weiner P, Kaye D. Association of lack of mitogen-induced lymphocyte proliferation with increased mortality in the elderly. Aging: Immunology and Infectious Disease. 1: 1–6, 1988.

Poon LW, Martin P, Clayton GM, Messner S, Noble CA, Johnson MA. The influences of cognitive resources on adaptation and old age. International Journal of Aging and Human Development. 34: 31–46, 1992.

Reichlin M. Autoantibodies to ubiquitous intracellular antigens interact with living cells. The Immunologist. 6: 76–78, 1998.

Thompson JS, Wekstein DR, Rhoades JL, Kirkpatrick C, Brown SA, Roszman T, Straus R, Tietz N. The immune status of healthy centenarians. Journal of the American Geriatrics Society. 32: 274–281, 1984.

Index

Infectious agent, identification of, 18
Infectious diseases
  bacterial infection
    gram-negative, 255
    gram-positive, 254–255
    intracellular, 255
  defenses
    immune system, 76–79
    innate, 68–70, 123
  viral infection
    Epstein-Barr virus, 262–263
    herpes zoster, 262
    human immunodeficiency virus (HIV),
      263–265
    latent, 261
    overview, 255–261
Inflammation, characteristics of, 15, 70–72
Inflammatory cells, 68
Inflammatory phase, 70
Insulin-dependent diabetes mellitus
  (IDDM), 250–253
Integrins, 73
Interdigitating dendritic cells, 20
Interferons, 256
Intimacy, 301–303
Intracellular adhesion molecule-1 (ICAM-1),
  96
Intracellular bacterial infection, 255
Ischemic stroke, 299

Joining chain (J chain), 61

Keyhole limpet hemocyanin (KLH),
  170–171, 316
Kibbutzes, 290
Kidney, glomerulonephritis, 92

Laboratory tests, 98
Latent viral infections, 261
Lateral medulla, 121
Lateral septal area, 121
Lateralization, brain, 148–150
Laughter, impact on immune system, 292
L chain, 58
Leu-enkaphalin, 210
Leukocyte
  adhesion molecules, 73
  defined, 15
  inhibition factor, 70

Leukotrienes, 89–90
Life span
  autoimmune disease and, 238–239
  self-perception and, 281–282
Locus coeruleus (LC), 122, 130–131, 142
L-selectin, 74
Lymph, defined, 15
Lymphatic fluid, 80
Lymphatic vessels, 80
Lymph node, 79–83, 117, 136
Lymphocytes, *see* Specific types of lymphocytes
  defined, 15–16
  early environment effects on, 319
  function tests, 160–161
Lymphocyte subset quantitation, *see* Flow
  cytometry
Lymphoid follicles, 81, 84
Lymphoid tissue
  catecholamine, effect on, 190
  diffuse, 84
  innervation in
    characteristics of, 132–136
    interruption of, effect on immune func-
      tion, 136–141
  lymph nodes, 79–83
  lymphoid follicles
    aggregated, 84
    defined, 81
    solitary, 84
  mucosal associated, 84–85
  spleen, 83–84
Lysis, 67
Lytic pathway, 66

Macrophage, 26–27
Major histocompatibility complex (MHC)
  autoimmune disease, initiation of, 233,
    238
  CD4 T lymphocytes, interaction with, 47
  function of, generally, 43–45, 78
  groupings of, 44
Malignant disease, 265–269
Marginal zone, 134
Marital status, significance of, 283, 288
Mast cells
  function of, generally, 26, 56–57
  IgE-mediated effect on, 88
  soluble mediators released by, 89